Hepatocellular Carcinoma

Kelly M. McMasters
Jean-Nicolas Vauthey
Editors

Hepatocellular Carcinoma

Targeted Therapy and Multidisciplinary Care

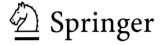 Springer

Editors
Kelly M. McMasters, MD, PhD
Department of Surgery
University of Louisville
Louisville, KY, USA
mcmasters@louisville.edu

Jean-Nicolas Vauthey, MD
Department of Surgical Oncology
University of Texas MD Anderson
  Cancer Center
Houston, TX, USA
jvauthey@mdanderson.org

ISBN 978-1-60327-521-7   e-ISBN 978-1-60327-522-4
DOI 10.1007/978-1-60327-522-4
Springer New York Dordrecht Heidelberg London

Library of Congress Control Number: 2010931163

Printed on acid-free paper

Springer is part of Springer Science+Business Media (www.springer.com)

Foreword

It is a great pleasure and an honor to write the preface for this outstanding book dedicated to the therapy of hepatocellular carcinoma (HCC). This tumor, which is a major health problem worldwide, has stimulated the energy of several disciplines. The liver is a massive and complex organ requiring an excellent knowledge of its anatomy and physiology, with an exquisite comprehension of its impact on cardiovascular, pulmonary, and renal function.

Initially, the treatment of HCC was limited to surgical approaches with liver resection being the only option with curative intent. The development of HCC in chronic liver disease was associated with a high risk of technical difficulties and a high morbidity/mortality rate. This has challenged liver surgeons to improve their knowledge regarding liver anatomy, assessment of liver function, use of intraoperative imaging, tolerance of vascular clamping, and better anticipation of postoperative liver recovery. As shown in several chapters of this book, progress in liver surgery for HCC has expanded its development, yielding a true specialty. Imaging of liver parenchyma was motivated by two different goals including an efficient screening along with an accurate evaluation of the tumor in a background of abnormal parenchyma. Interventional radiology was initially focused on the treatment of this tumor with substantial technical advances allowing an efficient destruction of larger tumors. In parallel, radiologists developed transarterial chemoembolization and radioembolization. Those two locoregional approaches can stabilize the tumors, allowing in some cases for subsequent resection or transplantation. These multiple therapeutic approaches have contributed to expand the indications for liver transplantation, which remains the best curative treatment for limited HCC in patients with advanced chronic liver disease. However, this luxury treatment is restricted to very few countries, with a discrepancy between the increasing number of candidates and the limited number of grafts. Therefore, there is a considerable need for alternative treatments which are extensively developed in this textbook.

There is no efficient treatment without an accurate comprehension of the development of HCC. Beyond viral infections of the liver, the role of other potential causes is emphasized in an important chapter. There is no doubt that etiologies of HCC will not be considered similarly in the future, given more attention to both environmental and chronic medical conditions. These emerging factors, such as metabolic syndrome, will probably highlight future targets relevant to the screening of high-risk patients.

The chapter on staging of HCC is very comprehensive. As such, J.N. Vauthey dedicated a great part of his initial studies to the stratification of patients with similar prognostic factors. The ongoing debate on transplant candidates confirms that stratification of patients is a prerequisite before considering any therapeutic modalities.

Indeed, our clinical experience shows that HCC is often a heterogeneous disease with variable outcomes. The chapter on pathologic considerations confirms that HCC has multiple histological components which will be clarified in the future by molecular classifications.

The last chapters of this remarkable book highlight that management of patients with HCC relies necessarily upon multidisciplinary effort involving the skills of radiologists, pathologists, oncologists, gastroenterologists, hepatologists, anesthesiologists, hepatobiliary, and transplant surgeons. In addition, these specific areas of knowledge and experience are guided by the important innovations from Asian countries and efficiency of medical treatment to an increasing degree. Of note in this book, supervised by eminent US authors, an entire chapter is devoted to the guidelines for treatment in Japan. Sorafenib has been approved as a standard of care for advanced HCC. Several studies evaluating other antiangiogenic agents and multi-target inhibitors are at various phases of their development with promising results. However, the most fascinating forthcoming issue will be the appropriate combination of medical treatment with surgical and radiological procedures. The improvement of resectability and survival observed in patients with colorectal liver metastasis treated by novel active chemotherapy was a major therapeutic step. Recent results in HCC strongly support that similar expectations might be achieved to improve outcome by including neoadjuvant or adjuvant therapy.

Jacques Belghiti   Clichy, France
                                                                         October 2010

Preface

Hepatocellular carcinoma (HCC) is a major cause of cancer mortality worldwide. Because early detection is rare, the overall prognosis is generally poor. Understanding of the etiology, epidemiology, pathophysiology, molecular biology, and clinical features of HCC is important in providing optimal patient care. In addition, understanding of the limitations of our current knowledge and therapeutic capabilities is essential in order to guide future research efforts. Management of patients with HCC is necessarily a multidisciplinary effort which involves the skill of radiologists, pathologists, gastroenterologists, anesthesiologists, surgeons, medical oncologists, radiation oncologists, nurses, and other health professionals. This book is dedicated to the researchers, clinicians, and support staff involved in the fight against HCC, with admiration and appreciation for the work that is done every day to prevent, detect, and treat this disease. Most of all, this book is dedicated to the patients we treat, in the hope that sharing the collective wisdom of this esteemed group of experts will stimulate and encourage collaborative efforts to combat this formidable cancer.

Kelly M. McMasters, MD, PhD   Louisville, Kentucky
Jean-Nicolas Vauthey, MD   Houston, Texas
                                                              January 2010

Acknowledgement

The authors thank Margaret Abby, Ruth J. Haynes and Antoine Brouquet for their assistance in editing the textbook.

Contents

Contributors

Eddie K. Abdalla, MD Department of Surgical Oncology, The University of Texas MD Anderson Cancer Center, Houston, TX, USA

Ghassan K. Abou-Alfa, MD Department of Gastrointestinal Oncology, Memorial Sloan-Kettering Cancer Center, New York, NY, USA

Costantine Albany, MD Department of Gastrointestinal Oncology, Memorial Sloan-Kettering Cancer Center, New York, NY, USA

Thomas A. Aloia, MD, FACS Department of Surgery, Weill-Cornell Medical College, The Methodist Hospital, Houston, TX, USA

Rony Avritscher, MD Interventional Radiology Section, Division of Diagnostic Imaging, The University of Texas MD Anderson Cancer Center, Houston, TX, USA

Maria Luisa Balmer, MD Department of Clinical Pharmacology and Visceral Research, University of Bern, Bern, Switzerland

Joseph F. Buell, MD Surgery and Pediatrics, Abdominal Transplant Institute, Hepatobiliary Surgery and Oncology, Tulane University, New Orleans, LA, USA

E. Ramsay Camp, MD Department of Surgery, Medical University of South Carolina, Charleston, SC, USA

Stewart Carter, MD Division of Surgical Oncology, Department of Surgery, University of Louisville School of Medicine, Louisville, KY, USA

Daniel Cherqui, MD Department of Surgery, New York-Presbyterian/Weill Cornell, New York, NY, USA

Carlo M. Contreras, MD The University of Texas MD Anderson Cancer Center, Houston, TX, USA

Steven A. Curley, MD Department of Surgical Oncology, The University of Texas MD Anderson Cancer Center, Houston, TX, USA

Jean-François Dufour, MD, MSC Department of Clinical Pharmacology and Visceral Research, University of Bern, Bern, Switzerland

Nestor F. Esnaola, MD, MPII Department of Surgery, Medical University of South Carolina, Charleston, SC, USA

Jonas W. Feilchenfeldt, MD Department of Gastrointestinal Medical Oncology, Memorial Sloan-Kettering Cancer Center, New York, NY, USA

A. Osama Gaber, MD Department of Surgery, Weill-Cornell Medical College The Methodist Hospital Houston, TX, USA

Christos Georgiades, MD, PhD Department of Radiology, Johns Hopkins University School of Medicine, Baltimore, MD, USA

Jean-Francois Geschwind, MD Department of Radiology, Johns Hopkins University School of Medicine, Baltimore, MD, USA

R. Mark Ghobrial, MD Department of Surgery, Weill-Cornell Medical College, The Methodist Hospital, Houston, TX, USA

Sanjay Gupta, MD Section of Interventional Radiology, Division of Diagnostic Imaging, The University of Texas MD Anderson Cancer Center, Houston, TX, USA

Kiyoshi Hasegawa, MD, PhD Hepato-Biliary-Pancreatic Surgery Division, Department of Surgery, University of Tokyo, Tokyo, Japan

Manal M. Hassan, MB BCH, MPH, PhD Department of Gastrointestinal Medical Oncology, The University of Texas MD Anderson Cancer Center, Houston, TX, USA

Alan W. Hemming, MD Division of Transplantation and Hepatobiliary Surgery, Department of Surgery, University of California, San Diego, CA, USA

Philip J. Johnson, MD Clinical Trials Unit, CRUK Institute for Cancer Studies, The University of Birmingham, Birmingham, UK

Ahmed O. Kaseb, MD Department of Gastrointestinal Medical Oncology, The University of Texas MD Anderson Cancer Center, Houston, TX, USA

Robin D. Kim, MD Division of Transplantation and Hepatobiliary Surgery, Department of Surgery, University of Florida College of Medicine, Gainesville, FL, USA

Norihiro Kokudo, MD, PhD Hepato-Biliary-Pancreatic Surgery Division, Department of Surgery, University of Tokyo, Hongo, Bunkyo-ku, Tokyo, Japan

Gregory Y. Lauwers, MD Department of Pathology, Massachusetts General Hospital, Boston, MA, USA

David C. Madoff, MD Interventional Radiology Section, Division of Diagnostic Imaging, The University of Texas MD Anderson Cancer Center, Houston, TX, USA

Robert C.G. Martin, II, MD, PhD Division of Surgical Oncology, Department of Surgery, University of Louisville School of Medicine, Louisville, KY, USA

Ryota Masuzaki, MD Department of Gastroenterology, The University of Tokyo, Hongo, Bunky-oku, Tokyo, Japan

Kelly M. McMasters, MD, PhD Department of Surgery, University of Louisville, Louisville, KY, USA

Ravi Murthy, MD Section of Interventional Radiology, Division of Diagnostic Imaging, The University of Texas MD Anderson Cancer Center, Houston, TX, USA

Pritesh Mutha, MD Section of Interventional Radiology, Division of Diagnostic Imaging, The University of Texas MD Anderson Cancer Center, Houston, TX, USA

Hari Nathan, MD Department of Surgery, The Johns Hopkins University School of Medicine, Baltimore, MD, USA

Eileen M. O'Reilly, MD Department of Gastrointestinal Medical Oncology, Memorial Sloan-Kettering Cancer Center, New York, NY, USA

Masao Omata, MD Department of Gastroenterology, University of Tokyo, Hongo, Bunkyo-ku, Tokyo, Japan

Daniel Palmer, BSc, MBChB, FRCP, PhD Clinical Trials Unit, CR UK Institute for Cancer Studies, University of Birmingham, Birmingham, United Kingdom

Timothy M. Pawlik, MD, MPH Division of Surgical Oncology, Department of Surgery, The Johns Hopkins School of Medicine, Baltimore, MD, USA

Kadiyala V. Ravindra, MD Department of Surgery, Duke University Medical Center, Durham, NC, USA

Charles R. Scoggins, MD, MBA Division of Surgical Oncology, Department of Surgery, University of Louisville School of Medicine Louisville, KY, USA

Melanie B. Thomas, MD, MS Division of Hematology/Oncology, Department of Medicine, Medical University of South Carolina, Hollings Cancer Center, Charleston, SC, USA

Guido Torzilli, MD, PhD Department of Surgery, Istituto Clinico Humanitas IRCCS, University of Milan, School of Medicine, Milan, Italy

Jean-Nicolas Vauthey, MD Department of Surgical Oncology, The University of Texas MD Anderson Cancer Center, Houston, TX, USA

Luca Viganò, MD Unit of Surgical Oncology, Institute for Cancer Research and Treatment, Candiolo, Turin, Italy

Charles E. Woodall, III, MD, MSc Surgical Oncology/Surgical Endoscopy, Ferrell Duncan Clinic General Surgery, CoxHealth, Springfield, MO, USA

Daria Zorzi, MD Department of Surgical Oncology, The University of Texas MD Anderson Cancer Center, Houston, TX, USA

Chapter 1
Epidemiology and Pathogenesis of Hepatocellular Carcinoma

Manal M. Hassan and Ahmed O. Kaseb

Keywords Hepatocellular carcinoma · HCC · HCC incidence · HCC risk factors · Diabetes mellitus · HBV · HCV

Liver cancer is the sixth most common cancer worldwide and the third most common cause of cancer mortality, with more than 500,000 deaths annually [1, 2]. Hepatocellular carcinoma (HCC), which comprises most primary liver cancer cases, is rarely detected early and is usually fatal within a few months of diagnosis [3]. A recently published study indicated that the incidence rates of HCC tripled in the United States from 1975 through 2005 [4].

Hepatocellular cancer has been shown to have wide variations in the geographic distribution, and there is a marked difference in the incidence between different races and genders. The highest incidence rates of HCC are in sub-Saharan Africa and Eastern Asia (>80% of all HCC), with China accounting for over 50% of the cases [5]. The low incidence countries include North and South America, Australia, and Northern Europe. HCC incidence varies among people of different ethnicity. For example, Chinese men have rates 2.7 times that of Indian men in Singapore [5]. In the United States, HCC rates are the highest in Asians, Hispanic, and African American middle-age men [4]. In most populations, the incidence of HCC is higher in males as compared to females. Surprisingly, the largest differences between the two genders are in the low-risk populations of central and southern Europe [6].

The peculiar pattern of HCC, that is the rise in the disease incidence among young persons and its varied incidence among different populations and races, suggests that this tumor is caused by several etiologic factors and that interactions among these factors may significantly increase the risk for HCC.

Many environmental and genetic factors have been identified as increasing one's risk for the development of HCC. Furthermore, the synergy between these factors has been shown to be significant in hepatocarcinogenesis. This chapter reviews the

M.M. Hassan (✉)
Department of Gastrointestinal Medical Oncology, The University of Texas MD Anderson Cancer Center, Houston, TX, USA

K.M. McMasters, J.-N. Vauthey (eds.), *Hepatocellular Carcinoma*, DOI 10.1007/978-1-60327-522-4_1, © Springer Science+Business Media, LLC 2011

available data on these risk factors and generally discusses the pathogenesis of HCC development.

Risk Factors of HCC

Hepatitis Virus Infection

Hepatitis B Virus

The hepatitis B virus (HBV) genome is a partially double-stranded, circular DNA molecule. Since the identification of hepatitis B surface antigen (HBsAg) and its importance as a marker of chronic HBV infection, several epidemiological studies have established the significant hepatocarcinogenicity of chronic infection with HBV in humans; all were summarized by the International Agency for Research on Cancer (IARC) of the World Health Organizations (WHO) [7]. The association between HBV and HCC is not restricted to those who are positive for HBsAg; other studies have shown that some patients with hepatitis B core antibodies (anti-HBc)-positive and HBsAg-negative continue to be at risk for HCC development [8]. Meanwhile, after the initiation of HBV vaccination, significant declines in the incidence of HCC have been documented in high-risk countries like Taiwan [9].

The mechanism whereby HBV may induce HCC has been investigated through different approaches. The HBV-DNA integration has been detected in hepatocytes prior to tumor development among patients positive for HBsAg, which may enhance chromosomal instability and facilitate HCC development [10, 11]. In addition, the oncogenic role of the HBs and HBx proteins has been documented. HBx protein has been shown to transactivate both HBV and cellular genes, which may alter host gene expression and lead to HCC development [12]. In addition, the direct necrotic and inflammatory effect of viral hepatitis with cirrhosis cannot be excluded [13].

By using the complete nucleotide sequence of the viral genome, eight genotypes of HBV have been identified (A–H) [14]. The prevalence of HBV genotypes varies by geographical areas [15]. Genotype A is common in Europe, India, and Africa. Genotypes B and C are common in China, Japan, and Southeast Asia. Genotype D is common in Mediterranean areas and in the Middle East [16]. Genotypes E–G are common in Central and South America [15]. In the United States, all types are present with prevalence of 35, 22, 31, 10, and 2 for genotypes A, B, C, D, E–G, respectively [15]. A study showed that patients with genotype C infection may develop advanced liver disease rather than with genotype B or D. Genotype B was associated with hepatitis B e antigen (HBeAg) seroconversion at earlier age and less active hepatic inflammation. In addition genotypes A and B are associated with higher rate of HBeAg seroconversion during interferon therapy [17].

Hepatitis C Virus

Hepatitis C virus (HCV) is a small, single-stranded RNA virus [18]. The prevalence of HCV infection varies widely according to geographical areas. It represents a major public health problem in the United States; approximately four million Americans are infected with HCV [19]. Several studies have demonstrated the significant role of HCV in the development of HCC. Antibodies against HCV (anti-HCV) can be detected in up to 90% of HCC patients [20]. A previously published meta-analysis of 21 case–control studies indicated that HCC risk was 17 times higher among HCV-positive individuals as compared to HCV-negative individuals [21]. HCV increases HCC risk by promoting progressive end-stage liver diseases. About 60–80% of anti-HCV-positive HCC patients were found to have liver cirrhosis [22].

It has been suggested that oxidative stress is one of the mechanisms involved in inflammation-related carcinogenesis in patients with chronic HCV infection [23]. In response to viral antigens, the activated macrophages and other recruited leukocytes release powerful reactive oxygen species (ROS) such as HOONO (from NO and O_2^-), HOCl, and H_2O_2, at sites of infection, causing areas of focal necrosis and compensatory cell division [24]. These oxidants not only kill target cells but may also overwhelm the antioxidant defenses of neighboring cells, leading to damage of important biomolecule, such as DNA, RNA, and proteins; if these relate to critical genes such as oncogenes or tumor suppressor genes, the initiation of cancer may result. In addition, ROS may serve as proinflammatory mediators [25].

Hepatocellular damage induced by oxidative stress may result in the recruitment of inflammatory cells and the activation of Kupffer cells and hepatic stellate cells (HSCs), which may enhance the inflammatory responses. Factors involved in this early phase are the release of proinflammatory and antiinflammatory cytokines [26, 27]. If oxidative stress persists, hepatic injury will also persist, and the activated HSCs will migrate and proliferate. As a consequence, extracellular matrix protein may accumulate in the damaged tissues, and the disease may progress to cirrhosis.

Like other RNA viruses, HCV displays a high genetic variability. On the basis of nucleotide sequence homology, whole-sequenced HCV isolates are classified as type I (1a), type II (1b), type III (2a), and type IV (2b). Provisionally, type V (3a) and type VI (3b) isolates were reported on the basis of data on partially sequenced genomes [28]. The geographic distribution of these genotypes demonstrated that genotypes I, II, and III are predominate in Western countries and the Far East, whereas type IV is predominant in the Middle East [29].

There is some evidence that the HCV genotype 1b is more aggressive and more closely associated with advanced chronic liver diseases such as liver cirrhosis and HCC [30, 31], although high prevalence of HCV type 1b has been reported among patients with HCC and no cirrhosis [32]. This information may indicate that in some cases the neoplastic transformation in type 1b infection may not require transition through the stage of cirrhosis. The observation that many HCC can develop in patients with HCV with no cirrhosis and that many of the HCV structural and non-structural proteins have not been entirely investigated indicates that the molecular mechanism of HCV in hepatocarcinogenesis is not well established.

Although HBV and HCV are the major etiologic factors for HCC development, approximately 60% of HCC patients are negative for HBV and HCV which implicates that other factors are involved (Fig. 1.1).

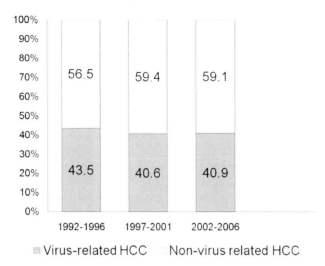

Fig. 1.1 Proportion of HCC related to hepatitis virus infection (HBV and HCV) and non-viral factors between 1992 and 2006 (Hassan M, unpublished data)

Environmental Risk Factors

Alcohol Consumption

Numerous studies included in a review by the international agency for research on cancer have concluded that alcohol consumption is important risk factor for HCC development [33]. The alcohol–liver disease relationship correlates with the quantity of alcohol consumed over a drinking lifetime, with heavy alcohol consumption being the main risk for HCC and not social drinking [34]. Previous European studies [35, 36] reported a steep dose-dependent increase in relative risk of alcohol-induced liver disease above a "threshold" of 7–13 drinks per week in women and 14–27 drinks per week in men. Association between alcohol consumption and chronic liver diseases including HCC is partially related to ethanol metabolism and its major oxidation product, acetaldehyde [37], which modifies macromolecules in the cell by acetylation, leading to generation of free radicals, possible chromosomal abnormalities, and DNA mutation.

Our results from a US case–control study demonstrated approximately three-fold increase in HCC risk among individuals who consumed more than 60 ml ethanol per day [38]. The association between heavy alcohol consumption and HCC was larger in women than in men, which may be partially attributable to the synergism between female sex and heavy alcohol consumption. A recent review by Mancinelli et al. [39] suggested that women may experience a more rapid progression of alcohol damage than men. The lower body mass index and body fluid content in women than men may contribute to lowered ethanol diffusion and high blood concentration in women [40]. Moreover, the activity of gastric alcohol dehydrogenase, which is responsible for the first-pass metabolism of ethanol in the stomach, is significantly lower in women than in men, which implies that large amounts of alcohol will be metabolized by hepatic alcohol dehydrogenase [41, 42]. It is also possible that genetic variations in carcinogen metabolism, inflammatory response, DNA repair, and cell cycle regulation play a role in determining individual susceptibility to alcohol carcinogenesis, which may partially explain variations in HCC risk by sex.

Seroepidemiological studies have demonstrated a high frequency of anti-HCV and HCV RNA in alcohol users and those among them who develop alcoholic liver diseases [43]. Despite this close relationship, there is little understanding of how HCV and alcohol may interact in the development of HCC. In most studies, anti-HCV in alcoholics was found to be closely associated with the presence of HCV RNA in serum, a marker of HCV replication [44], which may suggest that immunosuppression associated with chronic alcohol consumption may enhance HCV replication.

Smoking

Cigarette smoking is significantly associated with HCC development [45]. A meta-analysis on the association between smoking and liver cancer [46] concluded an overall OR of 1.6 (95% CI, 1.3–1.9) for current smokers and 1.5 (95% CI, 1.1–2.1) for former smokers. The recently released report by IARC had confirmed that smoking is considered a risk factor for liver cancer [47]. Despite evidence sufficient to judge the positive association between active smoking and liver cancer, smoking–HCC relationship in men and women separately has not been widely addressed. A US study suggested that smoking is more likely associated with HCC in men and not women [38]. Moreover, synergistic interactions between cigarette smoking and alcohol consumption, HBV, or HCV infection were reported by different studies [38, 48, 49]. Despite the significant association between cigarette smoking and the risk of HCC, passive smoking exposure is not associated with HCC development [38]. The use of chewing tobacco and snuff was also not related to HCC development in general or in nonsmokers [38].

The exact mechanism of tobacco hepatocarcinogenesis is unknown; however, of approximately 4,000 components identified in tobacco smoke, at least 55 are known carcinogens. The major chemical carcinogens include polycyclic aromatic hydrocarbons, such as benzo[a]pyrene; aromatic amines, such as 4-aminobiphenyl; and nitrosamines, such as 4-(methylnitrosamine)-1-(3-pyridyl)-1-butanone. A case–control study demonstrated that 4-aminobiphenyl DNA adducts contained in tobacco smoke is a liver carcinogen [50]. In addition, tobacco smoke contains volatile compounds (e.g., benzene), radioactive elements (e.g., polonium-210), and free radicals that may also play a role in hepatocarcinogenicity [51, 52]. Substantial evidence supports the notion that oxidative stress has been linked to tobacco use. In vitro studies demonstrated that the gas phase of cigarette smoke caused lipid peroxidation of human plasma, which was preventable by the addition of ascorbic acid

[53, 54]. This may support the smoking synergism with alcohol consumption and chronic viral hepatitis on HCC development.

Aflatoxin Exposure

Aflatoxins (AFs) are toxic secondary fungal metabolites (mycotoxins) produced by *Aspergillus flavus* and *A. parasiticus*. There are four AF compounds: B_1, B_2, G_1, and G_2 [55]. The most common and most toxic AF is AFB_1, and the most important target organ is the liver, where the toxicity can lead to liver necrosis and bile duct proliferation [55].

In order for AFB_1 to exert its toxic effects, it must be converted to its highly reactive 8,9-epoxide metabolite by the action of the mixed function monooxygenase enzyme systems in the liver (CYP450 dependent) [56, 57]. Therefore, the development of AF biomarkers is based on detection of the AFB_1 active metabolites, which can covalently interact with cellular molecules, including DNA, RNA, and protein. Epidemiologic research has documented a significant risk for HCC development among individuals who consumed highly AF-contaminated diets [58, 59].

Hormonal Intake

The use of oral contraceptive pills and risk for HCC development is inconclusive. A recent review of 12 case–control studies that included 739 HCC cases and 5,223 controls [60] yielded an overall adjusted OR of 1.6 (0.9–2.5); however, six studies, included in the analysis, showed a significant increase in HCC risk with longer duration of exposure of oral contraceptives (>5 years). The observed association between liver cancer and oral contraceptive in animals is believed to be related to the proliferative effect of estrogen on hepatocytes where estrogen receptors exist and are highly expressed in HCC [61]. On the other hand, a protective effect of hormonal replacement therapy on liver cancer was determined by some studies [62, 63].

Occupational Exposures

Meta-analyses of epidemiological studies indicated a slightly increased risk of HCC with high level of occupation exposure to vinyl chloride [64]. However, such risk elevation can be a function of disease misclassification bias, since HCC was not analyzed separately from other liver tumors. Reviewing the epidemiological and experimental studies for the association between vinyl chloride and HCC indicated no evidence of biological plausibility for the risk of vinyl chloride on HCC [65].

Chronic Medical Conditions

Diabetes Mellitus

Because the liver plays a crucial role in glucose metabolism, it is not surprising that diabetes mellitus is an epiphenomenon of many chronic liver diseases such as chronic hepatitis, fatty liver, liver failure, and cirrhosis. A recent systematic review of several cohort and case–control studies concluded that diabetes mellitus is significantly associated with HCC [66].

There are several lines of evidence suggesting that diabetes is in fact an independent risk factor for HCC development. This evidence includes (1) results from review and meta-analysis reports concluding that diabetes is a risk factor of HCC [66–69]; (2) findings that the positive association between diabetes and HCC is independent from underlying cirrhosis and chronic liver diseases [70, 71]; (3) findings that the association is positively correlated with disease duration [72–74]; (4) demonstration of the synergistic interaction between diabetes and other HCC risk factors [72, 75, 76]; (5) findings of HCC recurrence after liver resection and transplantation among patients with diabetes [77, 78]; (6) suggestion of a biological plausibility that underlies the association between diabetes and HCC [67, 68, 79]; and (7) the observation of risk of HCC development among patients with type 1 diabetes mellitus [76].

The key mechanism for liver cell damage induced by type 2 diabetes mellitus involves insulin resistance and hyperinsulinemia [69, 80]. HCC development related to hyperinsulinemia can be mediated through inflammation, cellular proliferation, inhibition of apoptosis, and mutation of tumor suppressor genes [69]. Increased insulin levels lead to reduced liver synthesis and blood levels of insulin growth factor binding protein-1 (IGFBP-1), which may contribute to increased bioavailability of insulin-like growth factor-1 (IGF-1), the promotion of cellular proliferation, and the inhibition of apoptosis [81]. Insulin also binds to the insulin receptor and activates its intrinsic tyrosine kinase, leading to phosphorylation of insulin receptor substrate-1 (IRS-1) [82]. HCC tumor cells have been shown to overexpress both IGF-1 and IRS-1 [83]. Overexpression of IRS-1 has been associated with the prevention of apoptosis mediated by transforming growth factor-β [84]. In addition, insulin is associated with lipid peroxidation and increased oxidative stress and the generation of ROS, which may contribute to DNA mutation [85].

Obesity

It is well established that obesity is significantly associated with a wide spectrum of hepatobiliary diseases, including fatty liver diseases, steatosis, and cryptogenic cirrhosis [68, 86]. Once steatosis has developed, cellular adaptations may occur to allow the cell to survive in the new stressful environment and enhance vulnerability to a second hit, or genetic and environmental factors, leading to necroinflammatory changes (non-alcoholic steatohepatitis) or non-alcoholic steatohepatitis (NASH) where different mediators are involved in such pathogenesis [87]. However, there is little information regarding the association between obesity and HCC. A recent meta-analysis 11 cohort studies reported a summary relative risks (95% CI) of 1.17 (1.02–1.34) and 1.89 (1.51–2.36) for overweight and obese individuals, respectively [88]. Nevertheless, the study did not separate HCC from other primary tumors of the liver nor control for the confounding effect of HCV, HBV, diabetes, and heavy alcohol consumption on HCC development.

Lipid peroxidation and free oxygen radicals may play a central role in NASH during which the initiation stage of HCC mechanism takes place. Proliferation of oval cells (the cells of origin for several types of liver cancer) and mutation of P53 tumor suppressor gene can also be potentiated. It is then suggested that the second stage (promotion) takes place as a result of balance in apoptotic and antiapoptotic factors; disturbance in growth factors such as TNF and TGF may facilitate oval cell proliferation [89]. Progression to HCC (stage 3) is suggested to be mediated through cyclooxygenase-2 (COX-2) gene expression by peroxisome proliferator-activated receptor (PPAR-β) nuclear receptors implicated in fatty acid oxidation, cell differentiation, inflammation, cell motility, and cell growth [90, 91]. It was suggested that PPAR-β promotes human HCC cell growth through induction of COX-2 expression and prostaglandins (PGE_2) synthesis. The produced PGE_2 phosphorylates and activates cytosolic phospholipase $A_2\alpha$ ($cPLA_2\alpha$), releasing arachidonic acid for further PPAR-β activation and PGE_2 synthesis via COX-2. This positive-forward loop between PPAR-β and PG pathway likely plays role in the regulation of human cell growth and HCC development (Fig. 1.2).

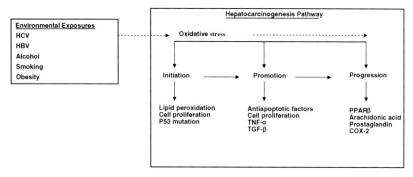

Fig. 1.2 Steps in hepatocarcinogenesis, modified from Xu et al. [90] and Bensinger and Tontonoz [91]

On the other hand, the association between obesity and HCC is hammered by the following obstacles: (1) categorizing HCC among patients with primary liver cancer, (2) inappropriate adjustment for the confounding effect of HCC risk factors specially type 2 diabetes mellitus, and (3) misclassification of obesity definition among patients with HCC. Relying on baseline body weight to estimate body mass index (BMI) at the time of HCC diagnosis could have led to patient misclassification because most HCC is associated with ascites, which can affect the BMI calculation and definition of obesity. Results from an ongoing case–control study indicated

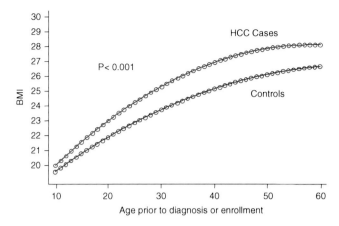

Fig. 1.3 Difference in BMI means between cases and controls at different age periods prior to HCC diagnosis or control enrolment: US case–control study (Hassan unpublished data)

means of BMIs at different age periods prior to HCC development were significantly larger for HCC patients as compared to healthy controls (Hassan, unpublished data) (Fig. 1.3).

Thyroid Diseases

Thyroid hormones play an essential role in lipid mobilization, lipid degradation, and fatty acid oxidation [92]. Patients with hypothyroidism may experience 15–30% weight gain [93] and insulin resistance [94, 95], which are significant factors of NASH. A recent study [96] reported that the prevalence of hypothyroidism in patients with NASH was significantly higher than in controls (15% vs 7.2%, respectively; $p = 0.001$). Such findings were later supported by Reddy and colleagues [97] from Mayo Clinic who assessed the association between hypothyroidism and HCC among 54 HCC patients of unknown etiology and 116 HCC patients related to HCV and alcohol. The study reported OR of 6.8 (95% CI, 1.1–42.1) for HCC development after adjusting for several confounding factors. Our recently published case–control study reported positive association between hypothyroidism and HCC among women [98].

Whether and why hypothyroidism causes HCC is not clear. However, the association between hypothyroidism and NASH can be explained by the underlying hyperlipidemia, decreased fatty acid oxidation, insulin resistance, and lipid peroxidation in patients with hypothyroidism. All of these conditions may enhance the susceptibility to chronic inflammation, DNA damage, and HCC development. Moreover, concurrent thyroid dysfunction among diabetic patients may exacerbate the coexisting diabetes-induced dyslipidemia and may explain our observation of HCC risk modification among patients with hypothyroidism and diabetes [98].

Obesity and hyperinsulinemia may increase the level of insulin-like growth factor-1, which in turn may reduce hepatic synthesis and blood concentration of sex hormone-binding globulin (SHBG) [99, 100], a glycoprotein produced in the liver with high-binding affinity for testosterone and lower affinity for estradiol. Independent of obesity, there is sufficient evidence that thyroid hormones have a positive effect on hepatic SHBG synthesis and that patients with hypothyroidism may experience a lower level of SHBG [101]. Thus, a decreased level of SHBG may lead to increased plasma testosterone and estradiol, both of which may promote cellular proliferation and inhibit apoptosis. Elevated levels of serum testosterone and testosterone to estradiol ratio have been proposed to be predictive of HCC development in Japanese men with cirrhosis [102]. Nevertheless, the fact that the association between hypothyroidism and HCC continued to be significant after adjustment for prior history of obesity suggested that other mechanisms of hepatocarcinogenesis were involved, especially among women.

Cholelithiasis (Gallbladder Stones)

The prevalence of gallstones in patients with cirrhosis is significantly higher than in the general population [103, 104]. This is partially attributed to the metabolic changes such as increased unconjugated bilirubin in bile secondary to hypersplenism, decreased cholesterol secretion, and decreased in apolipoprotein (apo) A-1 and AoA-II sections [105, 106]. A recent study reported significant association between gallbladder stones and HCC; the estimated OR (95% CI) was 14.75 (13.14–16.56) [107]. Nevertheless, the association between gallstones and HCC is difficult to assess from epidemiological studies due to recall bias among HCC patients and due to the subsequent cholecystectomy procedure with liver resection in patients with HCC. Therefore, it is not clear whether cholelithiasis is a risk factor for HCC or a consequence of the underlying chronic liver diseases in patients with HCC.

Dietary Factors

Most of the epidemiological evidence on diet and liver cancer is based on case–control studies and retrospective analysis. This type of assessment is subjective to recall bias due to the fact that patients with chronic liver diseases or cirrhosis may change their diet after being diagnosed with liver diseases. An example of the association between diet and HCC is HCC risk reduction (25–75%) among coffee drinkers who consume two to four cups of coffee per day as compared to non-coffee drinkers [108–110]. HCC risk reduction was also observed for the intake of eggs, milk, yogurt, vegetables, white meat, and fruits [111]. Moreover, the intake of dietary antioxidants, especially selenium and retinoic acid, showed a protective effect for HCC development in HBV carriers and cigarette smokers [112].

Genetic Risk Factors

Familial Aggregation

Familial aggregation of liver cancer has been reported. However, most of these studies were conducted among Asians, particularly in China [113–117]. Given the high prevalence of chronic infection with HBV and that vertical transmission of HBV is the major source for viral transmission among Asians, the reported association between a family history of liver cancer and HCC could be explained by clustering of HBV infection among members of the same family [118]. To avoid this obstacle, Yu et al. [117] matched 553 patients with HCC and 4,684 controls according to HBV infection status. They reported an OR of 2.4 (95% CI, 1.5–3.9) for HCC development in subjects with HBV and a family history of HCC as compared to subjects with HBV but no family history of HCC. A later study by the same investigators showed that familial segregation of HCC in HBsAg carriers is associated with familial clustering of liver cirrhosis [119].

A segregation analysis of Chinese HCC patients suggested that a Mendelian autosomal recessive major gene might also play role in HCC etiology [114]. In addition, first-degree family history of liver cancer in American and European populations is likely to be associated with HCC development independent of chronic infection with HBV and HCV [120]. Synergism between HBV/HCV and a family history of liver cancer was also noted by Hassan et al. [120] among Italian and American individuals.

Inherited Diseases

Hereditary Hemochromatosis

Hereditary hemochromatosis (HHC) is an autosomal recessive genetic disorder of iron metabolism that causes excessive intestinal absorption of dietary iron and deposition of iron in organs including the liver [121]. Recently, a major histocompatibility complex class I gene named *HLA-H* or *HFE* was cloned. Two mutations were described: Cys282Tyr (*C282Y*) and His63Asp (*H63D*) [122]. The *C282Y* mutation is more frequent in HHC [123]. There is growing evidence that even mildly increased amounts of iron in the liver can be damaging, especially when combined with other hepatotoxic factors such as alcohol consumption and chronic viral hepatitis. Iron enhances the pathogenicity of microorganisms, adversely affects the function of macrophages and lymphocytes, and enhances fibrogenic pathways [124, 125], all of which may increase hepatic injury caused by iron alone or by iron and other factors such as chronic HCV infection.

Indeed, a synergistic relationship between HCV and iron overload from hemochromatosis has been suggested [126]. In a study by Hayashi et al., iron depletion improved liver function tests in HCV-infected individuals [127]. In a study by Mazzella and colleague response of chronic HCV to interferon was shown to be related to hepatic iron concentration [128].

Possible factors contributing to the actions of iron in chronic viral hepatitis include enhancement of oxidative stress and lipid peroxidation, exacerbation of immune-mediated tissue inflammation, enhancement of the rate of viral replication, enhancement of the rate of viral mutation, possible impairment of cellular immunity or humoral immunity, and possible impairment of T-lymphocyte proliferation and maturation [129].

α_1 Antitrypsin Deficiency

α_1 antitrypsin deficiency (AATD) is an autosomal dominant genetic disorder characterized by a deficiency in a major serum protease inhibitor (Pi) [130]. AATD is caused by a mutation in the 12.2 kb α_1 antitrypsin gene on chromosome 14 [130]. Over 75 different Pi alleles have been identified, most of which not associated with disease [131]. A relationship exists between Pi phenotypes and serum concentrations of α_1 antitrypsin. Thus, the MM phenotype (normal) is associated with a serum concentration of 100%, MZ 60%, SS 60%, FZ 60%, M 50%, PS 40%, SZ 42.5%, ZZ 15%, and Z 0 to 10%. The most common deficiency variant, PiZ, in its homozygote state is often associated with liver cirrhosis and liver cancer [132]. The role of the heterozygous PiZ state in the development of primary liver cancer is controversial [133–135]. However, there is increasing evidence suggesting that chronic liver disease develops only when another factor such as HCV infection is present and acts as a promoter for the liver damage process. α_1 antitrypsin is an acute-phase reactant whose major role is to inhibit the actions of neutrophil elastase, proteases, and cathepsin G [136]. Any condition triggering the acute-phase response would be expected to stimulate the production of α_1 antitrypsin by the liver.

Therefore, it is suggested that chronic HCV infection could constantly stimulate the hepatocytes to produce the mutant α_1 antitrypsin, leading to more liver damage [137]. Other less frequent inherited disorders such as glycogen storage disorder disease type I (von Gierke's disease) [138], Porphyria Cutanea Tarda [139], and Wilson's disease [140] have been found to be complicated to HCC. However, the interactions between these diseases and other established risk factors such as HCV or HBV have not been studied.

References

1. Parkin DM, Bray F, Ferlay J, Pisani P (2005) Global cancer statistics, 2002. CA Cancer J Clin 55:74–108
2. Parkin DM, Bray F, Ferlay J, Pisani P (2001) Estimating the world cancer burden: Globocan 2000. Int J Cancer 94:153–156
3. Thomas MB, Zhu AX (2005) Hepatocellular carcinoma: the need for progress. J Clin Oncol 23:2892–2899
4. Altekruse SF, McGlynn KA, Reichman ME (2009) Hepatocellular carcinoma incidence, mortality, and survival trends in the United States from 1975 to 2005. J Clin Oncol 27:1485–1491
5. McGlynn KA, London WT (2005) Epidemiology and natural history of hepatocellular carcinoma. Best Pract Res Clin Gastroenterol 19:3–23

6. El-Serag HB, Rudolph KL (2007) Hepatocellular carcinoma: epidemiology and molecular carcinogenesis. Gastroenterology 132:2557–2576
7. International Agency for Research on Cancer (IARC) (1994) Monographs on the evaluation of carcinogenic risks to humans. Hepatitis Viruses 59:182–221
8. Kew MC, Welschinger R, Viana R (2008) Occult hepatitis B virus infection in Southern African blacks with hepatocellular carcinoma. J Gastroenterol Hepatol 23: 1426–1430
9. Zanetti AR, Van DP, Shouval D (2008) The global impact of vaccination against hepatitis B: a historical overview. Vaccine 26:6266–6273
10. Brechot C (1987) Hepatitis B virus (HBV) and hepatocellular carcinoma. HBV DNA status and its implications. J Hepatol 4:269–279
11. Brechot C, Pourcel C, Louise A, Rain B, Tiollais P (1980) Presence of integrated hepatitis B virus DNA sequences in cellular DNA of human hepatocellular carcinoma. Nature 286: 533–535
12. Rossner MT (1992) Review: hepatitis B virus X-gene product: a promiscuous transcriptional activator. J Med Virol 36:101–117
13. Simonetti RG, Camma C, Fiorello F, Cottone M, Rapicetta M, Marino L et al (1992) Hepatitis C virus infection as a risk factor for hepatocellular carcinoma in patients with cirrhosis. A case-control study. Ann Intern Med 116:97–102
14. Okamoto H, Tsuda F, Sakugawa H, Sastrosoewignjo RI, Imai M, Miyakawa Y et al (1988) Typing hepatitis B virus by homology in nucleotide sequence: comparison of surface antigen subtypes. J Gen Virol 69(Pt 10):2575–2583
15. Kidd-Ljunggren K, Miyakawa Y, Kidd AH (2002) Genetic variability in hepatitis B viruses. J Gen Virol 83:1267–1280
16. Kramvis A, Kew M, Francois G (2005) Hepatitis B virus genotypes. Vaccine 23:2409–2423
17. Alexopoulou A, Dourakis SP (2005) Genetic heterogeneity of hepatitis viruses and its clinical significance. Curr Drug Targets Inflamm Allergy 4:47–55
18. Choo QL, Richman KH, Han JH, Berger K, Lee C, Dong C et al (1991) Genetic organization and diversity of the hepatitis C virus. Proc Natl Acad Sci USA 88:2451–2455
19. Alter MJ, Kruszon-Moran D, Nainan OV, McQuillan GM, Gao F, Moyer LA et al (1999) The prevalence of hepatitis C virus infection in the United States, 1988 through 1994. N Engl J Med 341:556–562
20. Yoshizawa H (2002) Hepatocellular carcinoma associated with hepatitis C virus infection in Japan: projection to other countries in the foreseeable future. Oncology 62(Suppl 1):8–17
21. Donato F, Boffetta P, Puoti M (1998) A meta-analysis of epidemiological studies on the combined effect of hepatitis B and C virus infections in causing hepatocellular carcinoma. Int J Cancer 75:347–354
22. Freeman AJ, Dore GJ, Law MG, Thorpe M, Von OJ, Lloyd AR et al (2001) Estimating progression to cirrhosis in chronic hepatitis C virus infection. Hepatology 34: 809–816
23. Parola M, Robino G (2001) Oxidative stress-related molecules and liver fibrosis. J Hepatol 35:297–306
24. Cerutti PA (1994) Oxy-radicals and cancer. Lancet 344:862–863
25. Wiseman H, Halliwell B (1996) Damage to DNA by reactive oxygen and nitrogen species: role in inflammatory disease and progression to cancer. Biochem J 313(Pt 1):17–29
26. Marra F (1999) Hepatic stellate cells and the regulation of liver inflammation. J Hepatol 31:1120–1130
27. Poli G (2000) Pathogenesis of liver fibrosis: role of oxidative stress. Mol Aspects Med 21:49–98
28. Simmonds P (1995) Variability of hepatitis C virus. Hepatology 21:570–583
29. Dusheiko G, Schmilovitz-Weiss H, Brown D, McOmish F, Yap PL, Sherlock S et al (1994) Hepatitis C virus genotypes: an investigation of type-specific differences in geographic origin and disease. Hepatology 19:13–18

30. Nousbaum JB, Pol S, Nalpas B, Landais P, Berthelot P, Brechot C (1995) Hepatitis C virus type 1b (II) infection in France and Italy. Collaborative Study Group. Ann Intern Med 122:161–168

31. Silini E, Bono F, Cividini A, Cerino A, Bruno S, Rossi S et al (1995) Differential distribution of hepatitis C virus genotypes in patients with and without liver function abnormalities. Hepatology 21:285–290

32. De Mitri MS, Poussin K, Baccarini P, Pontisso P, D'Errico A, Simon N et al (1995) HCV-associated liver cancer without cirrhosis. Lancet 345:413–415

33. International Agency for Research on Cancer (IARC) (1988) Monographs on the evaluation of carcinogenic risks to humans. Alcohol Drinking 44(44):207–215

34. Batey RG, Burns T, Benson RJ, Byth K (1992) Alcohol consumption and the risk of cirrhosis. Med J Aust 156:413–416

35. Brechot C, Nalpas B, Feitelson MA (1996) Interactions between alcohol and hepatitis viruses in the liver. Clin Lab Med 16:273–287

36. Morgan TR, Mandayam S, Jamal MM (2004) Alcohol and hepatocellular carcinoma. Gastroenterology 127:S87–S96

37. Stewart S, Jones D, Day CP (2001) Alcoholic liver disease: new insights into mechanisms and preventative strategies. Trends Mol Med 7:408–413

38. Hassan MM, Spitz MR, Thomas MB, El-Deeb AS, Glover KY, Nguyen NT et al (2008) Effect of different types of smoking and synergism with hepatitis C virus on risk of hepatocellular carcinoma in American men and women: case-control study. Int J Cancer 123:1883–1891

39. Mancinelli R, Binetti R, Ceccanti M (2007) Woman, alcohol and environment: emerging risks for health. Neurosci Biobehav Rev 31:246–253

40. Ely M, Hardy R, Longford NT, Wadsworth ME (1999) Gender differences in the relationship between alcohol consumption and drink problems are largely accounted for by body water. Alcohol Alcohol 34:894–902

41. Baraona E, Abittan CS, Dohmen K, Moretti M, Pozzato G, Chayes ZW et al (2001) Gender differences in pharmacokinetics of alcohol. Alcohol Clin Exp Res 25:502–507

42. Frezza M, di PC, Pozzato G, Terpin M, Baraona E, Lieber CS (1990) High blood alcohol levels in women. The role of decreased gastric alcohol dehydrogenase activity and first-pass metabolism. N Engl J Med 322:95–99

43. Oshita M, Hayashi N, Kasahara A, Hagiwara H, Mita E, Naito M et al (1994) Increased serum hepatitis C virus RNA levels among alcoholic patients with chronic hepatitis C. Hepatology 20:1115–1120

44. Paronetto F (1993) Immunologic reactions in alcoholic liver disease. Semin Liver Dis 13:183–195

45. International Agency for Research on Cancer (2004) (IARC) Monographs on the evaluation of carcinogenic risks to humans. Tobacco Smoke and Involuntary Smoking 83:161–176

46. Gandini S, Botteri E, Iodice S, Boniol M, Lowenfels AB, Maisonneuve P et al (2008) Tobacco smoking and cancer: a meta-analysis. Int J Cancer 122:155–164

47. International Agency for Research on Cancer (IARC) (2004) Monographs on the evaluation of carcinogenic risks to humans. Tobacco Smoke and Involuntary Smoking 83: 161–176.

48. Franceschi S, Montella M, Polesel J, La VC, Crispo A, Dal ML et al (2006) Hepatitis viruses, alcohol, and tobacco in the etiology of hepatocellular carcinoma in Italy. Cancer Epidemiol Biomarkers Prev 15:683–689

49. Mori M, Hara M, Wada I, Hara T, Yamamoto K, Honda M et al (2000) Prospective study of hepatitis B and C viral infections, cigarette smoking, alcohol consumption, and other factors associated with hepatocellular carcinoma risk in Japan. Am J Epidemiol 151:131–139

50. Wang LY, Chen CJ, Zhang YJ, Tsai WY, Lee PH, Feitelson MA et al (1998) 4-Aminobiphenyl DNA damage in liver tissue of hepatocellular carcinoma patients and controls. Am J Epidemiol 147:315–323

51. Vineis P, Pirastu R (1997) Aromatic amines and cancer. Cancer Causes Control 8:346–355
52. Hecht SS (1998) Biochemistry, biology, and carcinogenicity of tobacco-specific N-nitrosamines. Chem Res Toxicol 11:559–603
53. Frei B, Forte TM, Ames BN, Cross CE (1991) Gas phase oxidants of cigarette smoke induce lipid peroxidation and changes in lipoprotein properties in human blood plasma. Protective effects of ascorbic acid. Biochem J 277(Pt 1):133–138
54. Miro O, Alonso JR, Jarreta D, Casademont J, Urbano-Marquez A, Cardellach F (1999) Smoking disturbs mitochondrial respiratory chain function and enhances lipid peroxidation on human circulating lymphocytes. Carcinogenesis 20:1331–1336
55. Ueno Y (1985) The toxicology of mycotoxins. Crit Rev Toxicol 14:99–132
56. Guengerich FP, Shimada T (1991) Oxidation of toxic and carcinogenic chemicals by human cytochrome P-450 enzymes. Chem Res Toxicol 4:391–407
57. Guengerich FP, Shimada T, Iwasaki M, Butler MA, Kadlubar FF (1990) Activation of carcinogens by human liver cytochromes P-450. Basic Life Sci 53:381–396
58. Bulatao-Jayme J, Almero EM, Castro MC, Jardeleza MT, Salamat LA (1982) A case-control dietary study of primary liver cancer risk from aflatoxin exposure. Int J Epidemiol 11: 112–119
59. Yeh FS, Yu MC, Mo CC, Luo S, Tong MJ, Henderson BE (1989) Hepatitis B virus, aflatoxins, and hepatocellular carcinoma in southern Guangxi, China. Cancer Res 49:2506–2509
60. Maheshwari S, Sarraj A, Kramer J, El-Serag HB (2007) Oral contraception and the risk of hepatocellular carcinoma. J Hepatol 47:506–513
61. De B, V, Welsh JA, Yu MC, Bennett WP (1996) p53 mutations in hepatocellular carcinoma related to oral contraceptive use. Carcinogenesis 17:145–149
62. Persson I, Yuen J, Bergkvist L, Schairer C (1996) Cancer incidence and mortality in women receiving estrogen and estrogen-progestin replacement therapy–long-term follow-up of a Swedish cohort. Int J Cancer 67:327–332
63. Fernandez E, Gallus S, Bosetti C, Franceschi S, Negri E, La VC (2003) Hormone replacement therapy and cancer risk: a systematic analysis from a network of case-control studies. Int J Cancer 105:408–412
64. Boffetta P, Matisane L, Mundt KA, Dell LD (2003) Meta-analysis of studies of occupational exposure to vinyl chloride in relation to cancer mortality. Scand J Work Environ Health 29:220–229
65. Dragani TA, Zocchetti C (2008) Occupational exposure to vinyl chloride and risk of hepatocellular carcinoma. Cancer Causes Control 19:1193–1200
66. El-Serag HB, Hampel H, Javadi F (2006) The association between diabetes and hepatocellular carcinoma: a systematic review of epidemiologic evidence. Clin Gastroenterol Hepatol 4:369–380
67. Bell DS, Allbright E (2007) The multifaceted associations of hepatobiliary disease and diabetes. Endocr Pract 13:300–312
68. Tolman KG, Fonseca V, Tan MH, Dalpiaz A (2004) Narrative review: hepatobiliary disease in type 2 diabetes mellitus. Ann Intern Med 141:946–956
69. Harrison SA (2006) Liver disease in patients with diabetes mellitus. J Clin Gastroenterol 40:68–76
70. Davila JA, Morgan RO, Shaib Y, McGlynn KA, El-Serag HB (2005) Diabetes increases the risk of hepatocellular carcinoma in the United States: a population based case control study. Gut 54:533–539
71. Veldt BJ, Chen W, Heathcote EJ, Wedemeyer H, Reichen J, Hofmann WP et al (2008) Increased risk of hepatocellular carcinoma among patients with hepatitis C cirrhosis and diabetes mellitus. Hepatology 47:1856–1862
72. Yuan JM, Govindarajan S, Arakawa K, Yu MC (2004) Synergism of alcohol, diabetes, and viral hepatitis on the risk of hepatocellular carcinoma in blacks and whites in the U.S. Cancer 101:1009–1017

73. Yu MC, Tong MJ, Govindarajan S, Henderson BE (1991) Nonviral risk factors for hepatocellular carcinoma in a low-risk population, the non-Asians of Los Angeles County, California. J Natl Cancer Inst 83:1820–1826
74. El-Serag HB, Tran T, Everhart JE (2004) Diabetes increases the risk of chronic liver disease and hepatocellular carcinoma. Gastroenterology 126:460–468
75. Chen CL, Yang HI, Yang WS, Liu CJ, Chen PJ, You SL et al (2008) Metabolic factors and risk of hepatocellular carcinoma by chronic hepatitis B/C infection: a follow-up study in Taiwan. Gastroenterology 135:111–121
76. Hassan MM, Hwang LY, Hatten CJ, Swaim M, Li D, Abbruzzese JL et al (2002) Risk factors for hepatocellular carcinoma: synergism of alcohol with viral hepatitis and diabetes mellitus. Hepatology 36:1206–1213
77. Komura T, Mizukoshi E, Kita Y, Sakurai M, Takata Y, Arai K et al (2007) Impact of diabetes on recurrence of hepatocellular carcinoma after surgical treatment in patients with viral hepatitis. Am J Gastroenterol 102:1939–1946
78. Ikeda Y, Shimada M, Hasegawa H, Gion T, Kajiyama K, Shirabe K et al (1998) Prognosis of hepatocellular carcinoma with diabetes mellitus after hepatic resection. Hepatology 27:1567–1571
79. Dellon ES, Shaheen NJ (2005) Diabetes and hepatocellular carcinoma: associations, biologic plausibility, and clinical implications. Gastroenterology 129:1132–1134
80. Bugianesi E (2005) Review article: steatosis, the metabolic syndrome and cancer. Aliment Pharmacol Ther 22(Suppl 2):40–43
81. Moore MA, Park CB, Tsuda H (1998) Implications of the hyperinsulinaemia-diabetes-cancer link for preventive efforts. Eur J Cancer Prev 7:89–107
82. Alexia C, Fallot G, Lasfer M, Schweizer-Groyer G, Groyer A (2004) An evaluation of the role of insulin-like growth factors (IGF) and of type-I IGF receptor signalling in hepatocarcinogenesis and in the resistance of hepatocarcinoma cells against drug-induced apoptosis. Biochem Pharmacol 68:1003–1015
83. Tanaka S, Mohr L, Schmidt EV, Sugimachi K, Wands JR (1997) Biological effects of human insulin receptor substrate-1 overexpression in hepatocytes. Hepatology 26:598–604
84. Tanaka S, Wands JR (1996) Insulin receptor substrate 1 overexpression in human hepatocellular carcinoma cells prevents transforming growth factor beta1-induced apoptosis. Cancer Res 56:3391–3394
85. Hu W, Feng Z, Eveleigh J, Iyer G, Pan J, Amin S et al (2002) The major lipid peroxidation product, trans-4-hydroxy-2-nonenal, preferentially forms DNA adducts at codon 249 of human p53 gene, a unique mutational hotspot in hepatocellular carcinoma. Carcinogenesis 23:1781–1789
86. Reddy JK, Rao MS (2006) Lipid metabolism and liver inflammation. II. Fatty liver disease and fatty acid oxidation. Am J Physiol Gastrointest Liver Physiol 290:G852–G858
87. Browning JD, Horton JD (2004) Molecular mediators of hepatic steatosis and liver injury. J Clin Invest 114:147–152
88. Larsson SC, Wolk A (2007) Overweight, obesity and risk of liver cancer: a meta-analysis of cohort studies. Br J Cancer 97:1005–1008
89. Caldwell SH, Crespo DM, Kang HS, Al-Osaimi AM (2004) Obesity and hepatocellular carcinoma. Gastroenterology 127:S97–S103
90. Xu L, Han C, Lim K, Wu T (2006) Cross-talk between peroxisome proliferator-activated receptor delta and cytosolic phospholipase A(2)alpha/cyclooxygenase-2/prostaglandin E(2) signaling pathways in human hepatocellular carcinoma cells. Cancer Res 66:11859–11868
91. Bensinger SJ, Tontonoz P (2008) Integration of metabolism and inflammation by lipid-activated nuclear receptors. Nature 454:470–477
92. Pucci E, Chiovato L, Pinchera A (2000) Thyroid and lipid metabolism. Int J Obes Relat Metab Disord 24(Suppl 2):S109–S112
93. Krotkiewski M (2000) Thyroid hormones and treatment of obesity. Int J Obes Relat Metab Disord 24(Suppl 2):S116–S119

94. Dimitriadis G, Parry-Billings M, Bevan S, Leighton B, Krause U, Piva T et al (1997) The effects of insulin on transport and metabolism of glucose in skeletal muscle from hyperthyroid and hypothyroid rats. Eur J Clin Invest 27:475–483

95. Sanyal AJ, Campbell-Sargent C, Mirshahi F, Rizzo WB, Contos MJ, Sterling RK et al (2001) Nonalcoholic steatohepatitis: association of insulin resistance and mitochondrial abnormalities. Gastroenterology 120:1183–1192

96. Liangpunsakul S, Chalasani N (2003) Is hypothyroidism a risk factor for non-alcoholic steatohepatitis? J Clin Gastroenterol 37:340–343

97. Reddy A, Dash C, Leerapun A, Mettler TA, Stadheim LM, Lazaridis KN et al (2007) Hypothyroidism: a possible risk factor for liver cancer in patients with no known underlying cause of liver disease. Clin Gastroenterol Hepatol 5:118–123

98. Hassan MM, Curley SA, Li D, Kaseb A, Davila M, Abdalla EK et al (2010) Duration of Diabetes and type of diabetes treatment, increase the risk of hepatocellular carcinoma. Cancer 116:1938–1946

99. Haffner SM (2000) Sex hormones, obesity, fat distribution, type 2 diabetes and insulin resistance: epidemiological and clinical correlation. Int J Obes Relat Metab Disord 24(Suppl 2):S56–S58

100. Hautanen A (2000) Synthesis and regulation of sex hormone-binding globulin in obesity. Int J Obes Relat Metab Disord 24(Suppl 2):S64–S70

101. Hampl R, Kancheva R, Hill M, Bicikova M, Vondra K (2003) Interpretation of sex hormone-binding globulin levels in thyroid disorders. Thyroid 13:755–760

102. Tanaka K, Sakai H, Hashizume M, Hirohata T (2000) Serum testosterone:estradiol ratio and the development of hepatocellular carcinoma among male cirrhotic patients. Cancer Res 60:5106–5110

103. Conte D, Fraquelli M, Fornari F, Lodi L, Bodini P, Buscarini L (1999) Close relation between cirrhosis and gallstones: cross-sectional and longitudinal survey. Arch Intern Med 159:49–52

104. Conte D, Barisani D, Mandelli C, Bodini P, Borzio M, Pistoso S et al (1991) Cholelithiasis in cirrhosis: analysis of 500 cases. Am J Gastroenterol 86:1629–1632

105. Fornari F, Civardi G, Buscarini E, Cavanna L, Imberti D, Rossi S et al (1990) Cirrhosis of the liver. A risk factor for development of cholelithiasis in males. Dig Dis Sci 35:1403–1408

106. Zhu JF, Shan LC, Chen WH (1994) [Changes in lipids, bilirubin and metal elements in the gallbladder bile in patients with cirrhosis of the liver]. Zhonghua Nei Ke Za Zhi 33:767–769

107. El-Serag HB, Engels EA, Landgren O, Chiao E, Henderson L, Amaratunge HC et al (2009) Risk of hepatobiliary and pancreatic cancers after hepatitis C virus infection: a population-based study of U.S. veterans. Hepatology 49:116–123

108. Gallus S, Bertuzzi M, Tavani A, Bosetti C, Negri E, La VC et al (2002) Does coffee protect against hepatocellular carcinoma? Br J Cancer 87:956–959

109. Gelatti U, Covolo L, Franceschini M, Pirali F, Tagger A, Ribero ML et al (2005) Coffee consumption reduces the risk of hepatocellular carcinoma independently of its aetiology: a case-control study. J Hepatol 42:528–534

110. Tanaka K, Hara M, Sakamoto T, Higaki Y, Mizuta T, Eguchi Y et al (2007) Inverse association between coffee drinking and the risk of hepatocellular carcinoma: a case-control study in Japan. Cancer Sci 98:214–218

111. Talamini R, Polesel J, Montella M, Dal ML, Crispo A, Tommasi LG et al (2006) Food groups and risk of hepatocellular carcinoma: a multicenter case-control study in Italy. Int J Cancer 119:2916–2921

112. Yu MW, Hsieh HH, Pan WH, Yang CS, Chen CJ (1995) Vegetable consumption, serum retinol level, and risk of hepatocellular carcinoma. Cancer Res 55:1301–1305

113. Demir G, Belentepe S, Ozguroglu M, Celik AF, Sayhan N, Tekin S et al (2002) Simultaneous presentation of hepatocellular carcinoma in identical twin brothers. Med Oncol 19:113–116

114. Cai RL, Meng W, Lu HY, Lin WY, Jiang F, Shen FM (2003) Segregation analysis of hepatocellular carcinoma in a moderately high-incidence area of East China. World J Gastroenterol 9:2428–2432

115. Zhang JY, Wang X, Han SG, Zhuang H (1998) A case-control study of risk factors for hepatocellular carcinoma in Henan, China. Am J Trop Med Hyg 59: 947–951
116. Sun Z, Lu P, Gail MH, Pee D, Zhang Q, Ming L et al (1999) Increased risk of hepatocellular carcinoma in male hepatitis B surface antigen carriers with chronic hepatitis who have detectable urinary aflatoxin metabolite M1. Hepatology 30:379–383
117. Yu MW, Chang HC, Liaw YF, Lin SM, Lee SD, Liu CJ et al (2000) Familial risk of hepatocellular carcinoma among chronic hepatitis B carriers and their relatives. J Natl Cancer Inst 92:1159–1164
118. Chen CH, Huang GT, Lee HS, Yang PM, Chen DS, Sheu JC (1998) Clinical impact of screening first-degree relatives of patients with hepatocellular carcinoma. J Clin Gastroenterol 27:236–239
119. Yu MW, Chang HC, Chen PJ, Liu CJ, Liaw YF, Lin SM et al (2002) Increased risk for hepatitis B-related liver cirrhosis in relatives of patients with hepatocellular carcinoma in northern Taiwan. Int J Epidemiol 31:1008–1015
120. Donato F, Gelatti U, Chiesa R, Albertini A, Bucella E, Boffetta P et al (1999) A case-control study on family history of liver cancer as a risk factor for hepatocellular carcinoma in North Italy. Brescia HCC Study. Cancer Causes Control 10:417–421
121. Piperno A (1998) Classification and diagnosis of iron overload. Haematologica 83:447–455
122. Feder JN, Gnirke A, Thomas W, Tsuchihashi Z, Ruddy DA, Basava A et al (1996) A novel MHC class I-like gene is mutated in patients with hereditary haemochromatosis. Nat Genet 13:399–408
123. Beutler E, Gelbart T, West C, Lee P, Adams M, Blackstone R et al (1996) Mutation analysis in hereditary hemochromatosis. Blood Cells Mol Dis 22:187–194
124. Bullen JJ, Rogers HJ, Griffiths E (1978) Role of iron in bacterial infection. Curr Top Microbiol Immunol 80:1–35
125. Bullen JJ, Ward CG, Rogers HJ (1991) The critical role of iron in some clinical infections. Eur J Clin Microbiol Infect Dis 10:613–617
126. Miller M, Crippin JS, Klintmalm G (1996) End stage liver disease in a 13-year old secondary to hepatitis C and hemochromatosis. Am J Gastroenterol 91:1427–1429
127. Hayashi H, Takikawa T, Nishimura N, Yano M (1995) Serum aminotransferase levels as an indicator of the effectiveness of venesection for chronic hepatitis C. J Hepatol 22: 268–271
128. Mazzella G, Accogli E, Sottili S, Festi D, Orsini M, Salzetta A et al (1996) Alpha interferon treatment may prevent hepatocellular carcinoma in HCV-related liver cirrhosis. J Hepatol 24:141–147
129. Bonkovsky HL, Banner BF, Rothman AL (1997) Iron and chronic viral hepatitis. Hepatology 25:759–768
130. Sifers RN, Finegold MJ, Woo SL (1992) Molecular biology and genetics of alpha 1-antitrypsin deficiency. Semin Liver Dis 12:301–310
131. Fabbretti G, Sergi C, Consales G, Faa G, Brisigotti M, Romeo G et al (1992) Genetic variants of alpha-1-antitrypsin (AAT). Liver 12:296–301
132. Eriksson S, Carlson J, Velez R (1986) Risk of cirrhosis and primary liver cancer in alpha 1-antitrypsin deficiency. N Engl J Med 314:736–739
133. Blenkinsopp WK, Haffenden GP (1977) Alpha-1-antitrypsin bodies in the liver. J Clin Pathol 30:132–137
134. Carlson J, Eriksson S (1985) Chronic 'cryptogenic' liver disease and malignant hepatoma in intermediate alpha 1-antitrypsin deficiency identified by a Pi Z-specific monoclonal antibody. Scand J Gastroenterol 20:835–842
135. Zhou H, Fischer HP (1998) Liver carcinoma in PiZ alpha-1-antitrypsin deficiency. Am J Surg Pathol 22:742–748
136. Teckman JH, Qu D, Perlmutter DH (1996) Molecular pathogenesis of liver disease in alpha1-antitrypsin deficiency. Hepatology 24:1504–1516

137. Banner BF, Karamitsios N, Smith L, Bonkovsky HL (1998) Enhanced phenotypic expression of alpha-1-antitrypsin deficiency in an MZ heterozygote with chronic hepatitis C. Am J Gastroenterol 93:1541–1545
138. Bianchi L (1993) Glycogen storage disease I and hepatocellular tumours. Eur J Pediatr 152(Suppl 1):S63–S70
139. Siersema PD, ten Kate FJ, Mulder PG, Wilson JH (1992) Hepatocellular carcinoma in porphyria cutanea tarda: frequency and factors related to its occurrence. Liver 12:56–61
140. Cheng WS, Govindarajan S, Redeker AG (1992) Hepatocellular carcinoma in a case of Wilson's disease. Liver 12:42–45

Chapter 2
Biology of Hepatocellular Carcinoma

Maria Luisa Balmer and Jean-François Dufour

Keywords Angiogenesis · Apoptosis · HCC · Metastasis · miRNA · Oncogene · Stem cells · Telomeres

From Genotype to Phenotype – Or What a Cell Needs to Become a Cancer Cell

Being a cancer cell is not easy. You have to maintain DNA replication and protein production under adverse conditions in the abnormal architecture of a tumour which often deprives you of oxygen and nutrients. Thus, survival requires a complete kit of stress response tools that you have to acquire before becoming a cancer cell.

From a more scientific point of view, we can see tumorigenesis as fast-track evolution in miniature edition where genetic alterations drive the progressive transformation of normal human cells into highly malignant derivates that seem to be advantageous to their normal counterparts. Investigations have been conducted at different molecular levels including DNA level, RNA level and protein level, with regard to chromosomal imbalance and genetic instability, epigenetic alteration, gene expression and gene regulation and translation [1]. Whatever the level, cancer cells need to acquire a combination of properties which typify their malignant phenotype in the end (Fig. 2.1). Six essential alterations in cell physiology that collectively dictate malignant growth have been proposed: self-sufficiency in growth signals, insensitivity to growth inhibition (antigrowth), evasion of programmed cell death (apoptosis), limitless replicative potential, sustained angiogenesis and tissue invasion and metastasis [2].

In this chapter we briefly discuss these six properties as they are common in most cancers, including HCC.

J.-F. Dufour (✉)
Department of Clinical Pharmacology and Visceral Research, University of Bern, Bern, Switzerland

K.M. McMasters, J.-N. Vauthey (eds.), *Hepatocellular Carcinoma*,
DOI 10.1007/978-1-60327-522-4_2, © Springer Science+Business Media, LLC 2011

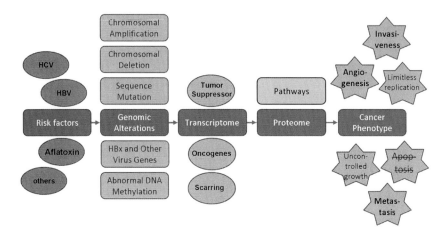

Fig. 2.1 The long and winding road to cancer

Growth signals are essential to move a cell from its quiescent state into an active proliferative state. Cancer cells generate many of their own growth signals, thereby reducing their dependence on stimulation from their normal tissue environment. This can happen by synthesis of their own growth signals (autocrine stimulation), growth factor receptor overexpression, ligand-independent signalling through structural alteration of receptors and alterations in components of the downstream cytoplasmic circuitry that receives and processes the signals emitted by ligand-activated growth factor receptors and integrins. Tumour development is not only the result of selection of a genetically mutated population of cells with advantageous capabilities but rather the result of a tiny communication between the altered cancer cell and its unaltered neighbours such as fibroblasts, endothelial cells and inflammatory cells which maintain tumour growth.

Within a normal tissue, multiple antiproliferative signals operate to maintain cellular quiescence and tissue homeostasis. These growth-inhibitory signals, like their positive counterparts, are received by transmembrane surface receptors coupled to intracellular signalling circuits. At the molecular level, many antiproliferative signals are funnelled through the retinoblastoma protein (pRb) and its two relatives, p107 and p130, which block proliferation by inhibiting progression from G1- into S-phase of the cell cycle [3]. The pRb signalling circuit, as governed by TGFβ and other extrinsic factors, can be disrupted in a variety of ways: some cancer cells display mutant, dysfunctional receptors while others lose TGFβ responsiveness through downregulation of their TGFβ receptor.

Apoptosis represents a physiological way to eliminate excess cells during both development and regeneration. Apoptosis can be triggered by an extrinsic pathway (death receptor associated) as well as an intrinsic pathway (mitochondria pathway), both of which might be inactivated during tumour development. Resistance to apoptosis can be acquired by cancer cells through a variety of strategies. Surely, the most commonly occurring loss of a pro-apoptotic regulator through mutation involves the *p53* tumour suppressor gene. The resulting functional inactivation of its product, the p53 protein, is seen in greater than 50% of human cancers and results in the removal of a key component of the DNA damage sensor that can induce the apoptotic effector cascade [4].

Many and perhaps all types of mammalian cells carry an intrinsic, cell-autonomous program that limits their multiplication and stops their growth. Tumour cells have to exhaust their endowment of allowed doublings and breach the mortality barrier to acquire unlimited replicative potential. Telomeres, which are composed of several thousand repeats of a short six base-pair sequence element, and which are shortened in each cell doubling, limit one cell's lifetime. Therefore, telomere maintenance either by upregulating expression of the telomerase enzyme [5] or by recombination-based interchromosomal exchanges of sequence information [6] is evident in virtually all types of malignant cells. By one or the other mechanism, telomeres are maintained at a length above a critical threshold, and this in turn permits unlimited multiplication of descendant cells.

The oxygen and nutrients supplied by the vasculature are critical for cell function and survival. Thus tumours need to induce blood vessel formation to maintain growth and viability. One common strategy is increased expression of angiogenesis inducers as vascular endothelial growth factor (VEGF) and fibroblast growth factor (FGF) or downregulation of angiogenesis inhibitors as thrombospondin-1 or β-interferon.

The development of cancer metastasis is a highly complex event, involving the generation of new blood and lymph vessels, growth, invasion with breakdown and cross talk of the host matrix, escape from immune surveillance, transport to other sites with adhesion, and subsequent invasion of the organ that hosts the metastasis. Several participants in this tightly orchestrated procedure are important, for instance cell-adhesion molecules, signalling pathways, immune cells, enzymes and receptors, acting all in concert to guide the tumour cell to its new home.

To reach the six capabilities necessary for survival, you have to be highly selected as a cancer cell. Genomic instability, altered transcription and translation, deregulated protein synthesis all act in concert to equip you with the necessary armamentarium to reach the cancer phenotype.

Biological Features of Liver Cancer – The Hallmark of Hepatocellular Carcinoma

Usually, HCC arises as a consequence of underlying liver diseases such as viral hepatitis and liver cirrhosis. Highly variable clinical phenotypes in HCC patients indicate that HCC comprises several biologically distinctive patterns. Patients can be categorized in subgroups by different grades of differentiation, proliferation rates, ability to invade vessels, potential for metastasis, sensitivity to chemotherapeutic agents, etc. [7]. When the liver gets injured by factors like HBV/HCV, alcohol or aflatoxin B1, necrosis will appear in the liver accompanied by the subsequent hepatocyte proliferation. After continuous cycles of destructive–regenerative process accumulate to some extent, the liver will suffer from cirrhosis. The main characteristic of cirrhosis is that abnormal nodules appear in the liver surrounded by collagens and scarring. Subsequently, the hyperplastic nodules will turn into dysplastic nodules (DNs) inducing a high risk of developing HCC for those patients [8]. DNs are classified into low grade and high grade according to cytological and architectural atypia on microscopic examination [9]. One-third of high-grade DNs will progress to HCC in 2 years, and the rate increases to 81% in 5 years [10].

Coming back to the introduced route of cancer development, HCC phenotype can result as a consequence of different alterations on different molecular levels. The observed genetic aberrations associated with HCC include the amplification or deletion of chromosomal regions, copy number changes of genes and abnormal epigenetic alterations. Chromosomal amplification regions often harbour oncogenes, whereas the chromosomal deletion regions often include tumour suppressor genes, both conferring a growth advantage for tumorigenesis in HCC [11]. These aberrations can be caused by different environmental factors like virus infection and alcohol and/or aflatoxin consumption [12, 13]. Epigenetic modifications refer to changes in DNA/chromatin that do not involve changes in the DNA sequence, for instance DNA methylation or histone modifications. A number of studies have indicated that promoter hypermethylation may be a key mechanism involved in the inactivation of some tumour suppressor genes in HCC [1]. Changes in the expression of many genes are also evident at both mRNA and protein levels. Such changes can be the consequences of the genetic aberrations and environmental interactions. As a complex disease, the genesis and development of HCC could not be decided by a single factor or a simple collection of single factors, but rather by interactions of multiple proteins, genes and miRNAs in biological pathways. Furthermore, significant and complex cross talks among the different pathways exist and are involved in different aspects of HCC development and progression. These cross talks, largely not understood at the molecular level, could potentially account for the resistance to molecularly targeted drugs, which are able to hit pathways only at one or few sites [14].

In this section, we discuss the hallmarks of liver cancer which are important for diagnosis and treatment of the disease.

Liver Stem Cells

Stem cells are generally characterized by their capacity for self-renewal through asymmetrical cell division, multipotency for producing progeny in at least two lineages, long-term tissue reconstitution, and serial transplantability [15]. When mature hepatocytes and cholangiocytes are damaged or inhibited in their replication a reserve compartment of hepatic progenitor cells located within the intrahepatic biliary tree is activated [16]. The activation of this stem cell compartment is observed in circumstances of prolonged necrosis, cirrhosis and chronic inflammatory liver disease. The liver is different from the skin and gastrointestinal tract with regard to transit-amplifying cells, in that the most highly differentiated cells, the hepatocytes, are not terminally differentiated and can respond to injury or loss by rapid, highly regulated proliferation. Thus, in the liver, differentiated hepatocytes per se can be viewed as the hepatic version of transit-amplifying cells. Given the postulated presence of a hepatic lineage of cells from periductal stem cells, to bipolar ductal progenitor cells, to hepatocytes, with each cell type proliferation competent, it would not be surprising to find that HCCs can arise from the stem cells, the bipolar ductal progenitor cells, or the hepatocytes [17]. The fact that stem cell activation precedes the development of HCC in almost all models of hepatocarcinogenesis and invariably accompanies chronic liver damage in humans makes it likely that the mature hepatocyte is not the cell of origin of all HCCs [18]. Detailed immunophenotyping of HCCs indicated that 28–50% of HCCs express markers of progenitor cells such as CK7 and CK19 [19]. But what transforms a stem cell into a cancer stem cell (CSC)? There are at least two proposed mechanisms of CSC origin: oncogenic mutations may inactivate the constraints on normal stem cell expansion or, alternatively, oncogenic mutations in a more differentiated cell generate continual proliferation of cells that no longer enter a postmitotic differentiated state, thereby creating a pool of self-renewing cells in which further mutations can accumulate [20]. Several pathways have been proposed to be implicated in stem cell proliferation: TGFβ, Notch, Wnt and Hedgehog are some examples [19]. The detailed mechanisms directing transformation of stem cells to cancer stem cells and hepatocellular cancer, however, remain still to be elucidated and definitive markers for these putative cancer stem cells have not yet been established.

Angiogenesis

HCC is one of the most vascular solid cancers, associated with a high propensity for vascular invasion. In fact, its active neovascularization can be visualized in angiography and is used as a diagnostic criterion for HCC. The development of neovasculature in the tumour provides two essential functions for the growth and metastasis of a cancer. First, the vessels provide a route for supply of nutrient and oxygen to sustain growth and excretion of metabolic waste. Second, the neovessels provide access for tumour cells to enter the circulation and spread as metastases. In fact, HCC is characterized by a high propensity for vascular invasion, and the angiogenic activity of HCC correlates with the risk of vascular invasion [21]. HCC typically develops from dysplastic nodules in a cirrhotic liver and the endothelial cells in these nodules undergo phenotypic changes during malignant transformation as demonstrated by changes in endothelial cell markers. The process of angiogenesis is a complex multistep process initiated by the release of angiogenic factors from tumour cells. The angiogenic factors bind to specific receptors of endothelial cells of preexisting blood vessels and activate the endothelial cells, which then secrete enzymes to degrade the underlying basement membrane. The activated endothelial cells then proliferate, migrate and assemble into new capillary tubes, followed by the synthesis of a new basement membrane. However, some recent studies suggested that some of the neovessels in tumours may be derived from circulating endothelial precursor cells that originate from the bone marrow [22, 23]. There is also evidence indicating that some tumours may be vascularized without significant angiogenesis, probably by using existing vessels through a process described as vascular co-option or even by forming vascular channels on their own through a nonendothelial cell process called 'vascular mimicry' [24]. Angiogenesis can be triggered by activation of oncogenes like *ras* or inactivation of tumour suppressor genes like *p53* [25, 26]. In addition, a number of cellular stress factors such as hypoxia, nutrient deprivation or inducers of reactive oxygen species are important stimuli of angiogenic signalling [27]. Many angiogenic and antiangiogenic factors have been studied in recent years.

Vascular endothelial growth factor (VEGF) is one of the first isolated angiogenic peptides and is the most well-studied angiogenic factor so far. It has a specific mitogenic effect on endothelial cells, and it also increases vascular permeability (hence also known as vascular permeability factor) and promotes extravasation of proteins from tumour vessels, leading to the formation of a fibrin matrix that supports the growth of endothelial cells and allows invasion of stromal cells into the developing tumour [28]. The expression of VEGF protein was found to correlate with clinicopathological factors such as proliferation, vascular invasion and tumour multiplicity and was reported to associate with not only invasion and metastasis of HCC but also postoperative recurrence [29]. Expression of VEGF is regulated by microenvironmental and genetic alterations in cancer cells. Hypoxia is a key microenvironmental factor of angiogenesis, and hypoxia-inducible factors (HIF) are known to stimulate VEGF expression [30, 31]. The upregulation of VEGF in HCC is controlled at transcriptional levels as well as by the mRNA stability of VEGF [32]. In addition, the *p53* tumour suppressor and *HBx* genes might regulate VEGF expression in HCC [33, 34].

Fibroblast growth factors (FGFs) are a family of heparin-binding growth factors that includes at least 22 structurally related members, of which acidic fibroblast growth factor (aFGF) and basic fibroblast growth factor (bFGF) are the best-known members. FGFs exert their pro-angiogenic activity by interacting with various endothelial cell surface receptors, including tyrosine kinase receptors FGFR1 and FGFR2, heparan sulphate proteoglycans and integrins [35]. bFGF appears to act synergistically with VEGF in the induction of angiogenesis [36]. Aside from its angiogenic effect, bFGF has also been shown to act as a mitogen for HCC cell proliferation via an autocrine mechanism [37].

Angiopoietins play an important role in angiogenesis. Angiopoietin-1 (Ang-1) is a survival signal for endothelial cells and it promotes recruitment of pericytes and smooth muscle cells to form mature blood vessels. In contrast to Ang-1, angiopoietin 2 (Ang-2) induces vascular regression in the absence of VEGF but increases vascular sprouting in its presence. It has been shown that the ectopic expression of Ang-2 in HCC cells promotes rapid development of tumour and aggravates its prognosis [38].

Other angiogeneic factors have also been shown to be involved in tumour angiogenesis including platelet-derived endothelial cell growth factor [39], tissue factor [40], cyclooxygenase-2 [41] and angiogenin [42].

Telomere Shortening

The progressive shortening of telomeres with each cell division serves in most somatic cells as a "mitotic clock," indicating cell age and cellular senescence. After a certain number of cell doublings, when a threshold level of telomeric length is reached, a signal is initiated to cease cell division and further progression to S-phase is prevented. Loss of telomeres initiates or drives chromosomal instability, which in turn results in chromosomal abnormalities such as end-to-end fusion and rearrangement. In carcinogenesis, certain cells such as those that have undergone viral transformation, irradiation or mutagenesis will continue to divide, have their telomeres further shortened and eventually die. However, prior to death, the resulting genomic instability causes a small number of these cells to undergo multiple mutations, including the regaining of telomerase activity which thereafter serves to maintain telomere length and genomic stability indefinitely [43]. Telomere shortening is accelerated in chronic liver disease and critically short telomeres characterize cirrhosis stage [44]. The cancer risk increases in response to telomere shortening during aging and chronic liver disease. Furthermore, telomerase activity has been detected in human HCC while it is absent in adjacent non-tumour tissues [43]. Studies in telomerase knockout mice have provided experimental evidence that telomere shortening influences stem cell function, aging and carcinogenesis. These mice exhibit an impaired maintenance and function of adult stem cells and reduced regenerative reserve in response to organ damage. Interestingly they show an increase in chromosomal instability and tumour initiation but impaired tumour progression [45]. Telomerase has been shown to be a critical component for in vivo progression of p53 mutant HCC with short telomeres in the chronically damaged liver. In this molecular context, telomerase limits the accumulation of telomere dysfunction, the evolution of excessive aneuploidy and the activation of p53-independent checkpoints suppressing hepatocarcinogenesis [46]. This dual role of telomeres may point to new treatment options in patients with HCC.

HCC in the Non-cirrhotic Liver

The incidence of HCC arising in the non-cirrhotic liver varies greatly between different studies, ranging from 10 to 50% [47–50]. These tumours have been characterized as often uninodular, encapsulated and expansive growing and they seem to be bigger than normal HCC [50]. All factors that can induce a HCC with cirrhosis can also lead to a non-cirrhotic HCC. Nevertheless, there are several conditions which are known to be associated predominantly with non-cirrhotic liver cancer: sexual steroids induce HCCs through the development of liver adenomas; patients with Alagille syndrome (arteriohepatic dysplasia) [51], hypercitrullinemia [51], α1-antitrypsin deficiency [52] and glycogenosis type 1 [53] often develop HCC without cirrhosis. Iron overload seems to be a general risk factor for developing a non-cirrhotic HCC [54], as well as clinically unapparent mutations in the *HFE* gene [55]. It has been estimated that up to 40% of hepatitis B virus (HBV)-related HCC occur in persons who do not have cirrhosis, while almost all cases of hepatitis C virus (HCV)-related HCC occur in the setting of cirrhosis [56, 57]. Direct oncogenic potential of HBV through chromosomal integration (*cis*-activation) or *trans*-activation of cellular genes seems to be an important feature in the pathogenesis of these cancers [58]. Nevertheless, the two major risk factors for developing an HCC without underlying liver cirrhosis seem to be the metabolic syndrome (MS) with fatty liver disease and liver adenomas. The association between diabetes, obesity, steatosis, non-alcoholic fatty liver disease (NAFLD) and the development of HCC is not well elucidated so far. Changes in fat metabolism, including expression of adipocyte-like gene pathways, appear to play a role both in hepatic regeneration and sometimes in neoplastic transformation [59, 60]. This relationship to fat metabolism appears to be important both in NAFLD-related cancer and in HCV, where steatosis, steatohepatitis and associated oxidative stress are increasingly recognized as significant risk or cofactors in HCC development [61]. Furthermore steatosis is an independent predictor of postoperative HCC recurrence in HCV-associated HCC [62]. Additional epidemiological data indicate a significantly increased risk of hepatocellular carcinoma among diabetic patients [63]. The pathophysiological components of this disorder, especially when steatohepatitis is present, include lipid peroxidation, stem cell proliferation, and increased growth factors, such as insulin and TGF. Proliferation of cells in the setting of oxidative stress and increased trophic factors associated with the metabolic syndrome such as hyperinsulinemia seems to be the hallmark of non-cirrhotic HCC in context with the metabolic syndrome [61]. Recently it has been shown that most of the tumours in context with the metabolic syndrome develop in nonfibrotic livers [64]. Wnt signalling pathway deregulation did not represent the main carcinogenic process involved in this context [64]. A significant percentage of HCCs that develop in the context of MS without significant fibrosis arises from malignant transformation of liver adenoma, especially the TA (telangiectatic) subtype.

It has been proposed that liver adenomas can transform into malignant liver tumours [53, 65–67]. However, the incidence and underlying molecular mechanisms still remain unclear. Moreover, the published data usually derive from patients without liver cirrhosis. This is rather due to the conceptual problem that adenomas are only diagnosed in non-cirrhotic livers and are labelled as macroregenerative nodules or adenomatous hyperplasias in patients with underlying liver cirrhosis, than due to a fundamentally different pathogenesis of these tumours. However, the conceptual adenoma-carcinoma sequence, as observed in other organs like the gut, seems to exist in a similar manner in HCC as well. Among the three genotypically identified subtypes of liver adenoma HNF1α inactivated (35–50% of cases), β-catenin activated (15–18% of cases) and inflammatory (40–55% of cases), the β-catenin-activated adenomas seem to be at higher risk of HCC [68].

Metastasis

HCC is characterized by early development of intrahepatic metastasis, whereas distant organs are usually late involved in the disease. In the diagnosis of intra-hepatic HCC metastases, one problem is to separate metastatic dissemination from multifocal tumours in the liver. The possibility that more than one nodule may be detected in patients with HCC has been known for more than 50 years [69]. This is not only semantic but of biological importance. 'Metastatic dissemination or multifocal tumour?' is not a Hamletic question, because the two possibilities are not mutually exclusive as cirrhotic liver can generate more than one cancer nodule with the same, still unknown mechanisms, during the history of the disease. However, the identification of these two distinct hypotheses seems to be an underestimated problem by clinicians, although a patient with a multifocal tumour has a better prognosis than a patient with a metastatic cancer [70, 71]. Multiple HCC nodules are an expression of metastasis rather than of multifocal cancer in more than 60% of cases [72], but more sensitive tests are needed to distinguish metastatic from multifocal HCC in the liver.

The process of metastasis involves an intricate interplay between altered cell adhesion, survival, proteolysis, migration, lymph/angiogenesis, immune escape mechanisms and homing on target organs. Not surprisingly, the molecular mechanisms that propel invasive growth and metastasis are also found in embryonic development and, however, to a less perpetual/chronic/aggressive/quantitatively different extent, in adult tissue maintenance (e.g. involving stem cell differentiation) and repair processes [73].

Several molecular examples and pathways are involved and all act in concert to guide the tumour cell to its new home (Table 2.1). All these players are tightly orchestrated and interact through several molecular pathways: The Wnt/β-catenin pathway links cell–cell adhesion and downstream signalling and mutations in β-catenin genes can be detected in 12–26% of human HCC; *p53* mutation is involved in determining dedifferentiation, proliferating activity and tumour progression [74]; is strongly related to the invasiveness of HCC and also influences the postoperative course (particularly recurrence within 1 year) [75]. The mitogen-activated protein kinase pathway (MAPK) and the Raf kinase inhibitor protein

Table 2.1 Molecular examples and pathways are involved and all act in concert to guide the tumour cell to its new home

Biological capability	Molecular examples/pathway entities
Survival	IGF survival factors
Adhesion and deadhesion	CAMs, cadherins, integrins
Migration	Met-SF/HGF signalling, FAK
Proteolysis/ECM remodelling	MMPs, uPA, ADAMs, heparanase
Immune escape	Downregulation of intrinsic immunogenicity, MHC loss
Lymph/angiogenesis	VEGF, PDGF, bFGF
Homing on target organs	Chemokines/chemokine receptors, CD44, osteopontin

(RKIP) as an inhibitor of this pathway revealed prominent roles during human HCC metastasis [76]. Signalling pathways in liver cancer metastasis are highly complex and little is known about the importance of every single cascade in metastasis development. A bioinformatics analysis of metastasis-related proteins in hepatocellular carcinoma resulted in a gigantic diversity of involved partners in metastasis development (506 proteins, 83 pathways) [77].

From a more macroscopic point of view, there are four proposed models of metastasis development: According to Chambers and coworkers, only a very small population of injected tumour cells in mice form micrometastases, although most of them are arrested in the liver. Furthermore, not all of the micrometastases persist, and the progressively growing metastases arise only from a small subset (0.02%) of cells [78]. Muschel and coworkers recently proposed a new model for pulmonary metastasis in which endothelium-attached tumour cells that survived the initial apoptotic stimuli proliferate intravascularly. Thus, a principal tenet of this new model is that the extravasation of tumour cells is not a prerequisite for metastatic colony formation and that the initial proliferation takes place within the blood vessels [79]. The unique ability of aggressive tumour cells to generate patterned networks, similar to the patterned networks during embryonic vasculogenesis, and concomitantly to express vascular markers associated with endothelial cells, their precursors and other vascular cells has been termed 'vasculogenic mimicry' by Hendrix and coworkers [80]. It has been shown that tumour cells can migrate as tumour emboli that conserve a tissue architecture reminiscent of the primary tumour. Tumour cells are thus protected from anoikis and direct immunological engagement during dissemination [81].

All of these mechanisms are supposed to have an impact on the pathogenesis of HCC metastasis and should be taken into account when planning new treatment strategies.

HCC in comparison to other solid tumours is a biologically highly multifaceted tumour in which a variety of different events have an impact on its development and characteristics. The epic voyage from genotype to phenotype includes chromosomal instability, altered transcription and translation, deregulated protein synthesis, miRNAs, altered signalling pathways and finally results in a tumour cell perfectly adapted to escape proliferation control and immune surveillance.

References

1. Pei Y, Zhang T, Renault V, Zhang X (2009) An overview of hepatocellular carcinoma study by omics-based methods. Acta Biochim Biophys Sin (Shanghai) 41:1–15
2. Hanahan D, Weinberg RA (2000) The hallmarks of cancer. Cell 100:57–70
3. Weinberg RA (1996) The retinoblastoma protein and cell cycle control. Cell 81:323–330
4. Harris CC (1996) p53 tumor suppressor gene: from the basic research laboratory to the clinic—an abridged historical perspective. Carcinogenesis 17:1187–1198
5. Bryan TM, Cech TR (1999) Telomerase and the maintenance of chromosome ends. Curr Opin Cell Biol 11:318–324
6. Bryan TM, Englezou A, Gupta J, Bacchetti S, Reddel RR (1995) Telomere elongation in immortal human cells without detectable telomerase activity. EMBO J 14:4240–4248

7. Lee JS, Heo J, Libbrecht L, Chu IS, Kaposi-Novak P, Calvisi DF, Mikaelyan A, et al (2006) A novel prognostic subtype of human hepatocellular carcinoma derived from hepatic progenitor cells. Nat Med 12:410–416

8. Farazi PA, DePinho RA (2006) Hepatocellular carcinoma pathogenesis: from genes to environment. Nat Rev Cancer 6:674–687

9. Borzio M, Bruno S, Roncalli M, Mels GC, Ramella G, Borzio F, Leandro G, et al (1995) Liver cell dysplasia is a major risk factor for hepatocellular carcinoma in cirrhosis: a prospective study. Gastroenterology 108:812–817

10. Nakamoto Y, Kaneko S, Fan H, Momoi T, Tsutsui H, Nakanishi K, Kobayashi K, et al (2002) Prevention of hepatocellular carcinoma development associated with chronic hepatitis by anti-fas ligand antibody therapy. J Exp Med 196:1105–1111

11. Huang J, Sheng HH, Shen T, Hu YJ, Xiao HS, Zhang Q, Zhang QH, et al (2006) Correlation between genomic DNA copy number alterations and transcriptional expression in hepatitis B virus-associated hepatocellular carcinoma. FEBS Lett 580:3571–3581

12. Pineau P, Marchio A, Battiston C, Cordina E, Russo A, Terris B, Qin LX, et al (2008) Chromosome instability in human hepatocellular carcinoma depends on p53 status and aflatoxin exposure. Mutat Res 653:6–13

13. Saigo K, Yoshida K, Ikeda R, Sakamoto Y, Murakami Y, Urashima T, Asano T, et al (2008) Integration of hepatitis B virus DNA into the myeloid/lymphoid or mixed-lineage leukemia (MLL4) gene and rearrangements of MLL4 in human hepatocellular carcinoma. Hum Mutat 29:703–708

14. Gramantieri L, Fornari F, Callegari E, Sabbioni S, Lanza G, Croce CM, Bolondi L, et al (2008) MicroRNA involvement in hepatocellular carcinoma. J Cell Mol Med 12:2189–2204

15. Morrison SJ, Kimble J (2006) Asymmetric and symmetric stem-cell divisions in development and cancer. Nature 441:1068–1074

16. Roskams T, Yang SQ, Koteish A, Durnez A, DeVos R, Huang X, Achten R, et al (2003) Oxidative stress and oval cell accumulation in mice and humans with alcoholic and nonalcoholic fatty liver disease. Am J Pathol 163:1301–1311

17. Sell S (2001) Heterogeneity and plasticity of hepatocyte lineage cells. Hepatology 33:738–750

18. Alison MR, Islam S, Lim S (2009) Stem cells in liver regeneration, fibrosis and cancer: the good, the bad and the ugly. J Pathol 217:282–298

19. Mishra L, Banker T, Murray J, Byers S, Thenappan A, He AR, Shetty K, et al (2009) Liver stem cells and hepatocellular carcinoma. Hepatology 49:318–329

20. Pardal R, Clarke MF, Morrison SJ (2003) Applying the principles of stem-cell biology to cancer. Nat Rev Cancer 3:895–902

21. Poon RT, Ng IO, Lau C, Zhu LX, Yu WC, Lo CM, Fan ST, et al (2001) Serum vascular endothelial growth factor predicts venous invasion in hepatocellular carcinoma: a prospective study. Ann Surg 233:227–235

22. Asahara T, Masuda H, Takahashi T, Kalka C, Pastore C, Silver M, Kearne M, et al (1999) Bone marrow origin of endothelial progenitor cells responsible for postnatal vasculogenesis in physiological and pathological neovascularization. Circ Res 85:221–228

23. Shi Q, Rafii S, Wu MH, Wijelath ES, Yu C, Ishida A, Fujita Y, et al (1998) Evidence for circulating bone marrow-derived endothelial cells. Blood 92:362–367

24. Ribatti D, Vacca A, Dammacco F (2003) New non-angiogenesis dependent pathways for tumour growth. Eur J Cancer 39:1835–1841

25. Kieser A, Weich HA, Brandner G, Marme D, Kolch W (1994) Mutant p53 potentiates protein kinase C induction of vascular endothelial growth factor expression. Oncogene 9:963–969

26. Rak J, Mitsuhashi Y, Bayko L, Filmus J, Shirasawa S, Sasazuki T, Kerbel RS (1995) Mutant ras oncogenes upregulate VEGF/VPF expression: implications for induction and inhibition of tumor angiogenesis. Cancer Res 55:4575–4580

27. North S, Moenner M, Bikfalvi A (2005) Recent developments in the regulation of the angiogenic switch by cellular stress factors in tumors. Cancer Lett 218:1–14

28. Dvorak HF, Nagy JA, Bersc B, Brown LF, Yeo KT, Yeo TK, Dvorak AM, et al (1992) Vascular permeability factor, fibrin, and the pathogenesis of tumor stroma formation. Ann N Y Acad Sci 667:101–111

29. El-Assal ON, Yamanoi A, Soda Y, Yamaguchi M, Igarashi M, Yamamoto A, Nabika T, et al (1998) Clinical significance of microvessel density and vascular endothelial growth factor expression in hepatocellular carcinoma and surrounding liver: possible involvement of vascular endothelial growth factor in the angiogenesis of cirrhotic liver. Hepatology 27:1554–1562

30. Sugimachi K, Tanaka S, Taguchi K, Aishima S, Shimada M, Tsuneyoshi M (2003) Angiopoietin switching regulates angiogenesis and progression of human hepatocellular carcinoma. J Clin Pathol 56:854–860

31. Yasuda S, Arii S, Mori A, Isobe N, Yang W, Oe H, Fujimoto A, et al (2004) Hexokinase II and VEGF expression in liver tumors: correlation with hypoxia-inducible factor 1 alpha and its significance. J Hepatol 40:117–123

32. von Marschall Z, Cramer T, Hocker M, Finkenzeller G, Wiedenmann B, Rosewicz S (2001) Dual mechanism of vascular endothelial growth factor upregulation by hypoxia in human hepatocellular carcinoma. Gut 48:87–96

33. Lee SW, Lee YM, Bae SK, Murakami S, Yun Y, Kim KW (2000) Human hepatitis B virus X protein is a possible mediator of hypoxia-induced angiogenesis in hepatocarcinogenesis. Biochem Biophys Res Commun 268:456–461

34. Tsukamoto A, Kaneko Y, Yoshida T, Ichinose M, Kimura S (1999) Regulation of angiogenesis in human hepatomas: possible involvement of p53-inducible inhibitor of vascular endothelial cell proliferation. Cancer Lett 141:79–84

35. Pang R, Poon RT (2006) Angiogenesis and antiangiogenic therapy in hepatocellular carcinoma. Cancer Lett 242:151–167

36. Yoshiji H, Kuriyama S, Yoshii J, Ikenaka Y, Noguchi R, Hicklin DJ, Huber J, et al (2002) Synergistic effect of basic fibroblast growth factor and vascular endothelial growth factor in murine hepatocellular carcinoma. Hepatology 35:834–842

37. Kin M, Sata M, Ueno T, Torimura T, Inuzuka S, Tsuji R, Sujaku K, et al (1997) Basic fibroblast growth factor regulates proliferation and motility of human hepatoma cells by an autocrine mechanism. J Hepatol 27:677–687

38. Mitsuhashi N, Shimizu H, Ohtsuka M, Wakabayashi Y, Ito H, Kimura F, Yoshidome H, et al (2003) Angiopoietins and Tie-2 expression in angiogenesis and proliferation of human hepatocellular carcinoma. Hepatology 37:1105–1113

39. Morinaga S, Yamamoto Y, Noguchi Y, Imada T, Rino Y, Akaike M, Sugimasa Y, et al (2003) Platelet-derived endothelial cell growth factor (PD-ECGF) is up-regulated in human hepatocellular carcinoma (HCC) and the corresponding hepatitis liver. Hepatogastroenterology 50:1521–1526

40. Poon RT, Lau CP, Ho JW, Yu WC, Fan ST, Wong J (2003) Tissue factor expression correlates with tumor angiogenesis and invasiveness in human hepatocellular carcinoma. Clin Cancer Res 9:5339–5345

41. Tang TC, Poon RT, Lau CP, Xie D, Fan ST (2005) Tumor cyclooxygenase-2 levels correlate with tumor invasiveness in human hepatocellular carcinoma. World J Gastroenterol 11:1896–1902

42. Hisai H, Kato J, Kobune M, Murakami T, Miyanishi K, Takahashi M, Yoshizaki N, et al (2003) Increased expression of angiogenin in hepatocellular carcinoma in correlation with tumor vascularity. Clin Cancer Res 9:4852–4859

43. Erlitzki R, Minuk GY (1999) Telomeres, telomerase and HCC: the long and the short of it. J Hepatol 31:939–945

44. Plentz RR, Park YN, Lechel A, Kim H, Nellessen F, Langkopf BH, Wilkens L, et al (2007) Telomere shortening and inactivation of cell cycle checkpoints characterize human hepatocarcinogenesis. Hepatology 45:968–976

45. Begus-Nahrmann Y, Lechel A, Obenauf AC, Nalapareddy K, Peit E, Hoffmann E, Schlaudraff F, et al.(2009) p53 deletion impairs clearance of chromosomal-instable stem cells in aging telomere-dysfunctional mice. Nat Genet 41:1138–1143

46. Lechel A, Holstege H, Begus Y, Schienke A, Kamino K, Lehmann U, Kubicka S, et al (2007) Telomerase deletion limits progression of p53-mutant hepatocellular carcinoma with short telomeres in chronic liver disease. Gastroenterology 132:1465–1475

47. Nzeako UC, Goodman ZD, Ishak KG (1996) Hepatocellular carcinoma in cirrhotic and non-cirrhotic livers. A clinico-histopathologic study of 804 North American patients. Am J Clin Pathol 105:65–75

48. Okuda K, Nakashima T, Kojiro M, Kondo Y, Wada K (1989) Hepatocellular carcinoma without cirrhosis in Japanese patients. Gastroenterology 97:140–146

49. Regimbeau JM, Colombat M, Mognol P, Durand F, Abdalla E, Degott C, Degos F, et al (2004) Obesity and diabetes as a risk factor for hepatocellular carcinoma. Liver Transpl 10: S69–S73

50. Trevisani F, D'Intino PE, Caraceni P, Pizzo M, Stefanini GF, Mazziotti A, Grazi GL, et al (1995) Etiologic factors and clinical presentation of hepatocellular carcinoma. Differences between cirrhotic and noncirrhotic Italian patients. Cancer 75:2220–2232

51. Okuda K (1997) Liver cancer. Churchill Livingstone, London

52. Zhou H, Ortiz-Pallardo ME, Ko Y, Fischer HP (2000) Is heterozygous alpha-1-antitrypsin deficiency type PIZ a risk factor for primary liver carcinoma? Cancer 88:2668–2676

53. Bianchi L (1993) Glycogen storage disease I and hepatocellular tumours. Eur J Pediatr 152(Suppl 1):S63–S70

54. Kowdley KV (2004) Iron, hemochromatosis, and hepatocellular carcinoma. Gastroenterology 127:S79–S86

55. Turlin B, Juguet F, Moirand R, Le Quilleuc D, Loreal O, Campion JP, Launois B, et al (1995) Increased liver iron stores in patients with hepatocellular carcinoma developed on a noncirrhotic liver. Hepatology 22:446–450

56. Lok AS (2009) Hepatitis B: liver fibrosis and hepatocellular carcinoma. Gastroenterol Clin Biol 33:911–915

57. But DY, Lai CL, Yuen MF (2008) Natural history of hepatitis-related hepatocellular carcinoma. World J Gastroenterol 14:1652–1656

58. Park NH, Song IH, Chung YH (2006) Chronic hepatitis B in hepatocarcinogenesis. Postgrad Med J 82:507–515

59. Terasaki S, Kaneko S, Kobayashi K, Nonomura A, Nakanuma Y (1998) Histological features predicting malignant transformation of nonmalignant hepatocellular nodules: a prospective study. Gastroenterology 115:1216–1222

60. Watanabe S, Horie Y, Kataoka E, Sato W, Dohmen T, Ohshima S, Goto T, et al (2007) Non-alcoholic steatohepatitis and hepatocellular carcinoma: lessons from hepatocyte-specific phosphatase and tensin homolog (PTEN)-deficient mice. J Gastroenterol Hepatol 22(Suppl 1):S96–S100

61. Caldwell S, Park SH (2009) The epidemiology of hepatocellular cancer: from the perspectives of public health problem to tumor biology. J Gastroenterol 44(Suppl 19):96–101

62. Takuma Y, Nouso K, Makino Y, Saito S, Takayama H, Takahara M, Takahashi H, et al (2007) Hepatic steatosis correlates with the postoperative recurrence of hepatitis C virus-associated hepatocellular carcinoma. Liver Int 27:620–626

63. Lagiou P, Kuper H, Stuver SO, Tzonou A, Trichopoulos D, Adami HO (2000) Role of diabetes mellitus in the etiology of hepatocellular carcinoma. J Natl Cancer Inst 92:1096–1099

64. Paradis V, Zalinski S, Chelbi E, Guedj N, Degos F, Vilgrain V, Bedossa P, et al (2009) Hepatocellular carcinomas in patients with metabolic syndrome often develop without significant liver fibrosis: a pathological analysis. Hepatology 49:851–859

65. Closset J, Veys I, Peny MO, Braude P, Van Gansbeke D, Lambilliotte JP, Gelin M (2000) Retrospective analysis of 29 patients surgically treated for hepatocellular adenoma or focal nodular hyperplasia. Hepatogastroenterology 47:1382–1384

66. Ferrell LD (1993) Hepatocellular carcinoma arising in a focus of multilobular adenoma. A case report. Am J Surg Pathol 17:525–529
67. Foster JH, Berman MM (1994) The malignant transformation of liver cell adenomas. Arch Surg 129:712–717
68. Bioulac-Sage P, Laumonier H, Couchy G, Le Bail B, Sa Cunha A, Rullier A, Laurent C, et al (2009) Hepatocellular adenoma management and phenotypic classification: the Bordeaux experience. Hepatology 50:481–489
69. Plopper H, Schaffner F (1957) Primary hepatic carcinomas. McGraw-Hill, New York, pp. 593–612
70. Nakano S, Haratake J, Okamoto K, Takeda S (1994) Investigation of resected multinodular hepatocellular carcinoma: assessment of unicentric or multicentric genesis from histological and prognostic viewpoint. Am J Gastroenterol 89:189–193
71. Yasui M, Harada A, Nonami T, Takeuchi Y, Taniguchi K, Nakao A, Takagi H (1997) Potentially multicentric hepatocellular carcinoma: clinicopathologic characteristics and post-operative prognosis. World J Surg 21:860–865
72. Ng IO, Guan XY, Poon RT, Fan ST, Lee JM (2003) Determination of the molecular relationship between multiple tumour nodules in hepatocellular carcinoma differentiates multicentric origin from intrahepatic metastasis. J Pathol 199:345–353
73. Dvorak HF (1986) Tumors: wounds that do not heal. Similarities between tumor stroma generation and wound healing. N Engl J Med 315:1650–1659
74. Itoh T, Shiro T, Seki T, Nakagawa T, Wakabayashi M, Inoue K, Okamura A (2000) Relationship between p53 overexpression and the proliferative activity in hepatocellular carcinoma. Int J Mol Med 6:137–142
75. Jeng KS, Sheen IS, Chen BF, Wu JY (2000) Is the p53 gene mutation of prognostic value in hepatocellular carcinoma after resection? Arch Surg 135:1329–1333
76. Guo K, Liu Y, Zhou H, Dai Z, Zhang J, Sun R, Chen J, et al (2008) Involvement of protein kinase C beta-extracellular signal-regulating kinase 1/2/p38 mitogen-activated protein kinase-heat shock protein 27 activation in hepatocellular carcinoma cell motility and invasion. Cancer Sci 99:486–496
77. Song PM, Zhang Y, He YF, Bao HM, Luo JH, Liu YK, Yang PY, et al (2008) Bioinformatics analysis of metastasis-related proteins in hepatocellular carcinoma. World J Gastroenterol 14:5816–5822
78. Chambers AF, Wilson SM, Kerkvliet N, O'Malley FP, Harris JF, Casson AG (1996) Osteopontin expression in lung cancer. Lung Cancer 15:311–323
79. Al-Mehdi AB, Tozawa K, Fisher AB, Shientag L, Lee A, Muschel RJ (2000) Intravascular origin of metastasis from the proliferation of endothelium-attached tumor cells: a new model for metastasis. Nat Med 6:100–102
80. Maniotis AJ, Folberg R, Hess A, Seftor EA, Gardner LM, Pe'er J, Trent JM, et al (1999) Vascular channel formation by human melanoma cells in vivo and in vitro: vasculogenic mimicry. Am J Pathol 155:739–752
81. Sugino T, Yamaguchi T, Hoshi N, Kusakabe T, Ogura G, Goodison S, Suzuki T (2008) Sinusoidal tumor angiogenesis is a key component in hepatocellular carcinoma metastasis. Clin Exp Metastasis 25:835–841

Chapter 3
Hepatocellular Cancer: Pathologic Considerations

Gregory Y. Lauwers

Keywords Histology · Prognostic factors · Precursor lesions

While the incidence of HCCs has been rising worldwide, there has been a steady stream of novel information related to the histologic characteristics of HCCs, including their pattern of spread, the risk factors for recurrence, and long-term prognosis. More particularly, a focus of great interest has been the diagnosis of early HCC. Understanding by histopathologists, surgeons, hepatologists, and oncologists of the nuances of the diagnosis of early HCC, as well as the importance of detailed pathologic analysis of surgical specimens, is crucial to developing appropriate therapeutic algorithms based on precise prognostic stratification.

Macroscopic Features of Hepatocellular Carcinoma

Variations in the morphology of HCC are related to the size of the tumor and whether the surrounding liver is cirrhotic.

Western series have emphasized that between 42 and 51% of HCCs arise in noncirrhotic livers [1, 2]. However, some of the "noncirrhotic" cases may be better characterized as associated with limited fibrosis. Differences in the multiplicity of tumors, incidence of encapsulation, and rate of venous invasion have been reported in this group of tumors. Also, HCCs in noncirrhotic livers may grow faster and in general are larger than those in cirrhotic livers [3, 4].

In cirrhotic livers, small HCCs may be well demarcated and surrounded by a fibrous capsule, whereas advanced tumors are expansive multinodular masses, frequently accompanied by intrahepatic metastases [5]. In noncirrhotic livers, HCCs usually present as single large tumors that may infiltrate both lobes [2, 3].

G.Y. Lauwers (✉)
Department of Pathology, Massachusetts General Hospital, Boston, MA, USA

K.M. McMasters, J.-N. Vauthey (eds.), *Hepatocellular Carcinoma*,
DOI 10.1007/978-1-60327-522-4_3, © Springer Science+Business Media, LLC 2011

    The risk of intrahepatic and extrahepatic spread is related to the size of the tumor
[6–8]. HCCs less than 5 cm in size are less likely to develop intrahepatic metastasis,
portal vein tumor thrombosis, or hematogenous metastasis [6, 8, 9]. Conversely, the
incidence of portal vein thrombosis rises from 40 to 75% when HCCs grow larger
than 5 cm, and the rate of intrahepatic metastasis rises dramatically (60% vs. 96%)
[6, 7].
    Most HCCs are soft neoplasms, often displaying hemorrhage and necrosis. Their
color ranges from tan-gray to green, the difference reflecting the degree of bile production [10]. Peritumoral capsule is found in 46% of HCCs measuring less than
2 cm and 84% of tumors between 2 and 5 cm in size. A capsule is present in only
45% of HCCs measuring more than 5 cm in diameter [11]. Peritumoral capsule is
associated with improved survival, lower rate of intrahepatic recurrence, and lower
incidence of venous invasion [1, 12].

Macroscopic Classification of HCCs

The different patterns of growth are associated with various risks of spread, both
intrahepatic and extrahepatic [6]. Eggel's classification, published in 1901, remains
widely used [13]. HCCs are divided into nodular, massive, and diffuse types. The
nodular type consists of well-circumscribed tumor nodules. *Massive HCCs* are
circumscribed, huge tumor masses occupying most or all of a hepatic lobe. This
type is commonly observed in patients without cirrhosis. The *diffuse* type is rare
and characterized by innumerable indistinct small nodules studding the entire liver.
Subsequently, the Liver Cancer Study Group of Japan has proposed a modification,
with the nodular category being divided into three subtypes: single nodular, single
nodular type with perinodular tumor growth, and the confluent multinodular subtype
[10] (Fig. 3.1)

HCC Is a Multicentric Disease

Multicentricity is noted in 16–74% of HCCs resected in cirrhotic liver [6, 11, 14–
17]. In contrast, multifocality is reported to be only 12% in noncirrhotic liver [3].
Tumor multiplicity can be explained by either the metachronous development of
tumors (i.e., multicentric carcinogenesis) or intrahepatic metastases via the portal system [18, 19]. Tumor nodules are considered metastatic if (a) they show a
portal vein tumor thrombus or grow contiguously with a thrombus, (b) multiple
small satellite nodules surround a larger main tumor, or (c) a single lesion is adjacent to the main tumor but is significantly smaller in size and presents the same
histology [18].

Intravascular and Biliary Growth

Malignant thrombosis of the portal vein system plays a role in the development
of intrahepatic metastases. Most patients develop recurrence within 1 year and die

Fig. 3.1 Macroscopic appearance of hepatocellular carcinoma (HCC). Example of large single nodular lesion involving most of a lobe. Note that the surrounding liver was not cirrhotic

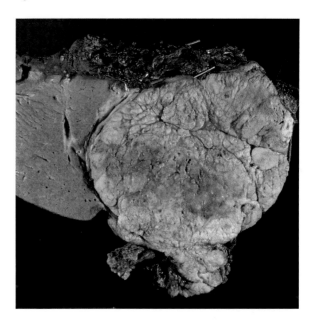

within 2 years after surgery [9, 20]. In some cases with thrombosis of the hepatic veins, the malignant thrombus may extend into the inferior vena cava and the right atrium [21].

Tumor extension into the hepatic duct or common bile duct or both is also rare. Patients may develop obstructive jaundice or hemobilia, at times leading to a misconstrued preoperative diagnosis of cholangiocarcinoma or choledocholithiasis [22, 23].

Microscopic Features of Hepatocellular Carcinoma

Neoplastic hepatocytes exhibit various degrees of hepatocellular differentiation. They usually are polygonal with abundant eosinophilic and granular cytoplasm surrounded by distinct cell membranes. Characteristically, the nucleus is round and vesicular with a distinct nucleolus. Various intracytoplasmic inclusions can be observed. Glycogen, fat, bile, fibrinogen (pale bodies), Mallory bodies (accumulation of keratin and p62 stress protein) and intracellular hyaline bodies (accumulations of p62 stress protein), α-fetoprotein (AFP), giant lysosomes, or α_1-antitrypsin have been reported [24, 25].

A trabecular arrangement mimicking normal hepatic cords is the basic architectural growth pattern of HCCs. The histologic appearance is variable, however.

Histologic Patterns of HCC

The World Health Organization classification recognizes five major histologic subtypes [24]. Except for the fibrolamellar pattern, their significance is more of diagnostic value than indicative of prognosis [24]. The four other subtypes, frequently found simultaneously, are *trabecular*, *pseudoglandular* (acinar), *compact*, and *scirrhous*.

The trabecular and acinar patterns are commonly observed in well to moderately differentiated HCCs. The trabeculae can vary from a few cells thick (microtrabecular pattern) to more than a dozen cells (macrotrabecular pattern) and are separated by sinusoid-like spaces lined by flat endothelial cells (Fig 3.2). In the acinar (pseudoglandular) variant, the cells are arranged in a rosette-like fashion with a central bile canaliculus (Fig 3.3). In the solid type, the sinusoids are compressed and obscured by the broad and compact trabeculae. Finally, the scirrhous pattern is characterized by abundant fibrous stroma separating cords of tumor cells. This pattern can be seen after radiation, chemotherapy, or infarction. Various degrees of the scirrhous pattern are found without any previous treatment in approximately 4% of cases [10, 24].

Histologic Grading of Hepatocellular Carcinomas

The Edmondson grading scheme is based on the degree of differentiation of the neoplastic cells [26]. Tumors with well-differentiated neoplastic hepatocytes arranged in thin trabeculae correspond to *grade I* (Fig 3.4). In *grade II*, the larger and more atypical neoplastic cells are sometimes organized in an acinar pattern. Architectural and cytologic anaplasia are prominent in *grade III*, but the neoplastic cells are readily identified as hepatocytic in origin. When composed of markedly anaplastic neoplastic cells not readily identified as hepatocytic origin, the tumor is *grade IV* (Fig. 3.5)

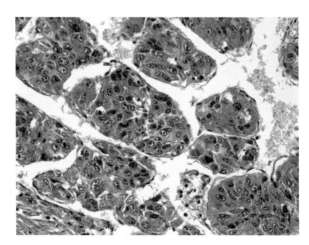

Fig. 3.2 Macrotrabecular growth pattern of hepatocellular carcinoma composed of wide anastomosing cords wrapped by endothelial cells

Fig. 3.3 Pseudoglandular (acinar) pattern of hepatocellular carcinoma. The neoplastic hepatocytes are moderately atypical (grade II), and bile plugs are identified in the lumen

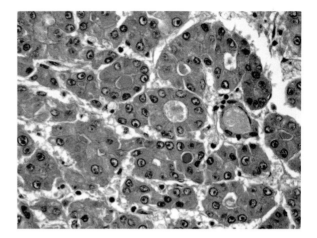

Fig. 3.4 Grade I (well-differentiated) hepatocellular carcinoma. The well-differentiated neoplastic hepatocytes show minimal cytologic and architectural atypia. Note the scattered acinar structures

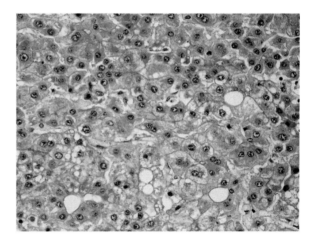

An alternate four-tier histologic grading scheme is advocated by the Liver Cancer Study Group of Japan [10]. In this classification, *well-differentiated HCCs* that commonly measure less than 2 cm in diameter demonstrate an increased cellular density. The small neoplastic cells are organized in irregular microtrabeculae, and focal acinar formation can be seen. Frequent fatty macrovesicular changes can be seen as well. Cellular and nuclear atypia are distinctly absent. *Moderately differentiated HCCs* are composed of neoplastic hepatocytes displaying abundant eosinophilic cytoplasm with round nuclei and distinct nucleoli. Notably, the nucleus to cytoplasm ratio is equal to that of the normal hepatocytes. These hepatocytes are organized in either trabeculae or pseudoglands.

Poorly differentiated HCCs usually grow in a solid sheet-like pattern. The hepatocytes show an increased nucleus to cytoplasm ratio. Cellular pleomorphism is noticeable, with mononucleated or multinucleated giant cells, or both.

Fig. 3.5 Spindle, sarcomatoid, high-grade variant of HCC. Spindle neoplastic cells mimicking a sarcoma are intermixed with bizarre multinucleated cells

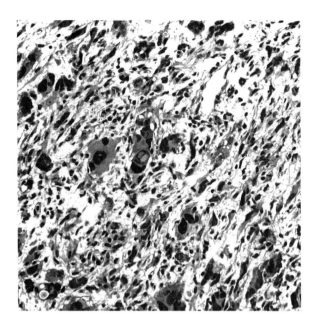

Undifferentiated HCCs are composed of tumor cells with little cytoplasm and short spindle-shaped or round nuclei. They grow in a solid or medullary pattern.

The prognostic value of histologic grading is debated. Some authors report better prognosis for low-grade HCC, whereas others contest a correlation between poor prognosis and high histologic grade [1, 27]. Edmondson–Steiner grading has not been found to be a predictor of intrahepatic recurrence by some, whereas a high histologic grade has been estimated by others to be a strong predictor of portal vein invasion [12, 28]. It has also been claimed that the odds of having a high-grade HCC are twice as high for cirrhotic patients compared to those without cirrhosis [1].

Cytologic Subtypes of HCC

The *clear cell variant* results from excessive intracytoplasmic deposits of glycogen [24]. Clear cells may be composed of only a limited portion of an otherwise typical HCC or the entire tumor. A reportedly favorable prognosis has not been confirmed [29, 30]. Pathologists should distinguish clear cell HCC from metastatic renal cell and adrenocortical carcinomas.

Pleomorphic HCCs display marked variations in shape and size of the neoplastic hepatocytes. Seemingly benign giant cells (osteoclast-type) or highly anaplastic bizarre cells can be observed [24]. *Spindle* (or sarcomatoid) tumor cells with features resembling fibrosarcoma, leiomyosarcoma, and malignant fibrous histiocytoma can be seen [24] (Fig. 3.5). Arterial chemotherapy has been implicated in the genesis of this phenotype [21]. Distinction from a sarcoma is largely dependent on the identification of foci morphologically typical for HCC. The differential diagnosis can be challenging, since epithelial markers (i.e., cytokeratin) are recognized in only 62% of cases [31].

Vascular Invasion is an important prognostic indicator, in part because intrahepatic metastases occur through portal vein invasion. In its absence, the patients experience a longer overall and disease-free survival [17, 27, 32, 33]. Risk factors for portal vein invasion include tumor diameter greater than 3 cm, high histologic grade, tumor multiplicity, and high mitotic activity (>4 mitoses per 10 HPF) [28, 34] (Fig. 3.6)

Fig. 3.6 Malignant tumor emboli in a small portal vein. Vascular invasion is a risk factor for intrahepatic metastasis and multicentricity

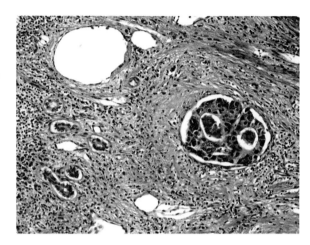

Histologic Variants of Hepatocellular Carcinoma

Fibrolamellar Carcinoma

Fibrolamellar HCC is a rare variant of HCC (less than 5% of all cases). These tumors occur at a young age and are not associated with common risk factors such as chronic hepatitis and cirrhosis [35–38] and thus are frequently amenable to surgical resection. The extended survival compared to that of usual HCCs is likely related to the absence of cirrhosis rather than distinct biologic characteristics [38–41]. Overall 5-year survival is estimated at between 35 and 76% for patients undergoing hepatic resection [38–41]. However, a recent series pointed out that with frequent vascular invasion (36%) and lymph node metastases (50%), late recurrences are common and the 5-year recurrence-free survival was only 18% [40]. Fibrolamellar carcinomas are firm, sharply demarcated, and usually single tumors. They range in size from 7 to 20 cm [36, 41]. The surrounding parenchyma is frequently unremarkable, with cirrhosis reported in less than 5% of cases [36]. The characteristic histologic features include large polygonal and deeply eosinophilic tumor cells embedded in hyalinized connective tissue commonly arranged in a lamellar fashion. The cells display single round vesicular nuclei with prominent nucleoli. They may also contain α_1-antitrypsin, seen as proteinaceous cytoplasmic inclusions, and fibrinogen containing *pale bodies*, presenting as pale ground-glass cytoplasmic inclusions [24, 36, 41].

Combined Hepatocellular Carcinoma and Cholangiocarcinoma

Combined HCC and cholangiocarcinomas (combined HCC–CC) contain unequivocal elements of both HCC and CC [24]. Two types are recognized: HCC-predominant (the most frequent) and CC-predominant variants [42] (Fig. 3.7). These tumors show variable combinations of characteristic features of HCC, i.e., bile production, intercellular bile canaliculi, or a trabecular growth pattern, as well as elements of cholangiocarcinoma, such as glandular structures lined by biliary type epithelium; intracellular mucin production; or immunoreactivity for MUC-1, CK 7, and CK19 [42–45]. AFP levels are usually low, whereas an increase in serum carcinoembryonic antigen and carbohydrate antigen 19-9 can be detected [42, 46]. Cirrhosis is associated with most cases of the HCC-predominant type (55% of cases) and only occasionally with the CC-predominant type (13% of cases) [42]. These combined neoplasms may be more common in the setting of genetic hemochromatosis. Reflecting the common embryologic origin of hepatocytes and cholangiocytes, two mechanisms of histogenesis have been hypothesized: (a) the CC component could differentiate from an initial pure HCC or (b) an intermediate "stem cell" cell could give rise to both HCC and CC components [42, 43, 47]. Support for the latter hypothesis includes the presence of hepatic progenitor cells as well as the detection

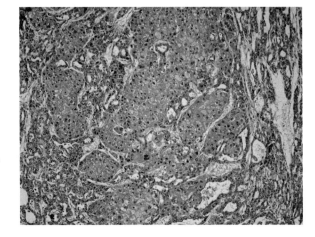

Fig. 3.7 Combined hepatocellular/cholangiocarcinoma. Note the large anastomosing trabeculae of HCC surrounded by anastomosing malignant ductular structures

of hepatocellular (albumin RNA) and biliary markers (keratin profile) in combined HCC [47, 48].

Precursor Lesions

A multistep carcinogenesis sequence of low- and high-grade dysplastic nodules and well-differentiated HCC is largely accepted as the morphologic process preceding the development of HCCs in cirrhotic livers.

Low-grade dysplastic nodules are distinct from surrounding cirrhotic nodules. Their size usually varies between 0.5 and 1.5 cm, although large examples have been reported. They are not encapsulated [49], but condensation of peripheral fibrous tissue is noted. These nodules are distinguishable from cirrhotic nodules by the presence of *dysplastic*, architectural, and cytologic features, i.e., mild increase in cellular density of monotonous hepatocytes, usually with no cellular atypia. Architecturally, *dysplasia* refers to the presence of minimally thick cell plates, but acinar formation or macrotrabeculae are absent [50]. Rare unpaired arteries can be seen. Large cell changes (formerly referred to as large cell dysplasia) can be seen. These consist of cellular enlargement with nuclear pleomorphism and frequent multinucleation [51]. Differences between simple macroregenerative and dysplastic nodules can be challenging, especially on needle biopsies. Subtle nuclear atypia with densely packed, smaller-than-normal hepatocytes with increased cellular density, sometimes twice normal as in the surrounding tissue, are helpful hints. Thickening of the nuclear membrane, higher nucleus to cytoplasm ratios, and rare mitoses are also seen [52–56]. Architectural atypia range from irregular trabecular patterns to minimally thickened trabeculae or pseudoglandular formation. *High-grade dysplastic nodules* can be either vaguely nodular or distinctly nodular lesions. Architectural and cytologic atypia are present but insufficient to merit a diagnosis of well-differentiated HCC. They commonly display increased cell density, cytoplasmic eosinophilia, and irregular thin trabeculae. Another notable feature is the increased number of unpaired muscularized arteries. However, differentiating these lesions is difficult, and significant overlap with *early HCCs* is seen (Fig. 3.8a,b).

Early HCCs may develop within dysplastic nodules, initially preserving a seemingly normal cytologic and architectural pattern. These HCCs, by definition, measure less than 2 cm, and most have only a vaguely nodular morphology [10, 57]. They are extremely well-differentiated, with little cellular and structural atypia [10, 58, 59]. Subtle diagnostic changes include increased cell density (more than twice that of surrounding tissue) and increased nucleus to cytoplasm ratio. Cytoplasmic eosinophilia, fatty or clear cell changes, or both, as well as iron-free foci, can also be noted [10, 58–60]. An irregular thin trabecular pattern, acinar patterns, or both can be seen [10, 58, 59] (Fig 3.9a,b). Another notable feature is the increased number of unpaired muscularized arteries [60]. Vascular invasion is uncommon,

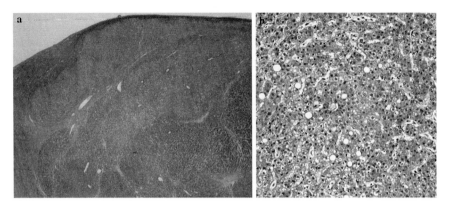

Fig. 3.8 (a) Vaguely nodular lesion characteristic of dysplastic nodules and early well-differentiated HCC. (b) The nodule is composed of hepatocytes with minimal cytologic atypia with slight increased cellular density and anastomosing one-cell-thick trabeculae with rare acinar structures

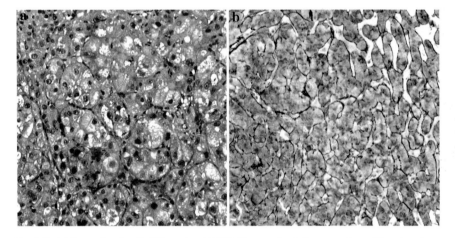

Fig. 3.9 (a) Example of well-differentiated HCC. The neoplastic hepatocytic proliferation shows cytoarchitectural atypia, highlighted in 9b. (b) Reticulin stain demonstrating focal loss and disarray of reticulin fibers

but "stromal invasion" of intratumoral portal spaces can be observed as the tumors enlarge [57, 59]. As they grow in size, fatty changes become uncommon and cellular dedifferentiation appears. The less differentiated component usually arises as a central subnodule expanding in a *nodule-in-nodule* fashion. It proliferates expansively, whereas the peripheral well-differentiated rim is compressed and eventually replaced [42, 58, 59, 61]. Approximately 40% of HCCs measuring between 1 and 3 cm consist of more than two patterns of varying differentiation [42] (Fig. 3.10).

Fig. 3.10 Nodule-in-nodule
growth pattern in early HCC.
The central nodule, less
differentiated, will entirely
replace the peripheral
well-differentiated lesion that
preceded it

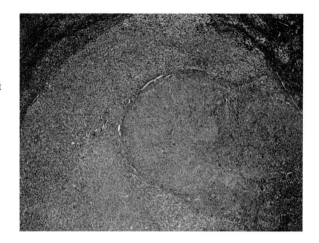

Ancillary Studies

Various techniques, including immunohistochemistry, cytogenetics, fluorescent in-
situ hybridization (FISH), and comparative genomic hybridization (CGH) [62, 63],
can be used to confirm a diagnosis of HCC, distinguishing it from a metastasis or
a peripheral cholangiocarcinoma (uncommonly), and, importantly, differentiating a
well-differentiated HCC from benign hepatocellular proliferations such as hepatocellular adenoma. We will focus on only a few ancillary tests in the context of the
usual clinical dilemmas.

Hepatocellular Carcinoma vs. Metastatic Adenocarcinoma and Cholangiocarcinoma

Mucin

Although mucin is noted in the lumen of acinar HCC [26], the intracytoplasmic demonstration of mucin generally rules out this diagnosis. In such cases, the
working differential diagnosis includes metastatic adenocarcinoma and cholangiocarcinoma. Using MUC antibodies against glycoprotein cores of mucin, HCCs are
uniformly negative for MUC-1, MUC-2, and MUC-5AC. Conversely, MUC-1 and
MUC-5AC are positive in 73 and 45% of cholangiocarcinomas respectively, as well
as in gastrointestinal cancers likely to metastasize to the liver [64].

Albumin

Albumin, exclusively synthesized by hepatocytes, is a highly specific marker of
hepatocytic lineage [65]. Unfortunately, immunohistochemistry is not a well-suited

detection tool, because of the abundance of the protein in the serum. Less commonly available, in-situ hybridization is a better technique, with albumin mRNA demonstrated in up to 96% of HCC [65].

Polyclonal CEA and CD10

Both polyclonal CEA and CD10 (neprilysin) antibodies have cross-reactivity with glycoprotein I and exhibit a canalicular distribution pattern. In both instances, their detection offers evidence of hepatocellular differentiation [66, 67].

Alpha-Fetoprotein

Alpha-fetoprotein, an oncofetal glycoprotein and established serologic marker of HCC, is not a useful immunohistochemical marker, with a low sensitivity (15–60%) [68–70]. However, its specificity is close to 100%, after exclusion of rare lesions such as yolk sac tumors [71–73].

Hepatocyte Paraffin 1 Antibody (HepPar1)

HepPar1 is a marker of both benign and neoplastic hepatocellular proliferations [74–76]. Its sensitivity is reported to be about 91%, with only 4% of non-hepatic tumors staining positively [76]. However, poorly differentiated HCCs can be negative, and occasional metastatic adenocarcinomas have been reported to be immunoreactive [76].

Cytokeratin

Low molecular weight keratins, including CAM 5.2 and cytokeratins 8 and 18, usually decorate neoplastic hepatocytes. Conversely, HCCs are negative for keratins 7 and 19, which stain cholangiocarcinomas. However, the diagnostic applicability of cytokeratin is limited by common overlap in the immunophenotype of HCC and CCs as well as metastases [71–73].

Adjunct Methods Used for Distinguishing Benign from Malignant Hepatic Tumors

CD 34

"Capillarization" of sinusoids, as expressed by various degrees of CD34 immunoreactivity, has been noted in hepatic adenoma, cirrhotic liver, adenomatous hyperplasia, and HCC [62, 77, 78]. Diffuse CD34 sinusoidal reactivity would support a diagnosis of HCC [79] and can help differentiate dysplastic nodules and early HCCs from macroregenerative nodules [80]. However, there is considerable overlap in the staining profiles of hepatocellular lesions (benign and malignant), and therefore caution is necessary. Of note, one series reported the lack of CD34 immunore-activity in a series of metastatic carcinomas to the liver, suggesting a role in this situation [81].

Novel immunohistochemical markers have been developed with the goal of supple-menting the morphologic evaluation of transforming hepatocyte nodules.

Heat Shock Protein 70

HSP70, a heat shock protein implicated in regulation of cellular apoptosis and cell cycle progression, is markedly upregulated in HCC.

HSP70 immunoreactivity has been reported in the majority of HCCs, particu-larly in early and well-differentiated tumors (90 and 72%, reportedly). However, the staining may be difficult to evaluate, as it can be patchy [82].

Glypican 3

Glypican 3 is a marker of the glypican family of hepatic sulfate proteoglycan linked to the cell surface. It is believed to play a negative role in cell proliferation and in inducing apoptosis. Glypican 3 is overexpressed in HCC with focal and weak staining in precursor lesions of HCC but diffuse staining in a large majority of HCC [82–86] (see Table 3.1 and Fig. 3.11).

In most cases, the use of a panel of several markers is best practice to avoid misconstrued conclusions. However, in closing, it is important to emphasize that these markers are best used to support a methodical histologic evaluation of small hepatocytic lesions, but do not supersede it.

Table 3.1 Glypican 3 expression in hepatocytic nodules [82–84, 86]

	% of positive cases	Number of cases tested
Benign		
Cirrhotic nodules	0–17	224
Macroregenerative nodules	0–17	127
Hepatocellular adenoma	0	22
Low-grade dysplastic nodules	0–8	47
Borderline and malignant		
High-grade dysplastic nodules	9–43	69
eHCC	50–60	40
Grade I HCC	56–90	63
Grade II HCC	64–83	166
Grade III HCC	57–89	77
Grade IV HCC	43	7

Fig. 3.11 Example of strong
glypican 3 positivity in grade
II HCC arising in cirrhotic
lines (negative background)

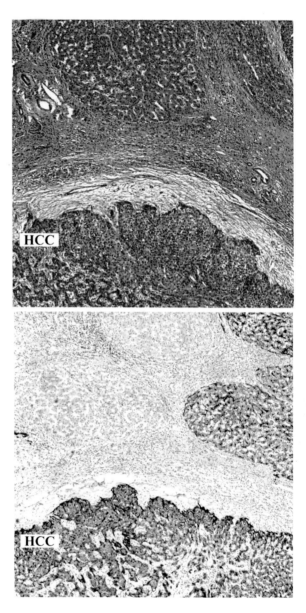

References

1. Nzeako UC, Goodman ZD, Ishak KG (1996) Hepatocellular carcinoma in cirrhotic and non-cirrhotic livers. A clinico-histopathologic study of 804 North American patients. Am J Clin Pathol 105:65–75
2. Smalley SR, Moertel CG, Hilton JF, Weiland LH, Weiand HS, Adson MA, Melton LJ, 3rd, Batts K (1988) Hepatoma in the noncirrhotic liver. Cancer 62:1414–1424

3. Bismuth H, Chiche L, Castaing D (1995) Surgical treatment of hepatocellular carcinomas in noncirrhotic liver: experience with 68 liver resections. World J Surg 19:35–41

4. Kishi K, Shikata T, Hirohashi S, Hasegawa H, Yamazaki S, Makuuchi M (1983) Hepatocellular carcinoma. A clinical and pathologic analysis of 57 hepatectomy cases. Cancer 51:542–548

5. Lauwers GY, Vauthey JN (1998) Pathological aspects of hepatocellular carcinoma: a critical review of prognostic factors. Hepatogastroenterology 45(Suppl 3):1197–1202

6. Yuki K, Hirohashi S, Sakamoto M, Kanai T, Shimosato Y (1990) Growth and spread of hepatocellular carcinoma. A review of 240 consecutive autopsy cases. Cancer 66: 2174–2179

7. Adachi E, Maeda T, Matsumata T, Shirabe K, Kinukawa N, Sugimachi K, Tsuneyoshi M (1995) Risk factors for intrahepatic recurrence in human small hepatocellular carcinoma. Gastroenterology 108:768–775

8. Liver Cancer Study Group of Japan (1990) Primary liver cancer in Japan. Clinicopathologic features and results of surgical treatment. Ann Surg 211:277–287

9. Izumi R, Shimizu K, Ii T, Yagi M, Matsui O, Nonomura A, Miyazaki I (1994) Prognostic factors of hepatocellular carcinoma in patients undergoing hepatic resection. Gastroenterology 106:720–727

10. Liver Cancer Study Group of Japan (1997) Classification of primary liver cancer. Kanehira & Co., Tokyo, p. 30 (in English)

11. Nagao T, Inoue S, Goto S, Mizuta T, Omori Y, Kawano N, Morioka Y (1987) Hepatic resection for hepatocellular carcinoma. Clinical features and long-term prognosis. Ann Surg 205:33–40

12. Arii S, Tanaka J, Yamazoe Y, Minematsu S, Morino T, Fujita K, Maetani S, Tobe T (1992) Predictive factors for intrahepatic recurrence of hepatocellular carcinoma after partial hepatectomy. Cancer 69:913–919

13. Eggel H (1901) Uber das primare carcinom der leber. Beitr Pathol Ann 30:506–604

14. Nagao T, Inoue S, Yoshimi F, Sodeyama M, Omori Y, Mizuta T, Kawano N, Morioka Y (1990) Postoperative recurrence of hepatocellular carcinoma. Ann Surg 211:28–33

15. Lai EC, You K-T, Ng IO, Shek TW (1993) The pathological basis of resection margin for hepatocellular carcinoma. World J Surg 17:786–791

16. Imamura H, Matsuyama Y, Tanaka E, Ohkubo T, Hasegawa K, Miyagawa S, Sugawara Y, Minagawa M, Takayama T, Kawasaki S, Makuuchi M (2003) Risk factors contributing to early and late phase intrahepatic recurrence of hepatocellular carcinoma after hepatectomy. J Hepatol 38:200–207

17. Lauwers GY, Terris B, Balis UJ, Batts KP, Regimbeau JM, Chang Y, Graeme-Cook F, Yamabe H, Ikai I, Cleary KR, Fujita S, Flejou JF, Zukerberg LR, Nagorney DM, Belghiti J, Yamaoka Y, Vauthey JN (2002) Prognostic histologic indicators of curatively resected hepatocellular carcinomas: a multi-institutional analysis of 425 patients with definition of a histologic prognostic index. Am J Surg Pathol 26:25–34

18. Sakamoto M, Hirohashi S, Tsuda H, Shimosato Y, Makuuchi M, Hosoda Y (1989) Multicentric independent development of hepatocellular carcinoma revealed by analysis of hepatitis B virus integration pattern. Am J Surg Pathol 13:1064–1067

19. Toyosaka A, Okamoto E, Mitsunobu M, Oriyama T, Nakao N, Miura K (1996) Pathologic and radiographic studies of intrahepatic metastasis in hepatocellular carcinoma; the role of efferent vessels. HPB Surgery 10:97–104

20. Ikai I, Yamaoka Y, Yamamoto Y, Ozaki N, Sakai Y, Satoh S, Shinkura N, Yamamoto M (1998) Surgical intervention for patients with stage IV-A hepatocellular carcinoma without lymph node metastasis: proposal as a standard therapy. Ann Surg 227: 433–439

21. Kojiro M, Sugihara S, Kakizoe S, Nakashima O, Kiyomatsu K (1989) Hepatocellular carcinoma with sarcomatous change: a special reference to the relationship with anticancer therapy. Cancer Chemother Pharmacol 23(Suppl):S4–S8

22. Kojiro M, Kawabata K, Kawano Y, Shirai F, Takemoto N, Nakashima T (1982) Hepatocellular carcinoma presenting as intrabile duct tumor growth: a clinicopathologic study of 24 cases. Cancer 49:2144–2147

23. Nakashima T, Kojiro M (1986) Pathologic characteristics of hepatocellular carcinoma. Semin Liver Dis 6:259–266

24. Ishak KG, Anthony PP, Sobin L (1994) Histological typing of tumours in the liver. Springer, Berlin

25. Denk H, Stumptner C, Fuchsbichler A, Muller T, Farr G, Muller W, Terracciano L, Zatloukal K (2006) Are the Mallory bodies and intracellular hyaline bodies in neoplastic and non-neoplastic hepatocytes related? J Pathol 208:653–661

26. Edmondson H, Steiner P (1954) Primary carcinoma of the liver; a study of 100 cases among 48,900 necropsies. Cancer 7:462–503

27. Haratake J, Takeda S, Kasai T, Nakano S, Tokui N (1993) Predictable factors for estimating prognosis of patients after resection of hepatocellular carcinoma. Cancer 72: 1178–1183

28. Adachi E, Maeda T, Kajiyama K, Kinukawa N, Matsumata T, Sugimachi K, Tsuneyoshi M (1996) Factors correlated with portal venous invasion by hepatocellular carcinoma: univariate and multivariate analyses of 232 resected cases without preoperative treatments. Cancer 77:2022–2031

29. Lai CL, Wu PC, Lam KC, Todd D (1979) Histologic prognostic indicators in hepatocellular carcinoma. Cancer 44:1677–1683

30. Yang SH, Watanabe J, Nakashima O, Kojiro M (1996) Clinicopathologic study on clear cell hepatocellular carcinoma. Pathol Int 46:503–509

31. Maeda T, Adachi E, Kajiyama K, Takenaka K, Sugimachi K, Tsuneyoshi M (1996) Spindle cell hepatocellular carcinoma. A clinicopathologic and immunohistochemical analysis of 15 cases. Cancer 77:51–57

32. Vauthey JN, Klimstra D, Franceschi D, Tao Y, Fortner J, Blumgart L, Brennan M (1995) Factors affecting long-term outcome after hepatic resection for hepatocellular carcinoma. Am J Surg 169:28–34

33. Nigam A, Zhurak M, Boitnott J, Goodman S, Abrams R, Sitzmann J (1995) Factors affecting survival in Western patients following curative resection for hepatocellular carcinoma [abstract]. Gastroenterology 108:A1235

34. Esnaola NF, Lauwers GY, Mirza NQ, Nagorney DM, Doherty D, Ikai I, Yamaoka Y, Regimbeau JM, Belghiti J, Curley SA, Ellis LM, Vauthey JN (2002) Predictors of microvascular invasion in patients with hepatocellular carcinoma who are candidates for orthotopic liver transplantation. J Gastrointest Surg 6:224–232; discussion 32

35. Craig JR, Peters RL, Edmondson HA, Omata M (1980) Fibrolamellar carcinoma of the liver: a tumor of adolescents and young adults with distinctive clinico-pathologic features. Cancer 46:372–379

36. Berman MA, Burnham JA, Sheahan DG (1988) Fibrolamellar carcinoma of the liver: an immunohistochemical study of nineteen cases and a review of the literature. Hum Pathol 19:784–794

37. El-Serag HB, Davila JA (2004) Is fibrolamellar carcinoma different from hepatocellular carcinoma? A US population-based study. Hepatology 39:798–803

38. Ringe B, Wittekind C, Weimann A, Tusch G, Pichlmayr R (1992) Results of hepatic resection and transplantation for fibrolamellar carcinoma. Surg Gynecol Obstet 175:299–305

39. Soreide O, Czerniak A, Bradpiece H, Bloom S, Blumgart L (1986) Characteristics of fibrolamellar hepatocellular carcinoma. A study of nine cases and a review of the literature. Am J Surg 151:518–523

40. Stipa F, Yoon SS, Liau KH, Fong Y, Jarnagin WR, D'Angelica M, Abou-Alfa G, Blumgart LH, DeMatteo RP (2006) Outcome of patients with fibrolamellar hepatocellular carcinoma. Cancer 106:1331–1338

41. Kakar S, Burgart LJ, Batts KP, Garcia J, Jain D, Ferrell LD (2005) Clinicopathologic features and survival in fibrolamellar carcinoma: comparison with conventional hepatocellular carcinoma with and without cirrhosis. Mod Pathol 18:1417–1423

42. Kojiro M (1997) Pathology of hepatocellular carcinoma. Churchill Livingstone, New York
43. Goodman ZD, Ishak KG, Langloss JM, Sesterhenn IA, Rabin L (1985) Combined hepatocellular-cholangiocarcinoma. A histologic and immunohistochemical study. Cancer 55:124–135
44. Maeda T, Adachi E, Kajiyama K, Sugimachi K, Tsuneyoshi M (1995) Combined hepatocellular and cholangiocarcinoma: proposed criteria according to cytokeratin expression and analysis of clinicopathologic features. Hum Pathol 26:956–964
45. Morcos M, Dubois S, Bralet MP, Belghiti J, Degott C, Terris B (2001) Primary liver carcinoma in genetic hemochromatosis reveals a broad histologic spectrum. Am J Clin Pathol 116: 738–743
46. Nakamura S, Suzuki S, Sakaguchi T, Serizawa A, Konno H, Baba S, Baba S, Muro H (1996) Surgical treatment of patients with mixed hepatocellular carcinoma and cholangiocarcinoma. Cancer 78:1671–1676
47. Theise ND, Yao JL, Harada K, Hytiroglou P, Portmann B, Thung SN, Tsui W, Ohta H, Nakanuma Y (2003) Hepatic 'stem cell' malignancies in adults: four cases. Histopathology 43:263–271
48. Tickoo SK, Zee SY, Obiekwe S, Xiao H, Koea J, Robiou C, Blumgart LH, Jarnagin W, Ladanyi M, Klimstra DS (2002) Combined hepatocellular-cholangiocarcinoma: a histopathologic, immunohistochemical, and in situ hybridization study. Am J Surg Pathol 26:989–997
49. International Working Party (1995) Terminology of nodular hepatocellular lesions. Hepatology 22:983–993
50. Borzio M, Fargion S, Borzio F, Fracanzani AL, Croce AM, Stroffolini T, Oldani S, Cotichini R, Roncalli M (2003) Impact of large regenerative, low grade and high grade dysplastic nodules in hepatocellular carcinoma development. J Hepatol 39:208–214
51. Anthony PP, Vogel CL, Barker LF (1973) Liver cell dysplasia: a premalignant condition. J Clin Pathol 26:217–223
52. Watanabe S, Okita K, Harada T, Kodama T, Numa Y, Takemoto T, Takahashi T (1983) Morphologic studies of the liver cell dysplasia. Cancer 51:2197–2205
53. Lee RG, Tsamandas AC, Demetris AJ (1997) Large cell change (liver cell dysplasia) and hepatocellular carcinoma in cirrhosis: matched case-control study, pathological analysis, and pathogenetic hypothesis. Hepatology 26:1415–1422
54. Borzio M, Borzio F, Croce A, Sala M, Salmi A, Leandro G, Bruno S, Roncalli M (1997) Ultrasonography-detected macroregenerative nodules in cirrhosis: a prospective study. Gastroenterology 112:1617–1623
55. Theise ND, Schwartz M, Miller C, Thung SN (1992) Macroregenerative nodules and hepatocellular carcinoma in forty-four sequential adult liver explants with cirrhosis. Hepatology 16:949–955
56. Terasaki S, Kaneko S, Kobayashi K, Nonomura A, Nakanuma Y (1998) Histological features predicting malignant transformation of nonmalignant hepatocellular nodules: a prospective study. Gastroenterology 115:1216–1222
57. Kojiro M (2004) Focus on dysplastic nodules and early hepatocellular carcinoma: an Eastern point of view. Liver Transpl 10:S3–S8
58. Kondo Y, Niwa Y, Akikusa B, Takazawa H, Okabayashi A (1983) A histopathologic study of early hepatocellular carcinoma. Cancer 52:687–692
59. Sakamoto M, Hirohashi S, Shimosato Y (1991) Early stages of multistep hepatocarcinogenesis: adenomatous hyperplasia and early hepatocellular carcinoma. Hum Pathol 22:172–178
60. Roncalli M (2004) Hepatocellular nodules in cirrhosis: focus on diagnostic criteria on liver biopsy. A Western experience. Liver Transpl 10:S9–S15
61. Arakawa M, Kage M, Sugihara S, Nakashima T, Suenaga M, Okuda K (1986) Emergence of malignant lesions within an adenomatous hyperplastic nodule in a cirrhotic liver. Observations in five cases. Gastroenterology 91:198–208
62. Wilkens L, Bredt M, Flemming P, Mengel M, Becker T, Klempnauer J, Kreipe H (2002) Comparative genomic hybridization (CGH) and fluorescence in situ hybridization (FISH) in the diagnosis of hepatocellular carcinoma. J Hepatobiliary Pancreat Surg 9:304–311

63. Chen ZM, Crone KG, Watson MA, Pfeifer JD, Wang HL (2005) Identification of a unique gene expression signature that differentiates hepatocellular adenoma from well-differentiated hepatocellular carcinoma. Am J Surg Pathol 29:1600–1608

64. Lau SK, Weiss LM, Chu PG (2004) Differential expression of MUC1, MUC2, and MUC5AC in carcinomas of various sites: an immunohistochemical study. Am J Clin Pathol 122: 61–69

65. Krishna M, Lloyd RV, Batts KP (1997) Detection of albumin messenger RNA in hepatic and extrahepatic neoplasms. A marker of hepatocellular differentiation. Am J Surg Pathol 21:147–152

66. Ma CK, Zarbo RJ, Frierson HF, Jr, Lee MW (1993) Comparative immunohistochemical study of primary and metastatic carcinomas of the liver. Am J Clin Pathol 99:551–557

67. Borscheri N, Roessner A, Rocken C (2001) Canalicular immunostaining of neprilysin (CD10) as a diagnostic marker for hepatocellular carcinomas. Am J Surg Pathol 25:1297–1303

68. Kondo Y (1985) Histologic features of hepatocellular carcinoma and allied disorders. Pathol Annu 20(Pt 2):405–430

69. Thung SN, Gerber MA, Sarno E, Popper H (1979) Distribution of five antigens in hepatocellular carcinoma. Lab Invest 41:101–105

70. Fucich LF, Cheles MK, Thung SN, Gerber MA, Marrogi AJ (1994) Primary vs metastatic hepatic carcinoma. An immunohistochemical study of 34 cases. Arch Pathol Lab Med 118:927–930

71. Hurlimann J, Gardiol D (1991) Immunohistochemistry in the differential diagnosis of liver carcinomas. Am J Surg Pathol 15:280–288

72. Johnson DE, Herndier BG, Medeiros LJ, Warnke RA, Rouse RV (1988) The diagnostic utility of the keratin profiles of hepatocellular carcinoma and cholangiocarcinoma. Am J Surg Pathol 12:187–197

73. Minervini MI, Demetris AJ, Lee RG, Carr BI, Madariaga J, Nalesnik MA (1997) Utilization of hepatocyte-specific antibody in the immunocytochemical evaluation of liver tumors. Mod Pathol 10:686–692

74. Kakar S, Muir T, Murphy LM, Lloyd RV, Burgart LJ (2003) Immunoreactivity of Hep Par 1 in hepatic and extrahepatic tumors and its correlation with albumin in situ hybridization in hepatocellular carcinoma. Am J Clin Pathol 119:361–366

75. Fan Z, van de Rijn M, Montgomery K, Rouse RV (2003) Hep par 1 antibody stain for the differential diagnosis of hepatocellular carcinoma: 676 tumors tested using tissue microarrays and conventional tissue sections. Mod Pathol 16:137–144

76. Lugli A, Tornillo L, Mirlacher M, Bundi M, Sauter G, Terracciano LM (2004) Hepatocyte paraffin 1 expression in human normal and neoplastic tissues: tissue microarray analysis on 3,940 tissue samples. Am J Clin Pathol 122:721–727

77. Scott FR, el-Refaie A, More L, Scheuer PJ, Dhillon AP (1996) Hepatocellular carcinoma arising in an adenoma: value of QBend 10 immunostaining in diagnosis of liver cell carcinoma. Histopathology 28:472–474

78. Kimura H, Nakajima T, Kagawa K, Deguchi T, Kakusui M, Katagishi T, Okanoue T, Kashima K, Ashihara T (1998) Angiogenesis in hepatocellular carcinoma as evaluated by CD34 immunohistochemistry. Liver 18:14–9

79. de Boer WB, Segal A, Frost FA, Sterrett GF (2000) Can CD34 discriminate between benign and malignant hepatocytic lesions in fine-needle aspirates and thin core biopsies? Cancer 90:273–278

80. Frachon S, Gouysse G, Dumortier J, Couvelard A, Nejjari M, Mion F, Berger F, Paliard P, Boillot O, Scoazec JY (2001) Endothelial cell marker expression in dysplastic lesions of the liver: an immunohistochemical study. J Hepatol 34:850–857

81. Gottschalk-Sabag S, Ron N, Glick T (1998) Use of CD34 and factor VIII to diagnose hepatocellular carcinoma on fine needle aspirates. Acta Cytol 42:691–696

82. Di Tommaso L, Franchi G, Park YN, Fiamengo B, Destro A, Morenghi E, Montorsi M, Torzilli G, Tommasini M, Terracciano L, Tornillo L, Vecchione R, Roncalli M (2007)

Diagnostic value of HSP70, glypican 3, and glutamine synthetase in hepatocellular nodules in cirrhosis. Hepatology 45:725–734

83. Shafizadeh N, Ferrell LD, Kakar S (2008) Utility and limitations of glypican-3 expression for the diagnosis of hepatocellular carcinoma at both ends of the differentiation spectrum. Mod Pathol 21:1011–1018

84. Baumhoer D, Tornillo L, Stadlmann S, Roncalli M, Diamantis EK, Terracciano LM (2008) Glypican 3 expression in human nonneoplastic, preneoplastic, and neoplastic tissues: a tissue microarray analysis of 4,387 tissue samples. Am J Clin Pathol 129:899–906

85. Wang XY, Degos F, Dubois S, Tessiore S, Allegretta M, Guttmann RD, Jothy S, Belghiti J, Bedossa P, Paradis V (2006) Glypican-3 expression in hepatocellular tumors: diagnostic value for preneoplastic lesions and hepatocellular carcinomas. Hum Pathol 37:1435–1441

86. Kandil DH, Cooper K (2009) Glypican-3: a novel diagnostic marker for hepatocellular carcinoma and more. Adv Ana Pathol 16:125–129

Chapter 4
Screening Program in High-Risk Populations

Ryota Masuzaki and Masao Omata

Keywords Screening · Surveillance · AFP · Ultrasonography

Introduction

Hepatocellular carcinoma (HCC) is one of the most common cancers worldwide [1–5]. The majority of patients with HCC have a background of chronic liver disease, especially chronic hepatitis due to hepatitis C virus (HCV) or hepatitis B virus (HBV) infection [6, 7]. Thus, at least some high-risk patients for HCC can be readily defined. Indeed, HCC surveillance is commonly performed as part of the standard clinical examination of patients with chronic viral hepatitis [8].

Ultrasonography and tumor marker tests, which play important roles in HCC surveillance in patients with chronic liver diseases, are widely used. However, insufficient evidence exists to suggest that surveillance by either of these methods improves the prognosis of patients with HCC or increases the chances of local therapies such as resection and local ablation therapy or even that of radical treatments such as liver transplantation. Similarly, the utility of computed tomography (CT) or magnetic resonance imaging (MRI) in the surveillance of HCC remains unclear.

The primary objective of screening and surveillance for HCC should be to reduce mortality as much as possible in patients who actually develop the cancer and in an acceptably cost-effective fashion. To attain this objective, two distinct issues deserve meticulous consideration: the target population and the mode of surveillance.

M. Omata (✉)
Department of Gastroenterology, University of Tokyo, Hongo, Bunkyo-ku, Tokyo, Japan

K.M. McMasters, J.-N. Vauthey (eds.), *Hepatocellular Carcinoma*,
DOI 10.1007/978-1-60327-522-4_4, © Springer Science+Business Media, LLC 2011

Target Population

HCC has been observed to show significant geographic regional clustering [9]. Moreover, HBV, HCV, and other environmental factors may play important roles in HCC development, with the relative importance of individual factors varying widely according to geographic area [7, 10–12]. In Japan, HCV infection is responsible for about 80% of HCC cases, whereas HBV infection is responsible for 10% and alcohol for about 5% [4, 13]. These values may differ substantially in other countries. For example, in China, HBV infection has a much higher prevalence and is therefore by far the predominant etiology behind HCC. In the United States, nonalcoholic steatohepatitis (NASH) is reportedly a major predisposing disease for HCC.

Surveillance is not recommended for the general population, given the low incidence of HCC among individuals with no risk factors. Thus, the first step in HCC screening should be the identification of patients at risk of HCC development. Since chronic viral hepatitis due to either HBV or HCV may be asymptomatic, mass screening for hepatitis virus infection of either the HBV or HCV type is justified if the prevalence of infection in the region is reasonably high. Indeed, mass screening of adults over 40 years of age for HBV and HCV infection has been performed in Japan since 2002, but the cost-effectiveness of this program has yet to be evaluated.

Persistent infection with HBV is a major risk factor for HCC. HBV carriers have a 223-fold higher risk of developing the cancer than noncarriers [14]. Among HBV carriers, those who are HBe-antigen positive are at a higher risk of HCC than those who are negative for the antigen (relative risk, 6.3) [15, 16]. The results of a recent large-scale, long-term cohort study conducted in Taiwan showed that serum HBV DNA levels are the strongest risk factor for both the progression to cirrhosis and the development of HCC among HBV-positive patients, independent of serum HBe-antigen/antibody status or alanine aminotransferase (ALT) levels [17]. With the advent of reliable quantitative assays, the determination of HBV DNA levels may replace that of HBe-antigen/antibody status as a risk indicator of HCC.

While the prevalence of chronic HBV infection is high in limited geographic areas, such as East and Southeast Asia and sub-Saharan Africa, the prevalence of chronic HCV infection has been increasing in many parts of the developed world, including Japan, southern Europe, and the United States. With chronic HCV infection, the risk of HCC increases with progression to liver fibrosis [6, 18], and patients with chronic HCV infection who have cirrhosis stand a very high risk of developing HCC [19]. In Japan, HCV infection spread throughout the country mainly in the 1950s and 1960s, and thus after the passing of a few decades required for progression to cirrhosis, it is currently by far the most predominant cause of HCC. The peak of viral spread in the United States took place a couple of decades later; accordingly, the incidence of HCV-related HCC is now rapidly increasing [20, 21]. In addition to the degree of liver fibrosis, male gender, older age, and heavy alcohol consumption are also known risk factors for HCV-related HCC. Human immunod-eficiency virus (HIV) coinfection is an important risk factor of rapid progression to liver fibrosis, which especially now in the United States constitutes a serious clinical problem.

Cirrhosis due to etiologies other than chronic viral hepatitis also presents a risk for HCC development. Major etiologies include alcoholic liver disease and NASH [22–24], the relative importance of which may differ geographically. Hassan et al. reported that alcoholic liver disease accounted for 32% of all cases of HCC in an Austrian cohort [25]. In the United States, the approximate hospitalization rate for HCC related to alcoholic cirrhosis is 8–9/100,000/year compared to about 7/100,000/year for hepatitis C [26]. NASH is a chronic liver disease that is gaining increasing importance due to its high prevalence worldwide and its potential pro-gression to cirrhosis, HCC, and liver failure. Although NASH has been described in cohorts of patients with HCC [27, 28], the incidence of HCC with respect to cirrho-sis due to NASH is not well known. In certain areas of the world, aflatoxin also may play a role in HCC development.

In brief, evaluation of the degree of liver fibrosis is of paramount importance in assessing the risk of HCC development in patients with chronic liver diseases of any etiology. Histological evaluation of liver biopsy samples has been consid-ered the gold standard for the assessment of liver fibrosis, but the invasiveness accompanying liver biopsy poses considerable limits to its clinical feasibility. In clinical practice, repeated assessment of liver fibrosis often will be required because a once non-cirrhotic liver may become cirrhotic over time, sometimes rather rapidly. Consequently, the noninvasive evaluation of liver fibrosis is currently one of the main interests of hepatology.

Results obtained from the recently developed technique of transient elastography correlate well with liver fibrosis stage, as determined histologically [29–31]. The cutoff value for the diagnosis of histological cirrhosis is 12.5–14.9 kPa [29, 31]. Higher values of liver stiffness may need proper attention as they indicate decom-pensation and HCC development. The fibrotest is based on the age and gender of the patient combined with measurements of five biochemical markers (total bilirubin, haptoglobin, gamma glutamyl transpeptidase, alpha-2 macroglobulin, and apolipoprotein A1) [32]. An index of 0–0.10 has a 100% negative predictive value, while an index of 0.60–1.00 has a greater than 90% positive predictive value for a Metavir score of F2 to F4. The APRI is the aspartate aminotransferase (AST) level/upper limit of normal divided by the platelet count (10^9/L) multiplied by 100 [33]. For a hypothetical patient with AST 90 IU/L (upper limit of normal, 45) and platelet count 100 ($\times 10^9$/L), the APRI score is 2.0, which means that the positive predictive value for significant fibrosis is 0.88. Nonetheless, the applicability of any of these methods for surveillance remains to be determined in prospective studies.

Patients who are considered to be at a non-negligible risk of developing HCC should participate in a surveillance program, as discussed below. Possible excep-tions may be patients with severe liver dysfunction who could not receive any treatment even if diagnosed with HCC or those with other life-threatening diseases.

Surveillance Methodology

Traditionally, two methodologies have been employed in HCC surveillance for high-risk patients: tumor marker determination, specifically serum alpha-fetoprotein (AFP) concentration, and diagnostic imaging via liver ultrasonography. The utility of a surveillance program should be evaluated based on its beneficial effects in terms of outcome of patients diagnosed with HCC relative to the cost. However, few prospective randomized trials have compared the outcome of patients with HCC enrolled or not in a surveillance program. Consequently, evidence regarding the benefits of surveillance on decreasing overall or disease-specific mortality has come mostly from retrospective or case–control studies.

Alpha-Fetoprotein (AFP)

The glycoprotein AFP has a molecular weight of 72 kDa. Its main physiologic function appears to be the regulation of fatty acids in both fetal and proliferating adult liver cells [34]. Since 1968, AFP has been used as a serum marker in the detection of human HCC [35], with a sensitivity of 39–65%, a specificity of 76–94%, and a positive predictive value of 9–50% (Table 4.1) [36–41]. Studies assessing the usefulness of AFP in HCC screening have varied widely in their design and in the characteristics of the targeted patients in terms of, for example, disease etiology and severity of background liver diseases. Moreover, the reported specificity and sensitivity values inevitably vary depending on the cutoff level chosen for the diagnosis of HCC.

An intrinsic disadvantage of AFP as a tumor marker is the fact that serum AFP levels can increase in patients who have active hepatitis, but not HCC; this is partly due to the accelerated cellular proliferation during liver regeneration. An AFP concentration of 20 ng/mL is often adopted as the upper limit of normal because this level is rarely exceeded in healthy people. However, slightly higher concentrations are hardly diagnostic of HCC among patients with chronic hepatitis, and the adoption of a cutoff value that is too low would result in an inappropriately low specificity. AFP levels above 400 ng/mL can be considered almost definitively diagnostic of HCC but sensitivity is inevitably lower at this higher cutoff value. Moreover, an additional disadvantage exists in using AFP for HCC surveillance. Small HCC tumors, the detection of which is the primary objective of surveillance, are less likely to be AFP producing, but even if the marker is expressed by these tumors, the levels may not be high enough to result in a diagnosis of HCC.

For this and other reasons, AFP determination has been frequently dismissed as a screening test for HCC, except when ultrasonography is either not available or of such poor quality that lesions smaller than 2 cm in diameter cannot be detected. Moreover, as shown in HCC screening of Alaskan carriers of hepatitis B, AFP testing allowed the detection of tumors at an earlier, treatable stage [42], but although screened patients survived longer than their historic controls, the difference could

Table 4.1 Surveillance studies for hepatocellular carcinoma

Author (Year)	Number screened	Incidence of HCC (%/year)	%HCV	%HBV	%Alcohol	AFP					Ultrasonography		
						Interval (months)	Cutoff (ng/mL)	Sensitivity (%)	Specificity (%)		Interval (months)	Sensitivity (%)	Specificity (%)
Oka (1990)	140	6.5		20	19	2	500	25	91.0		3	85	
Pateron (1994)	118	5.8		4.2	69.5	6	100	21	93		6	78	93
Sherman (1995)	1069	0.47	0	100		6	20	64.3	91.4		6	78.8	93.8
Bolondi (2001)	313	4.1	64.2	17.3		6	20	41.0	82				

be equally well explained by lead-time and length-time biases, which are inherent in retrospective studies on screening.

Ultrasonography

Ultrasonography has been applied to identify intrahepatic lesions since the early 1980s [43]. This imaging modality is appealing because it is almost completely noninvasive. Although both the ribs and the air in the lungs and gastrointestinal tract surround the liver and potentially hinder imaging, newer ultrasound devices and techniques have improved hepatic ultrasonography. The reported sensitivity of ultrasound imaging in the detection of HCC nodules is highly variable, ranging from 35 to 84% [44], depending on the expertise of the operator as well as on the ultrasound equipment used. Indeed, the current more sophisticated ultrasound instruments produce images with much better resolution, improving the detectability of small intrahepatic lesions. Note, however, that ultrasound diagnosis remains heavily operator dependent. A high level of skill and experience is required to record high-quality images and to make an accurate diagnosis. In addition, ultrasound diagnosis may not be possible due to the patient's physical condition, such as extreme obesity.

A previous study reported the sensitivity of ultrasonography for HCC detection to be as low as 20.5% [45] based on the detection of pathology in explanted livers removed from patients who underwent liver transplantation. Small HCC nodules less than or equal to 2 cm in diameter constituted 85% of the lesions that failed to be detected by ultrasonography [46]. This finding was confirmed in another study showing that the ultrasound detectability of HCC nodules depends on tumor size: nodules of >5.0, 3.1–5.0, 2.1–3.0, and 1.0–2.0 cm in diameter were detected at a rate of 92, 75, 20, and 13.6%, respectively [45].

Although these data are rather disappointing, other studies have found that the ability of ultrasonography to detect intrahepatic nodules is almost comparable to that of CT [47–50]. In a study on nodules that were 2 cm or smaller in diameter in patients with chronic hepatitis, the ability of ultrasonography to detect nodular lesions, adenomatous hyperplasia, and well-differentiated HCC was better than that of CT or MRI [51]. Thus, the noninvasiveness and relatively low cost of ultrasonography make it indispensable in HCC screening. Nonetheless, a definite diagnosis of HCC depends on the evaluation of tumor vascularity, which is not possible with conventional ultrasonography. Therefore, CT or MRI studies with contrast enhancement usually follow ultrasonography when the latter raises suspicion of HCC.

Ultrasonography, when conducted by less experienced operators, has blind spots. Moreover, the resolution may not be satisfactory in patients with cirrhosis who show rough echo patterns in the background liver. While it may be expected that the detection capability of HCC would improve with the use of CT or MRI in combination with ultrasonography, few studies have reported on HCC surveillance in which either one of these modalities was employed. In addition, their cost–benefit status remains unclear.

Recently, several contrast materials have been developed for ultrasonography. They are very useful in the differential diagnosis of intrahepatic nodules and the demarcation of intrahepatic lesions prior to percutaneous ablation, but their role in HCC screening has yet to be defined.

Combined Alpha-Fetoprotein Measurement and Ultrasonography

In HCC screening, serum AFP measurement is less sensitive than ultrasonography, but its specificity may be comparable if the appropriate cutoffs are used. Screening by a combination of ultrasonography and AFP may improve HCC detection, but the results described in previous reports were generally negative [37, 52–54]. However, in a nonrandomized study of patients with cirrhosis, the sensitivity of detection increased when both ultrasonography and AFP measurements were conducted as compared to either screening approach alone [52].

Recently, a randomized trial was carried out in which 18,000 Chinese patients with HBV infection were either screened every 6 months for HCC or not by AFP measurements and ultrasonography [55]. The results indicated that more cases of HCC were diagnosed in the screened group than in the non-screened group (86 vs. 67) and overall survival rate at 1,3, and 5 years were better: 65.9, 52.6, and 46.4 compared to 31.2, 7.2, and 0%, respectively.

A retrospective study assessed HCC screening in 367 patients aged 70 years or older, with AFP measurements and ultrasonography carried out every 6 or 12 months. Screening allowed more frequent diagnosis of HCC at an early stage, increased the proportion of patients able to be treated curatively, and improved the prognosis of these patients compared to those who had not been screened. The apparent survival benefit was restricted to the first 3 years after HCC detection, probably because of the shorter life expectancy of this elderly population [56].

New Serum Markers and New Methods

Recent developments in gene-expression microarrays, proteomics, and tumor immunology now permit thousands of genes and proteins to be screened simultaneously. Furthermore, new biomarkers are expected to be established in the next decade for the screening of many cancers, including HCC. To establish a formal framework to guide biomarker evaluation and development, a 5-phase program was adopted by the Early Detection Research Network (EDRN) of the National Cancer Institute [57]. Several newly identified markers, including des-gamma carboxyprothrombin (DCP), AFP-L3, glypican-3, IGF-1, and HGF, currently appear promising. They are to be evaluated further in phase 2 studies to determine their ability to detect early-stage HCC, followed by phase 3 studies, which will retrospectively determine whether these markers can detect preclinical diseases. If the preliminary results hold up in these trials, follow-up phase 4 studies will be needed to prospectively assess the ability of the markers to detect early HCC and phase 5 studies to confirm that marker-based surveillance reduces morbidity and mortality from HCC.

The detection sensitivities of dynamic CT and dynamic MRI are high for hyper-vascular HCC. Considering that patients with HCC undergo repeated imaging examinations and that the diagnostic capabilities of the two imaging modalities are almost the same, dynamic MRI, which does not involve X-ray exposure, may be more advantageous. However, MRI systems that allow high-quality dynamic studies are not yet as widely available as high-speed CT systems such that the number of institutions that can perform dynamic MRI is limited. Alternatively, high-speed dynamic CT, such as helical CT, or even more advanced systems such as multi-detector CT (MDCT) can be used to follow patients with HCC. The development of MDCT has dramatically accelerated scan acquisition in liver CT [58], allowing high-speed volume coverage of the entire liver in 4–10 s and the acquisition of two separate series of scans in the arterial phase (early and late arterial phase scans) [59, 60].

The tracer [18F]2-fluoro-D-2-deoxyglucose (FDG) is taken up by tumor cells during active glucose metabolism and is specifically accumulated by them. The accumulated fluorescence can then be visualized by positron emission tomography (FDG-PET). In a study evaluating the diagnosis of HCC based on a quantitative standardized uptake value (SUV) for FDG, the SUV for HCC was lower than that for metastatic liver cancer [61]. Nonetheless, FDG-PET is not recommended for the diagnosis of HCC because it is expensive and no better than conventional diagnostic imaging techniques such as CT and MRI.

Standardized Recall Procedures

Once patients are found to have an abnormal surveillance test, they need to be recalled for subsequent evaluation. However, none of the many recall algorithms described in the literature has been tested prospectively. Furthermore, the recall procedures for abnormal AFP values should differ from those for abnormal ultrasonography findings. Increases in serum AFP need to be interpreted against background liver diseases, as reactivated chronic hepatitis B is often accompanied by increased AFP levels. Pregnancy also may cause a temporary elevation in serum AFP, sometimes together with an increase in the proportion of the protein's L3 fraction. Thus, patients showing an increase in AFP levels require a detailed clinical evaluation to determine the cause of the increase.

Patients at risk for HCC in whom a low-echo lesion is detected in the liver by ultrasonography are strongly urged to undergo a complete evaluation. Typically, this involves further imaging by CT or MRI with contrast enhancement. The presence of hyperattenuation in the arterial phase with washout in the late phase is a definite sign of HCC [62]. In ambiguous cases, needle biopsy of the tumor under ultrasound guidance is recommended. However, whether all suspicious nodules should be subjected to liver tumor biopsy is discussed controversially because of concerns about the potential for tumor seeding.

Screening Intervals

Since the risk of HCC development does not usually diminish spontaneously in patients who are the typical targets of HCC screening, a surveillance program for HCC should consist of repeating screenings at determined intervals. Ultrasonography is superior to CT in this setting due to its noninvasiveness and cost-effectiveness. The guidelines of the American Association for the Study of Liver Diseases (AASLD) propose ultrasound surveillance for patients at high risk for HCC at 6-month intervals. The guidelines explicitly indicate that the surveillance interval should depend not on the degree of risk for HCC but exclusively on tumor doubling times, to detect cancer nodules while they are small enough to be cured.

In Japan, ultrasound surveillance at a shorter interval of 3–4 months is encouraged for extremely high-risk patients while a 6-month interval is recommended for those at high risk (Fig. 4.1) [63]. In Japanese patients with chronic hepatitis C marked by cirrhosis, the incidence of HCC is 6–8% per year; this group is therefore at an extremely high risk of tumor development. While theoretically, shorter surveillance intervals lead to the detection of smaller tumors, whether the potential difference in detected tumor size is large enough to affect prognosis in a cost-effective fashion is not known. Although no prospective comparison of different screening schedules has been performed, both a retrospective study on patients with cirrhosis and a mathematic model applied to HBV carriers suggested that a longer screening interval is just as effective as the 6-month interval in terms of survival.

Opinions also diverge as to whether AFP determination should be included in HCC surveillance programs. However, if AFP is to be measured, then measurements should be made repeatedly and an abnormal level of AFP must be interpreted not by simple comparison with a given cutoff value but in the context of a time series of values. An abrupt elevation of serum AFP levels in the absence of exacerbation of hepatitis is suggestive of the development of HCC, even if ultrasonography is apparently negative. In such cases, further evaluation with CT or MRI using contrast enhancement should be considered.

Cost-Effectiveness

According to a decision analysis model, the cost-effectiveness ratio of screening European patients with only Child–Pugh class A disease ranges from $48,000 to $284,000 for each additional life-year gained [64]. However, this study did not take into account liver transplantation as a treatment option. In a group of patients who could anticipate excellent survival, the cost-effectiveness ratio ranged from $26,000

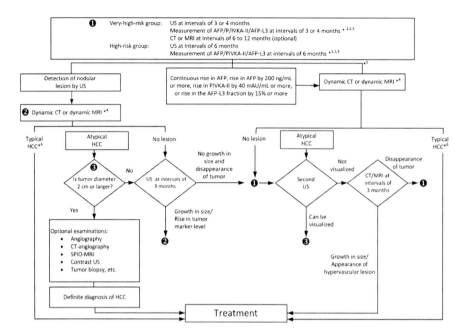

Fig. 4.1 Surveillance algorithm for hepatocellular carcinoma in Japan. Annotations: *1 The current health insurance policy in Japan covers the measurement of AFP or DCP level once per month. *2 AFP L3 can be measured only when patients are suspected of having hepatocellular carcinoma. *3 When AFP is 10 ng/mL or less, the AFP L3 fraction cannot be measured. *4 If patients have renal dysfunction or are suspected of being allergic to iodinated contrast media, dynamic MRI is recommended. *5 CT/MRI at regular intervals. *6 Tumor that is visualized as a high-intensity area in the arterial phase and relatively low-intensity area in the venous phase. *7 If patients are suspected of having other malignant tumors, such as cholangiocellular carcinoma or metastatic liver cancer, they proceed to thorough examination for the underlying disease

to $55,000. In another study, in which 313 Italian patients with cirrhosis underwent serum AFP measurement and liver ultrasonography every 6 months, the cost per one case of treatable HCC was $17,934, and the cost per year of life saved was $112,993 [40]. In the United States, the cost for each quality-adjusted life-year (QALY) gained through surveillance was estimated to range from $35,000 to $45,000 [64]. HCC screening in patients waiting for liver transplantation has been associated with a cost per year of life saved of $60,000–$100,000, depending on the screening modality used [65].

Note that the cost-effectiveness of HCC screening has thus far been assessed only by retrospective analysis or the use of decision-analysis models. Although retrospective studies suffer from selection bias, decision-analysis models are based on the simulation of costs and health outcomes. Consequently, their results may vary greatly according to the different assumptions made, such as the incidence of HCC in the screening population, the screening interval, the modality of diagnosis, the type of treatment after diagnosis, the tumor doubling time, and the tumor recurrence rate. If a screening is to be cost-effective at all, a feasible treatment should exist that can favorably affect the prognosis of patients.

Conclusions

High-risk populations for HCC have been clearly identified in many epidemiological studies and statistical analyses. HCC is a suitable disease for surveillance programs because it is relatively common, at least in patients with liver disease. The early detection and diagnosis of HCC allow patients to be treated curatively. Nonetheless, whether routine screening and surveillance for HCC actually improve outcome would be best determined by prospective randomized controlled trials.

References

1. Parkin DM, Bray F, Ferlay J, Pisani P (2001) Estimating the world cancer burden: Globocan 2000. Int J Cancer 94:153–156
2. Bosch FX, Ribes J, Diaz M, Cleries R (2004) Primary liver cancer: worldwide incidence and trends. Gastroenterology 127:S5–S16
3. Capocaccia R, Sant M, Berrino F, Simonetti A, Santi V, Trevisani F (2007) Hepatocellular carcinoma: trends of incidence and survival in Europe and the United States at the end of the 20th century. Am J Gastroenterol 102:1661–1670; quiz 1660, 1671
4. Kiyosawa K, Umemura T, Ichijo T, Matsumoto A, Yoshizawa K, Gad A, Tanaka E (2004) Hepatocellular carcinoma: recent trends in Japan. Gastroenterology 127:S17–26
5. El-Serag HB, Davila JA, Petersen NJ, McGlynn KA (2003) The continuing increase in the incidence of hepatocellular carcinoma in the United States: an update. Ann Intern Med 139:817–823
6. Yoshida H, Shiratori Y, Moriyama M, Arakawa Y, Ide T, Sata M, Inoue O, et al (1999) Interferon therapy reduces the risk for hepatocellular carcinoma: national surveillance program of cirrhotic and noncirrhotic patients with chronic hepatitis C in Japan. IHIT Study Group. Inhibition of hepatocarcinogenesis by interferon therapy. Ann Intern Med 131: 174–181
7. Shiratori Y (1996) Different clinicopathological features of hepatitis B- and C-related hepatocellular carcinoma. J Gastroenterol Hepatol 11:942–943
8. Bruix J, Sherman M (2005) Management of hepatocellular carcinoma. Hepatology 42: 1208–1236
9. Bosch FX, Ribes J, Borras J (1999) Epidemiology of primary liver cancer. Semin Liver Dis 19:271–285
10. Donato F, Tagger A, Chiesa R, Ribero ML, Tomasoni V, Fasola M, Gelatti U et al (1997) Hepatitis B and C virus infection, alcohol drinking, and hepatocellular carcinoma: a case-control study in Italy. Brescia HCC Study. Hepatology 26:579–584
11. Kew MC, Yu MC, Kedda MA, Coppin A, Sarkin A, Hodkinson J (1997) The relative roles of hepatitis B and C viruses in the etiology of hepatocellular carcinoma in southern African blacks. Gastroenterology 112:184–187
12. Sherlock S (1994) Viruses and hepatocellular carcinoma. Gut 35:828–832
13. Yoshizawa H (2002) Hepatocellular carcinoma associated with hepatitis C virus infection in Japan: projection to other countries in the foreseeable future. Oncology 62(Suppl 1):8–17
14. Beasley RP, Hwang LY, Lin CC, Chien CS (1981) Hepatocellular carcinoma and hepatitis B virus. A prospective study of 22 707 men in Taiwan. Lancet 2:1129–1133

15. Fattovich G, Giustina G, Schalm SW, Hadziyannis S, Sanchez-Tapias J, Almasio P, Christensen E, et al (1995) Occurrence of hepatocellular carcinoma and decompensation in western European patients with cirrhosis type B. The EUROHEP Study Group on Hepatitis B Virus and Cirrhosis. Hepatology 21:77–82

16. Tsukuma H, Hiyama T, Tanaka S, Nakao M, Yabuuchi T, Kitamura T, Nakanishi K et al (1993) Risk factors for hepatocellular carcinoma among patients with chronic liver disease. N Engl J Med 328:1797–1801

17. Chen CJ, Yang HI, Su J, Jen CL, You SL, Lu SN, Huang GT et al (2006) Risk of hepatocellular carcinoma across a biological gradient of serum hepatitis B virus DNA level. JAMA 295: 65–73

18. Takano S, Yokosuka O, Imazeki F, Tagawa M, Omata M. (1995) Incidence of hepatocellular carcinoma in chronic hepatitis B and C: a prospective study of 251 patients. Hepatology 21:650–655

19. Kato Y, Nakata K, Omagari K, Furukawa R, Kusumoto Y, Mori I, Tajima H et al (1994) Risk of hepatocellular carcinoma in patients with cirrhosis in Japan. Analysis of infectious hepatitis viruses. Cancer 74:2234–2238

20. Liang TJ, Jeffers LJ, Reddy KR, De Medina M, Parker IT, Cheinquer H, Idrovo V et al (1993) Viral pathogenesis of hepatocellular carcinoma in the United States. Hepatology 18: 1326–1333

21. Omata M, Yoshida H, Shiratori Y (2005) Prevention of hepatocellular carcinoma and its recurrence in chronic hepatitis C patients by interferon therapy. Clin Gastroenterol Hepatol 3:S141–143

22. Tanaka K, Hirohata T, Takeshita S, Hirohata I, Koga S, Sugimachi K, Kanematsu T et al (1992) Hepatitis B virus, cigarette smoking and alcohol consumption in the development of hepatocellular carcinoma: a case-control study in Fukuoka, Japan. Int J Cancer 51:509–514

23. Donato F, Tagger A, Gelatti U, Parrinello G, Boffetta P, Albertini A, Decarli A et al (2002) Alcohol and hepatocellular carcinoma: the effect of lifetime intake and hepatitis virus infections in men and women. Am J Epidemiol 155:323–331

24. Kuper H, Tzonou A, Kaklamani E, Hsieh CC, Lagiou P, Adami HO, Trichopoulos D et al (2000) Tobacco smoking, alcohol consumption and their interaction in the causation of hepatocellular carcinoma. Int J Cancer 85:498–502

25. Schoniger-Hekele M, Muller C, Kutilek M, Oesterreicher C, Ferenci P, Gangl A (2000) Hepatocellular carcinoma in Austria: aetiological and clinical characteristics at presentation. Eur J Gastroenterol Hepatol 12:941–948

26. El-Serag HB, Mason AC (2000) Risk factors for the rising rates of primary liver cancer in the United States. Arch Intern Med 160:3227–3230

27. Bugianesi E, Leone N, Vanni E, Marchesini G, Brunello F, Carucci P, Musso A et al (2002) Expanding the natural history of nonalcoholic steatohepatitis: from cryptogenic cirrhosis to hepatocellular carcinoma. Gastroenterology 123:134–140

28. Shimada M, Hashimoto E, Taniai M, Hasegawa K, Okuda H, Hayashi N, Takasaki K et al (2002) Hepatocellular carcinoma in patients with non-alcoholic steatohepatitis. J Hepatol 37:154–160

29. Castera L, Vergniol J, Foucher J, Le Bail B, Chanteloup E, Haaser M, Darriet M et al (2005) Prospective comparison of transient elastography, Fibrotest, APRI, and liver biopsy for the assessment of fibrosis in chronic hepatitis C. Gastroenterology 128:343–350

30. Sandrin L, Fourquet B, Hasquenoph JM, Yon S, Fournier C, Mal F, Christidis C et al (2003) Transient elastography: a new noninvasive method for assessment of hepatic fibrosis. Ultrasound Med Biol 29:1705–1713

31. Foucher J, Chanteloup E, Vergniol J, Castera L, Le Bail B, Adhoute X, Bertet J et al (2006) Diagnosis of cirrhosis by transient elastography (FibroScan): a prospective study. Gut 55: 403–408

32. Imbert-Bismut F, Ratziu V, Pieroni L, Charlotte F, Benhamou Y, Poynard T (2001) Biochemical markers of liver fibrosis in patients with hepatitis C virus infection: a prospective study. Lancet 357:1069–1075

33. Wai CT, Greenson JK, Fontana RJ, Kalbfleisch JD, Marrero JA, Conjeevaram HS, Lok AS (2003) A simple noninvasive index can predict both significant fibrosis and cirrhosis in patients with chronic hepatitis C. Hepatology 38:518–526

34. Taketa K (1990) Alpha-fetoprotein: reevaluation in hepatology. Hepatology 12:1420–1432

35. Alpert ME, Uriel J, de Nechaud B (1968) Alpha-1 fetoglobulin in the diagnosis of human hepatoma. N Engl J Med 278:984–986

36. Collier J, Sherman M (1998) Screening for hepatocellular carcinoma. Hepatology 27: 273–278

37. Sherman M, Peltekian KM, Lee C (1995) Screening for hepatocellular carcinoma in chronic carriers of hepatitis B virus: incidence and prevalence of hepatocellular carcinoma in a North American urban population. Hepatology 22:432–438

38. Trevisani F, D'Intino PE, Morselli-Labate AM, Mazzella G, Accogli E, Caraceni P, Domenicali M et al (2001) Serum alpha-fetoprotein for diagnosis of hepatocellular carcinoma in patients with chronic liver disease: influence of HBsAg and anti-HCV status. J Hepatol 34:570–575

39. Gambarin-Gelwan M, Wolf DC, Shapiro R, Schwartz ME, Min AD (2000) Sensitivity of commonly available screening tests in detecting hepatocellular carcinoma in cirrhotic patients undergoing liver transplantation. Am J Gastroenterol 95:1535–1538

40. Nguyen MH, Garcia RT, Simpson PW, Wright TL, Keeffe EB (2002) Racial differences in effectiveness of alpha-fetoprotein for diagnosis of hepatocellular carcinoma in hepatitis C virus cirrhosis. Hepatology 36:410–417

41. Tong MJ, Blatt LM, Kao VW (2001) Surveillance for hepatocellular carcinoma in patients with chronic viral hepatitis in the United States of America. J Gastroenterol Hepatol 16: 553–559

42. McMahon BJ, Bulkow L, Harpster A, Snowball M, Lanier A, Sacco F, Dunaway E et al (2000) Screening for hepatocellular carcinoma in Alaska natives infected with chronic hepatitis B: a 16-year population-based study. Hepatology 32:842–846

43. Takashima T, Matsui O, Suzuki M, Ida M (1982) Diagnosis and screening of small hepatocellular carcinomas. Comparison of radionuclide imaging, ultrasound, computed tomography, hepatic angiography, and alpha 1-fetoprotein assay. Radiology 145:635–638

44. Peterson MS, Baron RL (2001) Radiologic diagnosis of hepatocellular carcinoma. Clin Liver Dis 5, 123–144

45. Bennett GL, Krinsky GA, Abitbol RJ, Kim SY, Theise ND, Teperman LW (2002) Sonographic detection of hepatocellular carcinoma and dysplastic nodules in cirrhosis: correlation of pre-transplantation sonography and liver explant pathology in 200 patients. AJR Am J Roentgenol 179:75–80

46. Achkar JP, Araya V, Baron RL, Marsh JW, Dvorchik I, Rakela J (1998) Undetected hepatocellular carcinoma: clinical features and outcome after liver transplantation. Liver Transpl Surg 4, 477–482

47. de Ledinghen V, Laharie D, Lecesne R, Le Bail B, Winnock M, Bernard PH, Saric J et al (2002) Detection of nodules in liver cirrhosis: spiral computed tomography or magnetic resonance imaging? A prospective study of 88 nodules in 34 patients. Eur J Gastroenterol Hepatol 14:159–165

48. Libbrecht L, Bielen D, Verslype C, Vanbeckevoort D, Pirenne J, Nevens F, Desmet V et al (2002) Focal lesions in cirrhotic explant livers: pathological evaluation and accuracy of pretransplantation imaging examinations. Liver Transpl 8:749–761

49. Rode A, Bancel B, Douek P, Chevallier M, Vilgrain V, Picaud G, Henry L et al (2001) Small nodule detection in cirrhotic livers: evaluation with US, spiral CT, and MRI and correlation with pathologic examination of explanted liver. J Comput Assist Tomogr 25:327–336

50. Miller WJ, Federle MP, Campbell WL (1991) Diagnosis and staging of hepatocellular carcinoma: comparison of CT and sonography in 36 liver transplantation patients. AJR Am J Roentgenol 157:303–306

51. Horigome H, Nomura T, Saso K, Itoh M, Joh T, Ohara H (1999) Limitations of imaging diagnosis for small hepatocellular carcinoma: comparison with histological findings. J Gastroenterol Hepatol 14:559–565
52. Pateron D, Ganne N, Trinchet JC, Aurousseau MH, Mal F, Meicler C, Coderc E et al (1994) Prospective study of screening for hepatocellular carcinoma in Caucasian patients with cirrhosis. J Hepatol 20:65–71
53. Bolondi L, Sofia S, Siringo S, Gaiani S, Casali A, Zironi G, Piscaglia F et al (2001) Surveillance programme of cirrhotic patients for early diagnosis and treatment of hepatocellular carcinoma: a cost effectiveness analysis. Gut 48:251–259
54. Cottone M, Turri M, Caltagirone M, Parisi P, Orlando A, Fiorentino G, Virdone R et al (1994) Screening for hepatocellular carcinoma in patients with Child's A cirrhosis: an 8-year prospective study by ultrasound and alphafetoprotein. J Hepatol 21:1029–1034
55. Bo-Heng Z, Bing-Hui Y, Zhao-You T (2004) Randomized controlled trial of screening for hepatocellular carcinoma. J Cancer Res Clin Oncol 130:417–422
56. Trevisani F, Cantarini MC, Labate AM, De Notariis S, Rapaccini G, Farinati F, Del Poggio P et al (2004) Surveillance for hepatocellular carcinoma in elderly Italian patients with cirrhosis: effects on cancer staging and patient survival. Am J Gastroenterol 99:1470–1476
57. Pepe MS, Etzioni R, Feng Z, Potter JD, Thompson ML, Thornquist M, Winget M et al (2001) Phases of biomarker development for early detection of cancer. J Natl Cancer Inst 93:1054–1061
58. Foley WD, Mallisee TA, Hohenwalter MD, Wilson CR, Quiroz FA, Taylor AJ (2000) Multiphase hepatic CT with a multirow detector CT scanner. AJR Am J Roentgenol 175:679–685
59. Murakami T, Kim T, Takamura M, Hori M, Takahashi S, Federle MP, Tsuda K et al (2001) Hypervascular hepatocellular carcinoma: detection with double arterial phase multi-detector row helical CT. Radiology 218:763–767
60. Ichikawa T, Kitamura T, Nakajima H, Sou H, Tsukamoto T, Ikenaga S, Araki T (2002) Hypervascular hepatocellular carcinoma: can double arterial phase imaging with multidetector CT improve tumor depiction in the cirrhotic liver? AJR Am J Roentgenol 179:751–758
61. Iwata Y, Shiomi S, Sasaki N, Jomura H, Nishiguchi S, Seki S, Kawabe J et al (2000) Clinical usefulness of positron emission tomography with fluorine-18-fluorodeoxyglucose in the diagnosis of liver tumors. Ann Nucl Med 14:121–126
62. Torzilli G, Minagawa M, Takayama T, Inoue K, Hui AM, Kubota K, Ohtomo K et al (1990) Accurate preoperative evaluation of liver mass lesions without fine-needle biopsy. Hepatology 30:889–893
63. Makuuchi M, Kokudo N, Arii S, Futagawa S, Kaneko S, Kawasaki S, Matsuyama Y et al (2008) Development of evidence-based clinical guidelines for the diagnosis and treatment of hepatocellular carcinoma in Japan. Hepatol Res 38:37–51
64. Sarasin FP, Giostra E, Hadengue A (1996) Cost-effectiveness of screening for detection of small hepatocellular carcinoma in western patients with Child-Pugh class A cirrhosis. Am J Med 101:422–434
65. Everson GT (2000) Increasing incidence and pretransplantation screening of hepatocellular carcinoma. Liver Transpl 6:S2–10

Chapter 5
Staging of Hepatocellular Carcinoma

Hari Nathan and Timothy M. Pawlik

Keywords HCC staging · Okuda staging system · Cancer of the Liver Italian Program (CLIP) score · Barcelona Clinic Liver Cancer (BCLC) staging system · Liver Cancer Study Group of Japan (LCSGJ) staging system · Japanese Integrated Staging (JIS) score · Chinese University Prognostic Index (CUPI) · American Joint Committee on Cancer/International Union Against Cancer (AJCC/UICC) staging system

Introduction

Staging systems aim to stratify patients into groups with similar prognoses. As such, these staging systems may serve to guide choice of therapy, aid in patient counseling, allow comparisons of the end results of therapy, and facilitate patient selection and randomization for research protocols. Staging systems for hepatocellular carcinoma (HCC) are broadly divided into clinical and pathological staging systems. The clinical staging systems can be particularly useful in guiding choice of therapy and include the Okuda staging system [1], Cancer of the Liver Italian Program (CLIP) score [2], and Barcelona Clinic Liver Cancer (BCLC) staging system [3]. The pathologic staging systems are useful after resection or transplantation and include the Liver Cancer Study Group of Japan (LCSGJ) staging system [4], Japanese Integrated Staging (JIS) score [5], Chinese University Prognostic Index (CUPI) [6], and American Joint Committee on Cancer/International Union Against Cancer (AJCC/UICC) staging system [7, 8]. This chapter reviews these staging systems and highlights their relative strengths and weaknesses.

T.M. Pawlik (✉)
Division of Surgical Oncology, Department of Surgery, The Johns Hopkins School of Medicine, Baltimore, MD, USA

K.M. McMasters, J.-N. Vauthey (eds.), *Hepatocellular Carcinoma*,
DOI 10.1007/978-1-60327-522-4_5, © Springer Science+Business Media, LLC 2011

Clinical Staging Systems

Okuda Staging System

The Okuda scheme, proposed in 1985, was derived from an analysis of 850 Japanese patients who were treated with a range of surgical and non-surgical therapies [1]. In the Okuda system, patients are stratified based on the presence or absence of four factors: tumor involving >50% of the liver, ascites, serum albumin <3 g/dL, and serum bilirubin >3 mg/dL. Stage I disease was defined as having none of these features, Stage II as having one or two of these features, and Stage III as having three or four of these features. Although the Okuda staging system was once the most widely used, it has now fallen out of favor. There are two main criticisms of this system. First, it was derived in a cohort of patients with relatively advanced HCC and as such is less useful for prognostic discrimination at earlier stages of the disease. Second, it includes only one tumor-specific prognostic factor and therefore treats a wide range of tumors (all tumor sizes <50% of liver volume, solitary or multifocal, and with or without vascular invasion) as having comparable prognoses. Its usefulness in patients who do not have advanced disease is therefore limited.

Cancer of the Liver Italian Program Score

The CLIP score was conceived with the aim of allowing finer prognostic stratification than that provided by the Okuda system [2]. To this end, a scoring system with range 0–6 (Table 5.1) was developed using data on 435 Italian HCC patients treated with a range of surgical and non-surgical therapies [2]. A subsequent prospective validation in a cohort of 196 patients (over half of whom received no locoregional therapy) was also performed by the CLIP investigators [9]. Although the CLIP score in theory should allow the stratification of patients into seven separate groups by allotting points based on both tumor characteristics and liver function (Table 5.1), the CLIP investigators combined scores 5 and 6 for analysis in the original study [2] and scores 4–6 in their subsequent prospective validation [9]. Similarly, a Japanese validation study combined scores 5 and 6 [10], and a Canadian validation study combined scores 4–6 [11]. Nevertheless, all of these studies suggested that the CLIP score outperforms the Okuda staging system [2, 9–11].

Table 5.1 Cancer of the Liver Italian Program (CLIP) score

Variable	Points		
	0	1	2
Child–Pugh grade	A	B	C
Tumor morphology	Solitary and ≤50%	Multifocal and ≤ 50%	Massive or >50%
Serum α-fetoprotein	<400 ng/mL	≥400 ng/mL	
Portal vein thrombosis	Absent	Present	

While the CLIP score has been validated in patients with a wide range of HCC tumor burden who undergo a variety of locoregional therapies (including no therapy), it has several critical limitations. Like the Okuda system, it considers a wide range of early HCC tumors as a homogeneous group and therefore lacks sufficient sensitivity to discriminate between subgroups of patients with less advanced tumors. Although the CLIP score includes more tumor-specific prognostic factors than the Okuda system, it still groups a wide range of tumor sizes together and insufficiently accounts for the potential role of vascular invasion without clinically detectable sequelae such as portal vein thrombosis. At the other end of the disease spectrum, the CLIP score appears to poorly stratify patients with scores 4–6 [5]. As such, the CLIP score is limited in its ability to discriminate prognosis at both early and advanced stages of HCC.

Barcelona Clinic Liver Cancer Staging System

The BCLC staging system was proposed in 1999 both as a means of predicting prognosis and as a guide to selecting appropriate therapy [3]. It was intended to improve upon the prognostic performance of the Okuda system by incorporating factors related to liver function, tumor characteristics, and performance status (Table 5.2) [3, 12, 13]. In particular, the BCLC staging system sought to focus more precisely on prognosis in early stages of HCC, a deficiency of the Okuda system, because

Table 5.2 Barcelona Clinic Liver Cancer (BCLC) staging system

Stage	PST	Tumor extent	Liver disease	Proposed therapy
Stage A (early)				
A1	0	Solitary < 5 cm	No portal hypertension, normal bilirubin	Resection
A2	0	Solitary < 5 cm	Portal hypertension, normal bilirubin	Liver transplantation,
A3	0	Solitary < 5 cm	Portal hypertension, abnormal bilirubin	radiofrequency ablation, or ethanol
A4	0	Multifocal ≤ 3 *and* < 3 cm	Child–Pugh A–B	injection
Stage B (intermediate)	0	Multifocal >3 *or* ≥3 cm	Child–Pugh A–B	Transarterial (chemo)embolization
Stage C (advanced)[a]	1–2	Vascular invasion *or* extrahepatic spread	Child–Pugh A–B	Investigative therapy
Stage D (terminal)[a]	3–4	Any	Child–Pugh C	Palliation[b]

PST: Performance status [13]

[a] At least one of the conditions should be met

[b] Transplantation may be performed if not contraindicated by tumor extent

these patients are most likely to benefit from aggressive therapy. While the BCLC staging system has been demonstrated to work well as a prognostic tool [14–16], the BCLC treatment algorithm itself was based on a single institution's experience. Furthermore, the treatment algorithm is likely overly conservative with respect to the use of surgical therapy. For example, patients with large tumors would be excluded from surgical resection, although such patients have been shown to have 5-year survival of 25 to 39% after liver resection [17, 18]. Radiofrequency ablation and ethanol injection are recommended for patients with multifocal disease who fall within the Milan criteria [19] but have associated diseases. However, some patients with multifocal disease may indeed benefit from either transplantation or hepatic resection. In short, because it ties treatment decisions to prognostic factors, the BCLC is not a true staging system but rather a treatment algorithm. At the same time, its treatment recommendations may be overly conservative and in need of revision considering expanding indications for aggressive surgical therapy for HCC.

Pathologic Staging Systems

Liver Cancer Study Group of Japan Staging System

The LCSGJ 4th edition staging system was developed by a working group of the International Hepato-Pancreato-Biliary Association using data on 21,711 Japanese patients who underwent liver resection for HCC [4]. The LCSGJ system follows a tumor-node-metastasis (TNM) staging scheme. The tumor-specific factors considered are tumor number (solitary or not), size ($\leq$ 2 cm or not), and invasion of the portal vein, hepatic veins, or bile duct (present or not). T1 tumors exhibit all of these features, T2 tumors two of them, T3 tumors one of them, and T4 tumors none of them. Nodal disease is categorized as present (N1) or absent (N0), as is metastatic disease (M1 or M0). The TNM stage groupings are Stage I (T1N0M0), Stage II (T2N0M0), Stage III (T3N0M0), Stage IVA (T4N0M0 or any T, N1M0), and Stage IVB (any T, any N, M1).

There are several criticisms of the LCSGJ staging system. First, it places equal weight on each of the three tumor-specific factors. The resulting implication that, for example, tumor size of 3 cm has the same impact on prognosis as major vascular invasion is inconsistent with other published data [20]. Second, the LCSGJ system requires only macroscopic assessments of tumor extent and does not account for microscopic factors such as microvascular invasion. Finally, the LCSGJ system does not consider liver function and may therefore be inappropriate for patients whose prognoses are dominated by their liver dysfunction as opposed to their HCC tumor burden.

Japanese Integrated Staging Score

The JIS score specifically addresses the criticism that the LCSGJ TNM system ignores liver function [5]. By combining the Child–Pugh grade with the LCSGJ TNM stage, the JIS score allows prognostic stratification on a scale of 0–5

Table 5.3 Japanese Integrated Staging (JIS) score

Variable	Points			
	0	1	2	3
Child–Pugh grade	A	B	C	
LCSGJ TNM stage	I	II	III	IV

(Table 5.3). The JIS score was formulated to provide better stratification of patients with early HCC than that achieved by the CLIP score [5]. The original study that proposed this score suggested that the JIS score was superior to the CLIP score in a cohort of 722 Japanese patients undergoing a range of surgical and non-surgical therapies, but details of this cohort were sparse. In a subsequent validation study from the same group, 2502 of the 4525 patients analyzed did not have any histological confirmation of HCC [21]. Thus, although the JIS score appeared to outperform the CLIP score in this study, this finding may have been driven by the inappropriate inclusion of small dysplastic nodules in the group of very small (≤2 cm) HCC, spuriously improving the JIS score's discriminatory ability. With regard to its accounting for tumor characteristics, the JIS score shares the limitations of the LCSGJ TNM staging system.

Chinese University Prognostic Index

The CUPI was developed using a cohort of 926 Chinese patients, a minority (10%) of whom underwent surgical resection and a majority (58%) of whom received only supportive care and no locoregional therapy [6]. This staging system builds on the AJCC 5th edition TNM staging system but adds information on liver function to create a composite score, which in turn is used to stratify patients into low-risk, intermediate-risk, and high-risk groups (Table 5.4). No subsequent studies

Table 5.4 Chinese University Prognostic Index (CUPI)

Variable	Weight[a]
TNM stage	
Stage I or II	−3
Stage III	−1
Stage IV	0
Asymptomatic disease on presentation	−4
Ascites	3
α-Fetoprotein ≥500 ng/mL	2
Bilirubin	
< 2 mg/dL	0
2–3 mg/dL	3
>3 mg/dL	4
Alkaline phosphatase ≥200 IU/L	3

[a]Sum of weights: low risk (≤1), intermediate risk (2–7), or high risk (8–12)

comparing the CUPI to other staging systems have identified any particular advantages to the CUPI [14, 16, 22–25].

American Joint Committee on Cancer/International Union Against Cancer Staging System

The AJCC/UICC 6th edition TNM staging system was based on a study from the International Cooperative Study Group on Hepatocellular Carcinoma that included data on 591 patients from the United States, Japan, and France who all underwent surgical resection. A major strength of this study was the use of centralized pathological review. The AJCC 6th edition staging system represents a significant simplification over the AJCC 5th edition system, notably in that it eliminates a 2-cm size cutoff as a prognostic factor and instead recognizes size >5 cm as a prognostic factor only in patients with multifocal tumors. Thus, the 6th edition staging system focuses on tumor multifocality, size (only for multifocal tumors), and the presence of microvascular or major vascular invasion as the tumor characteristics of prognostic importance (Table 5.5). The 7th edition staging system of the AJCC/UICC has also recently been published. In the 7th edition, the staging system now distinguishes patients with invasion of major vessels from patients with multiple tumors of which any are >5 cm but lack major vessel invasion (Table 5.6). Ascertainment of the factors in the AJCC/UICC staging requires pathological review of resected specimens. As in the LCSGJ TNM system, nodal disease and metastatic disease are categorized as present (N1 or M1) or absent (N0 or M0).

Unlike the LCSGJ system, the AJCC/UICC staging system provides for the reporting of liver fibrosis and cirrhosis based on the Ishak histological grading scheme [26]. Fibrosis grades 0–4 (none to moderate fibrosis) are reported as fibrosis (F) score F0, and grades 5 and 6 (severe fibrosis/cirrhosis) are reported as F1. The F-score has additional prognostic value within each of the T1, T2, and T3 classifications with an effect on survival similar to that of upstaging to the next T classification

Table 5.5 American Joint Committee on Cancer/International Union Against Cancer (AJCC/UICC) 6th edition staging system [7]

T-classification		Stage grouping	
T1	Solitary with no vascular invasion	Stage I	T1N0M0
T2	Solitary with vascular invasion *or*	Stage II	T2N0M0
	multifocal ≤ 5 cm	Stage IIIA	T3N0M0
T3	Multifocal >5 cm *or* invasion of major	Stage IIIB	T4N0M0
	branch of portal/hepatic veins	Stage IIIC	N1M0 (any T)
T4	Invasion of adjacent organs[a] *or*	Stage IV	M1 (any T, any N)
	perforation of visceral peritoneum		

[a]Excluding gallbladder

Table 5.6 American Joint Committee on Cancer/International Union Against Cancer (AJCC/UICC) 7th edition staging system [8]

T-classification		Stage grouping	
T1	Solitary with no vascular invasion	Stage I	T1N0M0
T2	Solitary with vascular invasion *or*	Stage II	T2N0M0
	multifocal ≤ 5 cm	Stage IIIA	T3aN0M0
T3a	Multiple tumors >5 cm	Stage IIIB	T3bN0M0
T3b	Single tumor or multiple tumors of any	Stage IIIC	T4N0M0
	size involving a major branch of the	Stage IVA	Any T N1M0
	portal vein or hepatic vein	Stage IVB	Any T Any N M1
T4	Invasion of adjacent organs[a] *or*		
	perforation of visceral peritoneum		

[a]Excluding gallbladder

[20]. For example, patients with N0M0 disease have 5-year survival of 64% with T1 F0 disease, 49% with T1 F1 disease, and 46% with T2 F0 disease [20].

Although the AJCC/UICC staging system was developed using a cohort dominated by hepatitis C-related HCC, it has also been independently validated in a Chinese cohort with a high prevalence of hepatitis B [27]. Another advantage of the AJCC/UICC system is that it was based on a multivariate analysis of prognostic factors, which is important because of correlations between factors such as tumor size and vascular invasion. A potential limitation of the AJCC/UICC system is that it was developed using only resected patients. However, the 6th edition AJCC/UICC system also performs well in patients undergoing liver transplantation [28]. Its applicability to patients undergoing other non-surgical locoregional treatment modalities is questionable [16, 22], possibly due to the fact that prognosis in patients who are not candidates for liver resection may be highly influenced by underlying liver function.

The staging system for HCC has recently been updated in the 7th edition of the AJCC/UICC staging manual [8]. The T3 category has been sub-divided based on invasion of major vessels because of the markedly different prognosis conferred by this factor. Specifically, T3a now includes patients with multiple tumors, any of which is >5 cm. The T3b subgroup now includes tumors of any size involving a major portal vein or hepatic vein. The T4 category remains unchanged. Regarding the N category, inferior phrenic lymph nodes are now reclassified to regional lymph nodes (versus their classification as distant lymph nodes in the 6th edition of the AJCC/UICC staging). These T and N sub-category changes have resulted in a number of changes to the stage groupings. In the 7th edition AJCC/UICC staging manual, Stage IIIA now includes only T3a, while Stage IIIB now includes only T3b patients (i.e., those with tumors characterized by major vessel invasion). T4 is shifted to Stage IIIC. While Stage IV still includes all patients with metastasis, Stage IVA now includes those with nodal metastasis (N1), while Stage IVB now includes patients with distant metastasis (M1).

Choice of Appropriate Staging System

The "best" staging system for HCC depends in large part on the intended use of the system, the tumor characteristics, and the extent of underlying liver disease in the patient. The choice of staging system may be further complicated by the increasing use of multimodality therapy for HCC. Due in large part to differences in these factors, comparative studies of HCC staging systems have yielded variable results. For example, a single-institution study of 239 patients with cirrhosis and HCC suggested that the BCLC staging system outperformed the Okuda, CLIP, JIS, and CUPI systems (the AJCC/UICC system was not included) [14]. However, patients were treated according to an algorithm that was quite similar to that proposed by the BCLC system, so it is entirely unsurprising that the BCLC system performed well in this study [29]. Notably, only 4% of patients in this study underwent liver resection [14], calling into question the generalizability of the results.

A study of 195 HCC patients with less advanced disease (55% solitary, 71% ≤ 5 cm) suggested that the BCLC staging system was superior to the Okuda, CLIP, JIS, and 6th edition AJCC/UICC systems [15]. Importantly, while the study included a mix of patients who underwent ablation (42%), transplantation (21%), and resection (27%), the prognostic superiority of the BCLC system persisted even when evaluated specifically in the subgroup undergoing surgical therapy (transplantation or resection). Separate analyses for transplantation and resection were not reported. An advantage of this study is that the BCLC treatment algorithm was not applied, and it appears that surgical therapy was more aggressively applied than would be recommended by the BCLC system.

Other studies have suggested that the CLIP score has distinct advantages. Two Japanese studies found that the CLIP score was superior to the BCLC system [30, 31]. One of these found, however, that the JIS score was even better than the CLIP score [31]. A third Japanese study found that the CLIP score was superior to the JIS score as well as the LCSGJ and 6th edition AJCC/UICC TNM staging systems [32]. Interestingly, these studies consisted largely of patients with early HCC who underwent aggressive locoregional therapy, again emphasizing the sensitivity of such analyses to differences in patient cohorts and specifically highlighting the relationship of the BCLC system's performance to treatment decisions.

Several studies have focused specifically on patients undergoing liver resection. A study comparing the 6th edition AJCC/UICC system with the LCSJG system suggested that the 6th edition AJCC/UICC system was of greater utility in patients undergoing liver resection [27]. However, only 10% of patients in this study had tumors ≤ 2 cm, and 31% had tumors 2–5 cm. The Japanese system might have advantages in cohorts with smaller tumors. Another study found that the JIS score and the CLIP score were superior to the Okuda, BCLC, CUPI, and 6th edition AJCC/UICC systems in resected patients [23]. Specifically, the study suggested that the CLIP score should be used for patients undergoing major hepatectomy in a non-cirrhotic liver, while the JIS score should be used for patients undergoing minor hepatectomy in a cirrhotic liver. One interpretation of this finding is that the JIS score (based on the LCSGJ TNM system) performs well in patients with early HCC (who are usually amenable to aggressive locoregional therapy), which is entirely consistent with the characteristics of the cohorts in which it was developed and initially validated [5, 21]. Similarly, a Japanese study of resected patients, the majority of whom had early HCC, favored the JIS score and LCSGJ TNM system over the 6th edition AJCC/UICC TNM system, although the CLIP score outperformed all of these [32]. Patients with early HCC are the same ones in which a tumor size cutoff of 2 cm is most likely to have prognostic value – this is an important difference between the LCSGJ and 6th edition AJCC/UICC TNM systems. On the other hand, the relatively poor performance of the 6th edition AJCC/UICC system in these studies might also be related to the low proportion of patients with microvascular invasion (14% [23] and 19% [32]), which is a major prognostic factor in the AJCC/UICC system. Other comparative studies performed in resected cohorts have yielded divergent results. One favored the AJCC/UICC system over the Okuda, CLIP, and CUPI systems but did not analyze the LCSGJ or JIS systems [25]. The other study favored the JIS score over the CLIP, BCLC, and CUPI systems but did not analyze the 6th edition AJCC/UICC system [23]. In general, for patients who have undergone surgical resection/transplantation and who therefore have pathologic data available, the 6th edition AJCC/UICC staging system appears to provide the most accurate prognostic assessment. As noted, the 7th edition has undergone refinements in an attempt to improve further the prognostic accuracy of the AJCC/UICC staging system. Given that the staging system has only recently been introduced [8], future studies are needed to assess the performance of the revised AJCC/UICC staging system as compared with the performance of the 6th edition staging as well as other staging systems.

A few studies have addressed the comparative performance of these staging systems in cohorts undergoing other treatment modalities. For patients undergoing transarterial chemoembolization (TACE), the CLIP score may be particularly useful [33, 34], although one study suggested that the BCLC system might be better at very early stages [35]. One study has reported that the Child–Pugh nominal score is superior to both the CLIP and BCLC systems [22]. This study excluded patients in whom TACE allowed downstaging and subsequent surgical therapy, which may have created a cohort that was relatively homogeneous with respect to tumor biology such that underlying liver disease became the chief discriminating factor. While there is no clearly superior staging system for HCC treated by TACE, the CLIP score is most commonly used among interventional radiologists. Finally, one study has specifically addressed the performance of staging systems in patients undergoing radiofrequency ablation and concluded that the BCLC system performs best [16].

Conclusions

Various staging systems have been proposed and evaluated for HCC, and each has its merits. The evaluation of staging systems for HCC is more complex than for many other malignancies, as patient survival depends not only on tumor characteristics but also on the extent of underlying liver disease and the therapeutic modality or modalities used. For use in guiding therapy, clinical staging systems such as the CLIP score and BCLC algorithm may be useful, although each has its limitations. In those patients with advanced underlying cirrhosis, which will dominate the prognosis, tumor factors may be less important and clinical staging systems such as CLIP or BCLC may be more helpful. For patients in whom tumor resection allows pathological examination, the AJCC/UICC TNM staging system is the standard in the West. The AJCC/UICC TNM staging system has recently been further refined in the release of the 7th edition. Future studies will be needed to assess the relative improvement of the 7th edition AJCC/UICC staging system compared with the earlier version. The LCSGJ system (and related JIS score) may, however, have particular advantages in patients with early HCC. As the therapeutic modalities available for HCC and the indications for aggressive therapy expand, so too will the prognostic staging systems used. In particular, the increasing use of multimodality therapy can be expected to challenge our understanding of prognostic factors in HCC.

References

1. Okuda K, Ohtsuki T, Obata H et al (1985) Natural history of hepatocellular carcinoma and prognosis in relation to treatment. Study of 850 patients. Cancer 56:918–928
2. The Cancer of the Liver Italian Program (CLIP) investigators (1998) A new prognostic system for hepatocellular carcinoma: a retrospective study of 435 patients. Hepatology 28:751–755
3. Llovet JM, Bru C, Bruix J (1999) Prognosis of hepatocellular carcinoma: the BCLC staging classification. Semin Liver Dis 19:329–338
4. Makuuchi M, Belghiti J, Belli G et al (2003) IHPBA concordant classification of primary liver cancer: working group report. J Hepatobiliary Pancreat Surg 10:26–30
5. Kudo M, Chung H, Osaki Y (2003) Prognostic staging system for hepatocellular carcinoma (CLIP score): its value and limitations, and a proposal for a new staging system, the Japan Integrated Staging Score (JIS score). J Gastroenterol 38:207–215
6. Leung TW, Tang AM, Zee B et al (2002) Construction of the Chinese University Prognostic Index for hepatocellular carcinoma and comparison with the TNM staging system, the Okuda staging system, and the Cancer of the Liver Italian Program staging system: a study based on 926 patients. Cancer 94:1760–1769
7. Greene FL, Page DL, Fleming ID et al (2002) AJCC Cancer Staging Manual, 6th ed. New York, Springer-Verlag
8. Edge SB, Byrd DR, Compton CC et al (2010) AJCC Cancer Staging Manual, 7th ed. New York, Springer
9. The Cancer of the Liver Italian Program (CLIP) Investigators. (2000) Prospective validation of the CLIP score: a new prognostic system for patients with cirrhosis and hepatocellular carcinoma. Hepatology 31:840–845
10. Ueno S, Tanabe G, Sako K et al (2001) Discrimination value of the new western prognostic system (CLIP score) for hepatocellular carcinoma in 662 Japanese patients. Cancer of the Liver Italian Program. Hepatology 34:529–534
11. Levy I, Sherman M (2002) Staging of hepatocellular carcinoma: assessment of the CLIP, Okuda, and Child-Pugh staging systems in a cohort of 257 patients in Toronto. Gut 50:881–885
12. Bruix J, Llovet JM (2002) Prognostic prediction and treatment strategy in hepatocellular carcinoma. Hepatology 35:519–524

13. Sorensen JB, Klee M, Palshof T et al (1993) Performance status assessment in cancer patients. An inter-observer variability study. Br J Cancer 67:773–775
14. Marrero JA, Fontana RJ, Barrat A et al (2005) Prognosis of hepatocellular carcinoma: comparison of 7 staging systems in an American cohort. Hepatology 41:707–716
15. Cillo U, Vitale A, Grigoletto F et al (2006) Prospective validation of the Barcelona Clinic Liver Cancer staging system. J Hepatol 44:723–731
16. Guglielmi A, Ruzzenente A, Pachera S et al (2008) Comparison of seven staging systems in cirrhotic patients with hepatocellular carcinoma in a cohort of patients who underwent radiofrequency ablation with complete response. Am J Gastroenterol 103:597–604
17. Ng KK, Vauthey JN, Pawlik TM et al (2005) Is hepatic resection for large or multinodular hepatocellular carcinoma justified? Results from a multi-institutional database. Ann Surg Oncol 12:364–373
18. Pawlik TM, Poon RT, Abdalla EK et al (2005) Critical appraisal of the clinical and pathologic predictors of survival after resection of large hepatocellular carcinoma. Arch Surg 140: 450–458
19. Mazzaferro V, Regalia E, Doci R et al (1996) Liver transplantation for the treatment of small hepatocellular carcinomas in patients with cirrhosis. N Engl J Med 334:693–699
20. Vauthey JN, Lauwers GY, Esnaola NF et al (2002) Simplified staging for hepatocellular carcinoma. J Clin Oncol 20:1527–1536
21. Kudo M, Chung H, Haji S et al (2004) Validation of a new prognostic staging system for hepatocellular carcinoma: the JIS score compared with the CLIP score. Hepatology 40: 1396–1405
22. Georgiades CS, Liapi E, Frangakis C et al (2006) Prognostic accuracy of 12 liver staging systems in patients with unresectable hepatocellular carcinoma treated with transarterial chemoembolization. J Vasc Interv Radiol 17:1619–1624
23. Chen TW, Chu CM, Yu JC et al (2007) Comparison of clinical staging systems in predicting survival of hepatocellular carcinoma patients receiving major or minor hepatectomy. Eur J Surg Oncol 33:480–487
24. Kondo K, Chijiiwa K, Nagano M et al (2007) Comparison of seven prognostic staging systems in patients who undergo hepatectomy for hepatocellular carcinoma. Hepatogastroenterology 54:1534–1538
25. Lu W, Dong J, Huang Z et al (2008) Comparison of four current staging systems for Chinese patients with hepatocellular carcinoma undergoing curative resection: Okuda, CLIP, TNM and CUPI. J Gastroenterol Hepatol 23, 1874–1878
26. Ishak K, Baptista A, Bianchi L et al (1995) Histological grading and staging of chronic hepatitis. J Hepatol 22:696–699
27. Poon RT, Fan ST (2003) Evaluation of the new AJCC/UICC staging system for hepatocellular carcinoma after hepatic resection in Chinese patients. Surg Oncol Clin N Am 12: 35–50, viii
28. Vauthey JN, Ribero D, Abdalla EK et al (2007) Outcomes of liver transplantation in 490 patients with hepatocellular carcinoma: validation of a uniform staging after surgical treatment. J Am Coll Surg 204:1016–1028
29. Pawlik TM, Abdalla EK, Thomas M et al (2005) Staging of hepatocellular carcinoma. Hepatology 42:738–739; author reply 9–40
30. Tateishi R, Yoshida H, Shiina S et al (2005) Proposal of a new prognostic model for hepatocellular carcinoma: an analysis of 403 patients. Gut 54:419–425
31. Toyoda H, Kumada T, Kiriyama S et al (2005) Comparison of the usefulness of three staging systems for hepatocellular carcinoma (CLIP, BCLC, and JIS) in Japan. Am J Gastroenterol 100:1764–1771
32. Nanashima A, Omagari K, Tobinaga S et al (2005) Comparative study of survival of patients with hepatocellular carcinoma predicted by different staging systems using multivariate analysis. Eur J Surg Oncol 31:882–890

33. Testa R, Testa E, Giannini E et al (2003) Trans-catheter arterial chemoembolisation for hepa-tocellular carcinoma in patients with viral cirrhosis: role of combined staging systems, Cancer Liver Italian Program (CLIP) and Model for End-stage Liver Disease (MELD), in predicting outcome after treatment. Aliment Pharmacol Ther 17:1563–1569
34. Cho YK, Chung JW, Kim JK et al (2008) Comparison of 7 staging systems for patients with hepatocellular carcinoma undergoing transarterial chemoembolization. Cancer 112:352–361
35. Grieco A, Pompili M, Caminiti G et al (2005) Prognostic factors for survival in patients with early-intermediate hepatocellular carcinoma undergoing non-surgical therapy: comparison of Okuda, CLIP, and BCLC staging systems in a single Italian centre. Gut 54:411–418

Chapter 6
Multidisciplinary Care of the Hepatocellular Carcinoma Patient

Carlo M. Contreras, Jean-Nicolas Vauthey, and Kelly M. McMasters

Keywords HCC care · Hepatocellular carcinoma · Multidisciplinary care · HCC treatment

Introduction

Hepatocellular carcinoma (HCC) is a complex disease that requires the attention of physicians and surgeons from diverse backgrounds. This chapter will focus on the unique contributions of the hepatologist, radiologist, pathologist, medical oncologist, interventional radiologist, transplant surgeon, and the hepatobiliary surgeon. This chapter will conclude by illustrating how careful multidisciplinary care optimizes the long-term outcomes of patients with HCC.

Hepatologist

The hepatologist has particular expertise in the management of chronic cirrhosis and viral hepatitis and in implementing HCC screening protocols. The hepatologist is also essential in assessing a patient's candidacy for and optimizing a patient's medical comorbidities prior to initiating appropriate liver-directed therapies.

Randomized, controlled trials have established the efficacy of antiviral medication such as pegylated interferon ± ribavirin for the treatment of hepatitis C virus (HCV) infection. These studies also have detailed which patient factors are associated with a sustained viral response to antiviral therapy. Though genotype 1 is more prevalent in the USA, HCV subtypes 2 and 3 are much more likely to respond to

J.-N. Vauthey (✉)
Department of Surgical Oncology, The University of Texas MD Anderson Cancer Center, Houston, TX, USA

K.M. McMasters, J.-N. Vauthey (eds.), *Hepatocellular Carcinoma*,
DOI 10.1007/978-1-60327-522-4_6, © Springer Science+Business Media, LLC 2011

interferon ± ribavirin-based therapies [1]. Detailed treatment algorithms for patients with HCV are published by the National Institutes of Health [2].

Predictors of response for patients with hepatitis B virus (HBV) infection have also been identified. Response to pegylated interferon alpha-2b is associated with the HBV genotype (A>B>C>D) [3]. Options for initial antiviral HBV therapy now include pegylated interferon alpha-2b as well as a number of oral agents such as entecavir, lamivudine, and adefovir.

Chronic hepatocyte injury, viral or otherwise, is a well-established risk factor for the development of hepatocellular carcinoma. Many guidelines recommend screening an at-risk population to improve the detection of early HCC and thereby extend the HCC-specific mortality. To date, only one randomized study has demonstrated a 37% decrease in HCC-specific mortality, even though the study group completed only 58% of the screening exams offered. In this study, over 18,000 Chinese patients with chronic HBV or a history of chronic hepatitis were offered biannual liver ultrasonography and serum AFP levels [4]. The success of this screening program has been attributed to a high HCC incidence within the target population and to a favorable percentage of patients completing resection for the detected HCC lesions. The US population differs from the Chinese population in terms of the etiology of chronic liver injury and the prevalence of HCC within the at-risk population. The American Association for the Study of Liver Diseases has published indications for HCC screening [5].

To date, each of the available HCC staging systems has significant shortcomings. The TNM staging system has been validated in both eastern and western centers in patients who have undergone hepatic resection or transplantation [6–12]. When pathological data are not available from a surgical specimen, the Barcelona Clinic Liver Cancer (BCLC) staging system is commonly used. The development of a more comprehensive HCC staging system that can be applied to all patients is necessary to standardize inclusion criteria into clinical trials and to more accurately assess a patient's long-term risk when considering HCC treatment options.

Finally, as the liver specialist who is also broadly trained in internal medicine, the hepatologist is often the health-care provider who is relied upon to manage antiviral medications and treat the sequelae of chronic liver disease. The hepatologist is instrumental in optimizing and preparing the patient for the appropriate liver-directed therapies such as resection, ablation, transplantation, or transarterial chemoembolization (TACE).

Radiologist

The radiologist plays an obvious role in the detection and characterization of tumor masses and their relationship to important vascular and biliary structures. The radiologist recommends the optimal imaging modality depending on particular patient characteristics and the clinical indication for the examination. Due to its portability, ease of use, low cost, and absence of ionizing radiation, ultrasound is currently the imaging modality of choice for screening purposes. We will focus on the challenges of imaging small nodules suspicious for HCC and innovations in MR contrast media and on volumetric liver measurements.

Early HCC detection improves the probability that a patient will be a candidate for resection with curative intent. Accurate characterization of small arterial-enhancing lesions can be difficult. Such lesions can represent potentially premalignant dysplastic nodules or HCC. The radiologist is essential in recommending the optimal imaging modality in these situations. Identification of the optimal modality depends on multiple factors including the specifications of the ultrasound, CT and MR equipment, and the sequence protocols (which can vary from institution to institution) that are used to acquire the images. For lesions that are determined to be benign, it is uncertain how often repeat imaging should be performed. Current practice patterns are loosely based on an empiric 3-month UNOS guideline for hepatic re-imaging for listed patients awaiting transplantation [13].

New MR contrast media such as gadolinium benzyloxypropionictetraacetate and superparamagnetic iron oxide are the focus of ongoing research due to their differential uptake by certain types of cell lines within the liver tissue (i.e., hepatocytes versus reticuloendothelial cells) [14]. Use of agents with these properties may result in enhancements in MR imaging which could improve the detection of small HCC tumors.

Prior to hepatectomy for HCC, a minority of patients will require portal vein embolization to induce hypertrophy in the future liver remnant (FLR) in order to reduce the risk of post-hepatectomy hepatic insufficiency. The radiologist is instrumental in the measurement of detailed segmental liver volumes, or volumetry. These volumetric calculations involve the sum of multiple cross-sectional areas of each liver segment based on thin-section axial computed tomographic images. Ribero et al. have detailed the calculation process and the clinical application of volumetric data for patients undergoing hepatic resection [15].

Pathologist

Distinguishing between hepatocellular carcinoma, regenerative, and dysplastic nodules remains a challenge. Recent data indicate that gene expression profiles may aid in differentiating dysplastic nodules from HCC [16, 17]. Once a diagnosis of HCC has been established, histological review of both tumor-bearing and non-tumor-bearing tissue is crucial to ensure accurate stage classification. The following factors are independent predictors of death in patients undergoing resection for HCC: major vascular invasion, microvascular invasion, severe fibrosis/cirrhosis, multiple tumors, and tumors >5 cm [18]. The pathologist is particularly essential in characterizing the type and degree of both vascular invasion and fibrosis/cirrhosis if these features are present. Alpha-fetoprotein is still the most commonly utilized tumor marker but other relevant biomarkers are being identified. Though primarily a research tool, a gene expression signature has been developed, which has been associated with increased survival in patients undergoing HCC resection [19].

Finally, the pathologist is essential in identifying the fibrolamellar variant of HCC. Identifying this variant is important because hilar and portal lymphadenectomy is recommended at the time of hepatic resection due to the increased frequency of lymph node metastasis [20].

Medical Oncologist

Within the multidisciplinary team, the medical oncologist is the best resource for discussions regarding the use of systemic therapy for HCC. Systemic chemotherapy is generally ineffective against HCC, with response rates to doxorubicin of about 10%, and 20% for a combination regimen of cisplatin, interferon α-2b, doxorubicin, and fluorouracil [21]. The molecular targeted therapies hold considerably more promise. Most notable is sorafenib, an oral multikinase inhibitor with activity against various tyrosine and serine/threonine kinases, including vascular endothelial growth factor. Phase III data show that the median survival was 3 months longer in Child–Pugh Class A patients taking sorafenib compared to placebo [22]. A number of other targeted molecular therapies for HCC are currently being evaluated in clinical trials [23].

Interventional Radiologist

The interventional radiologist assists in a variety of liver-directed procedures for patients with HCC. These include preoperative portal vein embolization (PVE), ablative procedures, and TACE. The goal of preoperative PVE is to embolize the tumor-bearing lobe of the liver with the intent of causing ipsilateral lobar atrophy and contralateral hypertrophy with the intent of enlarging the volume of liver that will remain after HCC resection. The degree of hypertrophy following PVE is useful in predicting postoperative hepatic insufficiency [15]. When performing right portal vein embolization, extending the procedure to involve segment IV branches improves the hypertrophy in segments II and III compared to patients without segment IV embolization [24]. The use of PVE prior to major liver resection (≥3 segments) for HCC is associated with a lower rate of major operative complication compared to patients who did not undergo preoperative PVE [25].

Three main ablative modalities are available to patients who are not eligible for resection – radiofrequency, microwave, and cryoablation. A description of the indications and relative advantages of each technique is beyond the scope of this chapter [26]. TACE utilizes precisely delivered, high-dose chemotherapy via a lipiodol carrier that is preferentially retained by hepatocytes, thus minimizing the toxic effects of systemic administration. Meta-analysis and subsequent sensitivity analysis of 14 randomized arterial embolization trials showed that cisplatin or doxorubicin-based TACE was associated with an improved 2-year survival compared to patients who underwent conservative therapy for unresectable HCC [27].

Transplant Surgeon

The indications for resection versus transplantation of HCC remain controversial. Through technical improvements in both transplantation and resection, both fields continue to mature which contributes to the current lack of consensus. Adequate graft availability remains a practical constraint that also limits the availability of liver transplantation. Patients who have been treated for extrahepatic cancers are generally advised to successfully complete a disease-free surveillance period before undergoing liver transplantation for HCC, 5 years for solid malignancy or 2 years for a hematologic malignancy. Such waiting periods are not required prior to liver resection for HCC.

The universally accepted candidate for liver transplantation is a patient with poorly compensated cirrhosis or portal hypertension whose HCC tumor burden meets the Milan or University of California San Francisco (UCSF) criteria. The Milan criteria specify the presence of 1 tumor ≤5 cm or ≤3 tumors each ≤3 cm [28]. The UCSF criteria specify a single tumor ≤6.5 cm, a maximum of three total tumors ≤4.5 cm, and a cumulative tumor size ≤8 cm [29]. Including the transplant

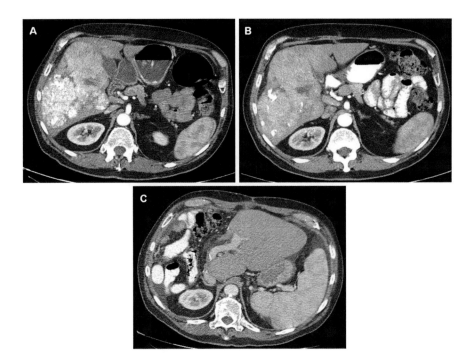

Fig. 6.1 A 70-year-old male with elevated transaminases is found to have HCC of the right liver and undergoes hepatic artery embolization (panel **a**). Due to abutment of the middle hepatic vein and an insufficient FLR, he underwent right portal vein embolization with hypertrophy to 32% of the total liver volume (panel **b**). The patient then underwent extended right hepatectomy (panel **c**)

surgeon in the multidisciplinary team can also help identify which patients will over the long term likely require liver transplantation. Select patients are then candidates for bridging procedures such as resection, TACE, or RFA which attempt to control the HCC until the point when the patient requires transplantation and a suitable graft is available.

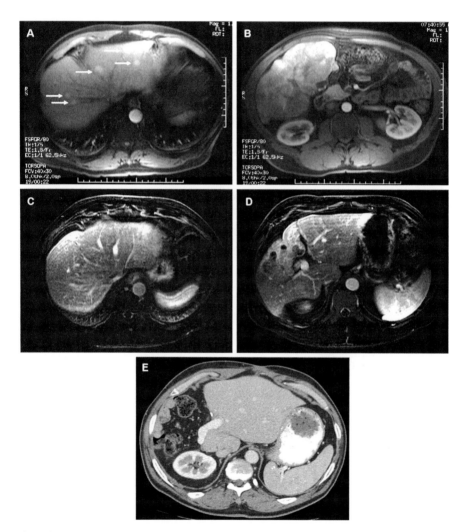

Fig. 6.2 A 54-year-old male presents with multiple bilateral liver nodules (panels **a** and **b**), initially deemed unresectable. Biopsy shows well-differentiated HCC. After five cycles of TACE, there was resolution of the nodules in the left liver (panel **c**), but persistent right-sided disease (panel **d**). Hepatic steatosis prompted right portal vein embolization with segment IV extension to induce hypertrophy of the FLR. The patient underwent extended right hepatectomy with common bile duct resection (panel **e**). He was alive without recurrence 3 years after the procedure

Hepatobiliary Surgeon

Together with the other members of the multidisciplinary team, an experienced hepatobiliary surgeon can help decide whether a patient's HCC is resectable. Innovations in surgical technique and perioperative care have expanded the inclusion criteria for which patients are offered curative resection. Impediments to *initial* resectability include poorly controlled cirrhosis, multiple medical comorbidities, metastatic deposits, insufficient future liver remnant, or overwhelming involvement of critical vascular or biliary structures. The multidisciplinary conference is the ideal forum in which to discuss these concerns and to develop the most oncologically appropriate treatment strategy. The following case presentations (Figs. 6.1 and 6.2) illustrate how the multidisciplinary team maximizes efficient, high-quality care for patients with HCC.

References

1. Zeuzem S, Feinman SV, Rasenack J et al (2000) Peginterferon alfa-2a in patients with chronic hepatitis C. N Engl J Med 343:1666–1672
2. Chronic Hepatitis C: Current Disease Management Hepatitis, vol. (2009) Bethesda: National Digestive Diseases Information Clearinghouse, 2006: NIH Publication No. 07–4230.
3. Dienstag JL (2008) Drug therapy: hepatitis B virus infection. N Engl J Med 359:1486–1500
4. Zhang BH, Yang BH, Tang ZY (2004) Randomized controlled trial of screening for hepatocellular carcinoma. J Cancer Res Clin Oncol 130:417–22
5. Bruix J, Sherman M (2005) Management of hepatocellular carcinoma. Hepatology 42: 1208–1236
6. Poon RTP, Fan ST (2003) Evaluation of the new AJCC/UICC staging system for hepatocellular carcinoma after hepatic resection in Chinese patients. Surg Oncol Clin N Am 12:35–50
7. Ramacciato G, Mercantini P, Cautero N et al (2005) Prognostic evaluation of the new American joint committee on cancer/international union against cancer staging system for hepatocellular carcinoma: Analysis of 112 cirrhotic patients resected for hepatocellular carcinoma. Ann Surg Oncol 12:289–297
8. Varotti G, Ramacciato G, Ercolani G et al (2005) Comparison between the fifth and sixth editions of the AJCC/UICC TNM staging systems for hepatocellular carcinoma: Multicentric study on 393 cirrhotic resected patients. Eur J Surg Oncol 31:760–767
9. Wu CC, Cheng SB, Ho WM et al (2005) Liver resection for hepatocellular carcinoma in patients with cirrhosis. Br J Surg 92:348–355
10. Lei HJ, Chau GY, Lui WY et al (2006) Prognostic value and clinical relevance of the 6th Edition 2002 American Joint Committee on Cancer staging system in patients with resectable hepatocellular carcinoma. J Am Coll Surg 203:426–435
11. Kee KM, Wang JH, Lee CM et al (2007) Validation of clinical AJCC/UICC TNM staging system for hepatocellular carcinoma: analysis of 5,613 cases from a medical center in southern Taiwan. Int J Cancer 120:2650–2655
12. Vauthey JN, Ribero D, Abdalla EK et al (2007) Outcomes of liver transplantation in 490 patients with hepatocellular carcinoma: validation of a uniform staging after surgical treatment. J Am Coll Surg 204:1016–1027
13. Pomfret EA, Washburn K, Wald C et al (2010) Report of a national conference on liver allocation in patients with hepatocellular carcinoma in the United States. Liver Transpl 16:262–278

14. Ariff B, Lloyd CR, Khan S et al (2009) Imaging of liver cancer. World J Gastroenterol 15:1289–1300
15. Ribero D, Abdalla EK, Madoff DC et al (2007) Portal vein embolization before major hepatectomy and its effects on regeneration, resectability and outcome. Br J Surg 94:1386–1394
16. Llovet JM, Chen Y, Wurmbach E et al (2006) A molecular signature to discriminate dysplastic nodules from early hepatocellular carcinoma in HCV cirrhosis. Gastroenterology 131:1758–1767
17. Wurmbach E, Chen Y-B, Khitrov G et al (2007) Genome-wide molecular profiles of HCV-induced dysplasia and hepatocellular carcinoma. Hepatology 45:938–947
18. Vauthey JN, Lauwers GY, Esnaola NF et al (2002) Simplified staging for hepatocellular carcinoma. J Clin Oncol 20:1527–1536
19. Hoshida Y, Villanueva A, Kobayashi M et al (2008) Gene expression in fixed tissues and outcome in hepatocellular carcinoma. N Engl J Med 359:1995–2004
20. Vauthey JN, Klimstra D, Franceschi D et al (1995) Factors affecting long-term outcome after hepatic resection for hepatocellular carcinoma. Am J Surg 169:28–34
21. Yeo W, Mok TS, Zee B et al (2005) A randomized phase III study of doxorubicin versus cisplatin/interferon {alpha}-2b/doxorubicin/fluorouracil (PIAF) combination chemotherapy for unresectable hepatocellular carcinoma. J Natl Cancer Inst 97:1532–1538
22. Llovet JM, Ricci S, Mazzaferro V et al (2008) Sorafenib in advanced hepatocellular carcinoma. N Engl J Med 359:378–390
23. Llovet JM, Bruix J (2008) Novel advancements in the management of hepatocellular carcinoma in 2008. J Hepatol 48(Suppl 1):S20–S37
24. Kishi Y, Madoff DC, Abdalla EK et al (2008) Is embolization of segment 4 portal veins before extended right hepatectomy justified? Surgery 144:744–751
25. Palavecino M, Chun YS, Madoff DC et al (2009) Major hepatic resection for hepatocellular carcinoma with or without portal vein embolization: perioperative outcome and survival. Surgery 145:399–405
26. Lencioni R, Cioni D (2007) Percutaneous methods for ablation of hepatic neoplasms. In: Blumgart L (ed) Surgery of the Liver, Biliary Tract, and Pancreas, 4th edn. Elsevier, New York, pp 1269–1277
27. Llovet JM, Bruix J (2003) Systematic review of randomized trials for unresectable hepatocellular carcinoma: chemoembolization improves survival. Hepatology 37:429–442
28. Mazzaferro V, Regalia E, Doci R et al (1996) Liver transplantation for the treatment of small hepatocellular carcinomas in patients with cirrhosis. N Engl J Med 334:693–699
29. Yao FY, Ferrell L, Bass NM et al (2001) Liver transplantation for hepatocellular carcinoma: expansion of the tumor size limits does not adversely impact survival. Hepatology 33:1394–403

Chapter 7
Evidence-Based Guidelines for Treatment of Hepatocellular Carcinoma in Japan

Kiyoshi Hasegawa and Norihiro Kokudo

Keywords Evidence-based medicine · Clinical practice guidelines · Randomized controlled trial · Treatment algorithm

Hepatocellular carcinoma (HCC) has five characteristics that are strikingly different from those of other malignant tumors of the digestive system: (1) a strong causal relationship with hepatitis viruses (especially type B and type C), (2) a major impact of the status of hepatic functional reserve and liver damage on the choice of treatment and the prognosis, (3) a high recurrence rate, with many of the recurrences developing within the liver, and the existence of two major routes of recurrence, i.e., multicentric carcinogenesis and intrahepatic metastasis, (4) the possibility of performing effective treatment, if confined to the liver and liver functional reserve permits, and (5) the existence of a clear outcome determinant as vascular invasion. Because of these characteristics, choosing the method of treatment for HCC is not easy, although several useful methods are available to treat HCC.

Three methods of treatment are currently recognized as effective against HCC: surgery, including liver resection and liver transplantation, percutaneous ablation therapy as represented by radiofrequency ablation (RFA) and percutaneous ethanol injection (PEI), and transcatheter arterial chemoembolization (TACE). Because almost all cases of HCC are associated with chronic liver damage in some degree, liver function conditions must be taken into consideration at the same time as tumor conditions when choosing treatment. Thus, treatment selection conditions are complicated. Especially, it is difficult to select surgery or percutaneous ablation therapy. Because studies that have evaluated the results of treatment scientifically have been inadequate, whenever it has been possible to select more than one method of treatment under certain tumor and liver function conditions, the choice has often ultimately depended on

N. Kokudo (✉)
Hepato-Biliary-Pancreatic Surgery Division, Department of Surgery, University of Tokyo, Hongo, Bunkyo-ku, Tokyo, Japan

K.M. McMasters, J.-N. Vauthey (eds.), *Hepatocellular Carcinoma*,
DOI 10.1007/978-1-60327-522-4_7, © Springer Science+Business Media, LLC 2011

the skill and convictions of the attending physician, customary practice at the institution, etc.

The Clinical Practice Guidelines for Hepatocellular Carcinoma published in 2005 [1] were devised to allow the attending physician and the patient to select evidence-based care as much as possible. The methods to construct the guidelines are described in detail elsewhere [2], and their main body can be read in English on the web site of the Japanese Society of Hepatology (http://www.jsh.or.jp/). The essential features of the guidelines have been summarized in two figures, one for a hepatocellular carcinoma surveillance algorithm and the other for a hepatocellular carcinoma treatment algorithm. At present, 4 years after their release, both algorithms have come into widespread use in clinical settings of Japan. Here we will focus on the hepatocellular carcinoma treatment algorithm and outline how treatment methods should be selected according to the algorithm.

Explanation of the Treatment Algorithm

As shown in Fig. 7.1 [1], the algorithm related to the treatment of HCC has been simplified based on three factors: degree of liver damage (Table 7.1) [3], number of tumors, and tumor diameter. The treatment methods that are recommended have been narrowed down to one or two, and the more highly recommended method

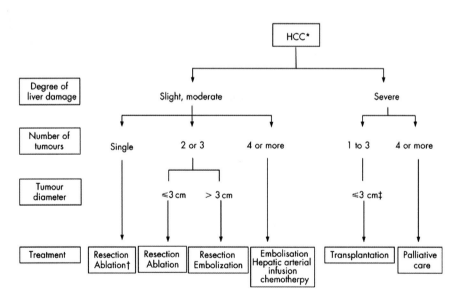

Fig. 7.1 Treatment algorithm for HCC (Reproduced with permission from [1]). *Presence of vascular invasion or extrahepatic metastasis to be indicated separately. †Selected when the severity of liver damage is class B and the tumor diameter is ≤2 cm. ††Tumor diameter ≤5 cm, when there is only one tumor

Table 7.1 Liver damage

Items	Liver damage		
	A	B	C
Ascites	None	Responsive	Unresponsive
Serum bilirubin (mg/dL)	<2.0	2.0–3.0	>3.0
Serum albumin (g/dL)	>3.5	3.0–3.5	<3.0
ICG R15 (%)	<15	15–40	>40
Prothrombin time (%)	>80	50–80	<50

If more than one item is applicable to the patient, the clinical stage with the worst degree of all involved items should be recorded. ICG R15, indocyanine green retention rate at 15 min
Reproduced with permission from [3]

is printed above. Since including the treatment of advanced cases associated with extrahepatic lesions and portal vein tumor thrombus into the algorithm would have made it too complicated, it has been omitted and will be described in other part of the guidelines [1]. There have been very few evidences for effective treatments in those subgroups of patients.

Selection of the Three Important Factors for the Algorithm

Degree of liver damage is similar to Child–Pugh class except the inclusion of ICG test. Although several Japanese hepatologists have asserted that Child–Pugh class should be chosen as a determinant of the treatment algorithm, degree of liver damage is selected, because ICG test is indispensible to decide a surgical indication and an operative procedure for HCC in Japan [4]. ICG test enables a liver surgeon to more accurately evaluate liver function of a HCC carrying patient, i.e., in a case with Child–Pugh A class cirrhosis, liver resection is never selected, if a result of ICG test indicates poor liver function. On the other hand, in the BCLC and AASLD guidelines [5, 6], presence or absence of portal hypertension is a key factor for decision making in the treatment of HCC. However, a recent report from Japan showed that patients with portal hypertension or multiple tumors may have survival benefit by liver resection although their outcomes are inferior to that of patients without portal hypertension or with single tumors [7]. Thus, we regard degree of liver damage including ICG test as more important than presence or absence of portal hypertension.

Number of tumors and tumor diameter are also chosen as determinants of the treatment algorithm. Vascular invasion would be the strongest prognostic factor as have been suggested in many previous reports; however, its presence or absence is difficult to be accurately assumed by the currently available diagnostic modalities before treatments. To the contrary, number of tumors and tumor diameter have much advantage in that they can be easily known and have been included to other staging systems [5, 6, 8]. Thus, both are included in the treatment algorithm, but not vascular invasion.

Degree of Liver Damage A and B

When the degree of liver damage is A and B, liver function is good, and there is only a solitary liver tumor, as a rule liver resection is the treatment of first choice regardless of tumor diameter. The basis for this recommendation is that when the long-term results of liver resection and PEI were compared using data from a nation-wide follow-up study by the Liver Cancer Study Group of Japan, they showed that liver resection was significantly superior to PEI in several conditions [9]. However, because there were no differences in the results of liver resection and PEI when the degree of liver damage was B and the tumor was solitary and no more than 2 cm in diameter, percutaneous ablation therapy is also recommended. Although not stated in the algorithm, because realistically it is difficult to treat tumors greater than 3 cm in diameter curatively by percutaneous ablation treatment methods (including RFA), liver resection is the sole recommended method of treatment.

When there are two or three tumors and their diameters do not exceed 3 cm, liver resection or percutaneous ablation treatment is recommended. When tumor diameter exceeds 3 cm, it is beyond percutaneous ablation treatment, and TACE is recommended instead. The results of a randomized controlled trial (RCT) by Llovet et al. that showed the efficacy of TACE are the basis for this recommendation [10].

When there are four or more tumors, TACE or hepatic arterial infusion therapy is recommended. There is no convincing evidence for hepatic arterial infusion therapy, and it has a recommendation degree of C1 (it is acceptable to consider performing it, but there is no scientific basis for it). Nevertheless, in view of the fact that it has been widely adopted in Japan and new treatment methods, such as combination with interferon, are anticipated, it has become the second recommendation.

Degree of Liver Damage C

Because liver function is poor in degree of liver damage C, treatment by any other means than liver transplantation, which can be expected to restore normal liver function as well as treat the HCC, is dangerous. The Milan criteria, which are the most widely recognized criteria worldwide, have been adopted as indications for liver transplantation. More specifically, liver transplantation is recommended if the HCC is solitary and no larger than 5 cm or if there are no more than three tumors and each tumor is no larger than 3 cm. Because of the high risk of recurrence after liver transplantation and the high risk of liver failure when other methods of treatment are used, none of them are recommended when there are four or more tumors, and best supporting care should be considered.

Advanced Cancer

Advanced HCC, in which there is extrahepatic metastasis or portal vein tumor thrombus, is not included in the algorithm. It has a poor prognosis, and no treatment that can be recommended has ever been established. Nevertheless, since there is a report that an improvement in outcome can be expected by combined use of TACE and liver resection [11], if liver function is good, "Liver resection is sometimes selected in cases with degree A liver damage" has been stated separately. Chemotherapy is often considered when there is extrahepatic metastasis, but since no anticancer drugs had been demonstrated to be effective against HCC at the time the guidelines were drawn up, the guidelines only state, "Chemotherapy is sometimes selected in cases with degree of liver damage A."

How to Use the Algorithm

The algorithm has been prepared by envisioning a scenario in which the attending physician selects the method of treatment while presenting it to the patient and discussing it in a clinical setting. In the Hepato-Biliary-Pancreatic Surgery Division of the University of Tokyo Hospital, an explanation in which the algorithm is presented is routinely provided both at the time of the initial examination (outpatient clinic) and before surgery (after hospital admission). According to the results of a questionnaire survey, the explanation has generally been favorably evaluated as easy to understand.

Nevertheless, it must be borne in mind that treatment methods that do not conform to the algorithm can be devised in individual cases. Since the evidence was compiled and generalized at the time the algorithm was drawn up, naturally it sometimes may not apply because of differences in a variety of conditions. These types of clinical practice guidelines are generally said to apply to 60–95% of all cases [12]. There is no problem per se with adding judgments based on physicians' experience or trials of the most advanced treatment methods. However, when recommending a method of treatment that differs from the guidelines to a patient, it would seem necessary to thoroughly explain at least two points to the patient, i.e., that the treatment differs from the recommendation in the guidelines and the reason for venturing to propose a different treatment, and then to obtain the patient's consent.

Evaluation of the Algorithm

A questionnaire survey regarding the guidelines was conducted in March 2006, approximately 1 year after they were published [13]. Survey sheets were distributed to 2,279 members of the Liver Cancer Study Group of Japan, and replies were obtained from 843 (37%) of them. Of those who replied, 55.4% were hepatologists and 38% were liver surgeons, and more than 70% of those who replied were practicing at institutions that were also engaged in education, such as university hospitals. The same questionnaire was sent to 689 general internists responsible for primary care in Osaka Prefecture and Hyogo Prefecture, and replies were received from 332 (48.2%) of them. First, 71.9% of the hepatologists, 75.6% of the liver surgeons, and 61% of the general internists knew about the guidelines. Both the hepatologists and the liver surgeons often referred to medical journals, the literature, guidelines, and the opinions of their colleagues in regard to clinical problems related to HCC, whereas the general internists tended to attach greater importance to the opinions of specialists or their colleagues (Fig. 7.2a) [13]. Although 19–21% of the hepatologists and liver surgeons changed their clinical practice patterns as a result of the release of the guidelines, 50–52% had not changed them at all. It was learned that 43% of the general internists followed the recommendations of the guidelines and had changed their clinical practice patterns (Fig. 7.2b) [13]. The results of the questionnaire survey showed that 1 year after the guidelines were released, they had reached both specialists and general practitioners, and that they were being used to decide on clinical practice policy as originally intended.

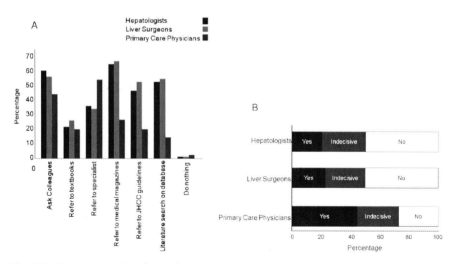

Fig. 7.2 From the results of questionnaire surveys about the treatment algorithm for HCC (Reproduced with permission from [1], cited from [13]). (**a**) What are your possible actions when you have clinical questions or problems in regard to the management of patients with hepatocellular carcinoma (HCC)? (a multiple-choice question). (**b**) Have you changed your practice pattern for HCC after reading the JHCC guidelines? (Responders who did not acknowledge the guidelines were excluded)

Revisions of the Guidelines Based on the Latest Knowledge

There have been remarkable advances in the management of HCC recently, and the content of parts of the 2005 version of the guidelines, which was based on the literature as of 2002, has become outdated. The work of adding new knowledge and evidence discovered in the period 2003–2007 and revising them is currently under way at present.

The widespread adoption of RFA would seem to be the greatest change that can contribute to the treatment algorithm since 2003. RFA enables reliable treatment of a larger area via a single puncture and was introduced in Japan around 1999. Since then it has been widely adopted and becoming covered by Japanese national health insurance in April 2004 provided an added boost, so that now it can be said to have replaced PEI. Moreover, the results of RCTs comparing RFA and PEI have been published [14, 15], and the superiority of RFA over PEI appears to have been established as evidence level Ib. Accordingly, not only the answers to the research question group related to percutaneous ablation treatment cited in the 2005 version but the research questions themselves may become the targets of revision.

Evaluation of the efficacy of treatment by liver resection and percutaneous ablation treatment has also had an impact on the widespread adoption of RFA. The 2005 version of the treatment algorithm is based on the results of treatment by liver resection and PEI, but now that the superiority of RFA over PEI has been established, a comparison between liver resection and percutaneous ablation treatment should be performed based on the results of RFA. The results of two RCTs in 2005–2006 have been reported [16, 17], and both of them concluded that the results of liver resection and percutaneous ablation treatment were equivalent. However, there were major problems with both of them, including in their design, and neither of them could be regarded as providing adequate evidence [18]. A paper comparing the outcome of liver resection, RFA, and PEI based on a nationwide follow-up survey by the Liver Cancer Study Group of Japan has recently been published [19]. Although the results showed that liver resection was significantly better in cases of recurrence, the differences in survival were not significant; however, the short follow-up period was a problem. The conduct of a high-quality RCT that is able to rigorously evaluate the outcome of RFA and liver resection is awaited in the future.

The recommendations of the Japanese guideline about liver transplantation are based on the results of deceased liver transplantation outside Japan. There is a rapid increase in the number of living-donor liver transplantations for HCC in Japan since 1999 [20]. Thus, the recommendations should be amended in an algorithm that reflects their results.

Moreover, the results of an RCT that showed the efficacy of a multikinase inhibitor (Sorafenib) against advanced HCC were reported in 2008 [21]. Since there has never been a drug whose efficacy against HCC was demonstrated by a statistically significant difference in as sufficient a number of cases as in this study, it generated considerable interest.

Conclusion

Because many effective methods are available to treat HCC and the balance between tumor status and liver function status must be taken into consideration, the judgment of skilled specialists is required to make the choice of treatment. On the other hand, the principle of treatment selection based on the hopes and preferences of patients, socioeconomic circumstances, etc., is also important. The treatment algorithm of the Japanese guideline extracts evidence at and above a certain level and reflects it, and it is useful for explaining the complex decision-making process to patients in a way that is easy to comprehend, and for obtaining their understanding in clinical settings, where time is limited.

References

1. Makuuchi M, Kokudo N (2006) Clinical practice guidelines for hepatocellular carcinoma: the first evidence based guidelines from Japan. World J Gastroenterol 12:828–829
2. Makuuchi M, Kokudo N, Arii S et al (2008) Development of evidence-based clinical guidelines for the diagnosis and treatment of hepatocellular carcinoma in Japan. Hepatol Res 38:37–51
3. Liver Cancer Study Group of Japan (1997) Classification of primary liver cancer. Kanehara & Co., Ltd., Tokyo p. 21
4. Makuuchi M, Kosuge T, Takayama T et al (1993) Surgery for small liver cancers. Semin Surg Oncol 9:298–304
5. Llovet JM, Brú C, Bruix J (1999) Prognosis of hepatocellular carcinoma: the BCLC staging classification. Semin Liver Dis 19:329–338
6. Bruix J, Sherman M (2005) Management of hepatocellular carcinoma. Hepatology 42:1208–1236
7. Ishizawa T, Hasegawa K, Aoki T et al (2008) Multiple tumors and concomitant portal hypertension are not operative contraindications for hepatocellular carcinoma. Gastroenterology 134:1908–1916
8. Vauthey JN, Lauwers GY, Esnaola NF et al (2002) Simplified staging for hepatocellular carcinoma. J Clin Oncol 20:1527–1536
9. Arii S, Yamaoka Y, Futagawa S et al (2000) Results of surgical and nonsurgical treatment for small-sized hepatocellular carcinomas: a retrospective and nationwide survey in Japan. Hepatology 32:1224–1229
10. Llovet JM, Real MI, Montaña X et al (2002) Arterial embolisation or chemoembolisation versus symptomatic treatment in patients with unresectable hepatocellular carcinoma: a randomized controlled trial. Lancet 359:1734–1739
11. Minagawa M, Makuuchi M, Takayama T et al (2001) Selection criteria for hepatectomy in patients with hepatocellular carcinoma and portal vein tumor thrombus. Ann Surg 233:379–384
12. Eddy DM (1990) Clinical decision making: from theory to practice. Designing a practice policy. Standards, guidelines, and options. JAMA 263:3077, 3081, 3084
13. Kokudo N, Sasaki Y, Nakayama T et al (2007) Dissemination of evidence-based clinical practice guidelines for hepatocellular carcinoma among Japanese hepatologists, liver surgeons, and primary care physicians. Gut 56:1020–1021
14. Lencioni RA, Allgaier HP, Cioni D et al (2003) Small hepatocellular carcinoma in cirrhosis: randomized comparison of radio-frequency thermal ablation versus percutaneous ethanol injection. Radiology 228:235–240

15. Shiina S, Teratani T, Obi S et al (2005) A randomized controlled trial of radiofrequency abla-
    tion with ethanol injection for small hepatocellular carcinoma. Gastroenterology 129:122–130
16. Huang GT, Lee PH, Tsang YM et al (2005) Percutaneous ethanol injection versus surgical
    resection for the treatment of small hepatocellular carcinoma: a prospective study. Ann Surg
    242:36–42
17. Chen MS, Li JQ, Zheng Y et al (2006) A prospective randomized trial comparing percuta-
    neous local ablative therapy and partial hepatectomy for hepatocellular carcinoma. Ann Surg
    243:321–328
18. Hasegawa K, Kokudo N, Makuuchi M (2008) Surgery or ablation for hepatocellular carci-
    noma? Ann Surg 247:557–558
19. Hasegawa K, Makuuchi M, Takayama T, et al. for the Liver Cancer Study Group of
    Japan (2008) Surgical resection vs. percutaneous ablation for hepatocellular carcinoma: a
    preliminary report of the Japanese nationwide survey. J Hepatol 49:589–594
20. Todo S, Furukawa H, Tada M; Japanese Liver Transplantation Study Group (2007) Extending
    indication: role of living donor liver transplantation for hepatocellular carcinoma. Liver
    Transpl 13(11 Suppl 2): S48–S54
21. Llovet JM, Ricci S, Mazzaferro V, et al. for SHARP Investigators Study Group (2008)
    Sorafenib in advanced hepatocellular carcinoma. N Engl J Med 359:378–390

Chapter 8
Hepatocellular Carcinoma Arising in the Non-viral, Non-alcoholic Liver

Charles E. Woodall, Robert C.G. Martin, Kelly M. McMasters, and Charles R. Scoggins

Keywords HCC risk factors · HCC in the non-fibrotic liver · Non-cirrhotic hepatoma · Fibrolamellar carcinoma (FLC) · Hereditary hemochromatosis (HH) · Non-alcoholic fatty liver disease (NAFLD)

Hepatocellular carcinoma is one of the five most common cancers worldwide and is one of the top three in regard to annual mortality. Greater than 80% occur in either sub-Saharan Africa or East Asia, and most of these cases are attributed to viral hepatitis. Increased public awareness and educational campaigns have led to decreasing incidences in these endemic areas. However, the rate of HCC in a number of areas with traditionally low rates of viral hepatitis, including Australia, the United States, Canada, and the United Kingdom, has increased significantly. This rising incidence cannot be easily explained by changes in immigration, hepatitis C virus, or ethanol.

Risk Factors for Hepatocellular Carcinoma

It is widely known that chronic hepatitis B and C virus infection remains the most dominant risk factor in HCC incidence. Other well-known hepatocellular carcinoma risk factors include alcoholic cirrhosis and carcinogen exposure. The universal belief has always been that cirrhosis precedes the development of HCC, even in the United States where continued reports state that approximately 95% of HCC arises in the background of cirrhosis [1]. Indeed, most cases of HCC occur in the setting of cirrhosis, thus impacting the treatment modalities available.

However, some cases of HCC arise in a normal liver in patients with no history of alcoholism and negative viral serologies. A certain proportion of these cases are

R.C.G. Martin (✉)
Division of Surgical Oncology, Department of Surgery, University of Louisville School of Medicine, Louisville, KY, USA

K.M. McMasters, J.-N. Vauthey (eds.), *Hepatocellular Carcinoma*,
DOI 10.1007/978-1-60327-522-4_8, © Springer Science+Business Media, LLC 2011

associated with rare etiologies such as non-alcoholic fatty liver disease, hemochromatosis, aflatoxin exposure, or variant subtypes of hepatoma not associated with cirrhosis. Recently, epidemiologic research has generated data demonstrating the emergence of HCC in the absence of underlying liver disease. These data may partially explain why there has been a two-fold increase in the age-adjusted incident rate of HCC in the United States between 1985 and 2002 [2]. This incidence has caused an increase of 1.3 per 100,000 during 1978–1980 to 3.3 per 100,000 during 1999–2001 [3]. Interestingly, the largest increase during this period has occurred in Caucasians (including Hispanics) while the lowest increase has been within the Asian population. More recent reports have demonstrated that as many as 40% of the HCC diagnosed in the United States is of unknown cause (i.e., no alcohol, hepatitis, or cirrhosis) [3] (Fig. 8.1).

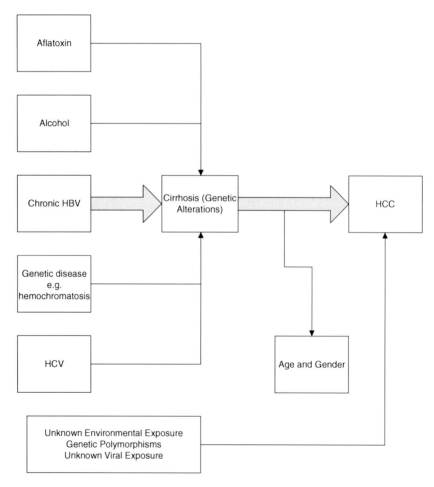

Fig. 8.1 Potential causes of non-cirrhotic hepatocellular cancer

HCC in the Non-fibrotic Liver

The etiology of HCC in patients without chronic hepatitis infection or chronic cirrhosis from other causes remains unclear. To date, because of the overwhelming data demonstrating that most cases of HCC arise in the cirrhotic liver (either associated with viral hepatitis or alcohol-related damage), there has been little attention on the increasing incidence of HCC in patients who lack fibrosis. Recent data from centers in the central United States have shed some light onto the rising incidence of HCC in the absence of fibrosis. It is quite possible that national increase in the incidence of HCC reflects similar increases in HCC among patients without hepatitis or cirrhosis in other regions [4]. Why some patients with apparently normal liver tissue would develop HCC is poorly understood.

One reason for the increased incidence of HCC may be related to changes in the diagnostic criteria used in epidemiologic databases. In the 1970s and early 1980s, the SEER database only recorded histologically confirmed cases of HCC. While this is highly specific, it may underestimate the true incidence of HCC. The average yearly age-adjusted incidence rates of all HCC captured by the SEER database irrespective of the method of diagnosis have increased approximately 30%. Because the diagnosis of HCC now can occur without histologic confirmation, based on the presence of underlying cirrhosis, nodular mass seen CT or MRI, and an elevated AFP level, the corresponding increased incidence in the SEER database may be partially related to these changes in diagnostic criteria.

Similarly, with the rapid rise in hepatic resections now being performed at all age groups, some patients who were initially diagnosed and treated for cancer of unknown primary are now being appropriately being diagnosed as having HCC. Perhaps the true incidence of HCC is not rising as quickly as previously described; instead, there might be some shift in the diagnosis, with the incidence of carcinoma of unknown primary decreasing as our ability to appropriately diagnose these patients as having either HCC or intrahepatic cholangiocarcinoma improves. A more liberal policy of resection in appropriate patients who were initially diagnosed as unknown primary cancers has led to more precise diagnoses, some of which are HCC. This type of policy may also contribute to the higher regional incidence of the non-cirrhotic hepatoma [4].

Other potential etiologies for the increasing incidence of the non-cirrhotic hepatoma may include the ever-increasing age of the US population. The elderly (defined as people aged 65 years or older) will account for over 61% of all new cancer cases and 70% of all annual cancer deaths [5]. It has been recently estimated that the elderly patient population has 11 times the cancer risk of people under the age of 65 years. It has also been estimated that in 2030 approximately 20% of the US population will be older than 65 years of age [6]. These changes alone coupled with environmental exposure and potential genetic effects along with other potential causes are the reason for these rising incidence rates.

This reasoning is further solidified by the significant differences in the clinical, radiologic, and pathologic features of the patients with non-cirrhotic hepatoma (Table 8.1) when compared to the common cirrhotic patient with HCC (Fig. 8.2).

Table 8.1 Features of the non-cirrhotic hepatoma

Patient	– Advanced age
	– Higher incidence of women
	– Non-alcohol related
	– Generally tolerate major hepatectomy well
Liver	– No fibrosis
	– Large, solitary tumor
Serum	– Low to normal AFP level
	– Absence of evidence for viral hepatitis
	– Preserved hepatic synthetic function

AFP, alpha fetoprotein

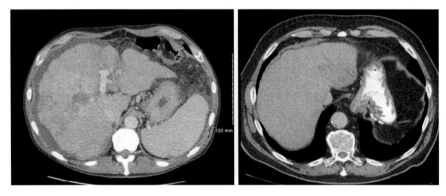

Fig. 8.2 Radiologic presentation of a cirrhotic HCC (*left*) with shrunken liver, ascites, and invasive lesion and non-cirrhotic HCC (*right*) with normal size liver, sharp liver borders, and non-evidence of nodularity

The non-cirrhotic hepatoma patients are significantly older, more commonly female, less often smokers, have a greater incidence of a normal alpha-fetoprotein level, larger sized tumors, and a smaller number of tumors (most commonly a single liver tumor). These more favorable features have led to an ability to be more surgically aggressive in these patients because of their underlying normal hepatic parenchyma. This variant histology responds well to aggressive surgical resection with a lower risk for hepatic failure postoperatively [4].

In a review of Kentucky's patients with HCC, we have seen a fourfold increase in age-specific HCC diagnosis, with the most rapid increase seen in the 60- to 69-year-old age group. We also have frequently observed the phenomenon in older patients, without hepatitis or cirrhosis, who have large solitary tumors and normal AFP levels. We have described these as "Kentucky hepatomas" because of the unique disease presentation that differs from most other regions with a greater endemic hepatitis population. In the University of Louisville database of hepatobiliary cancer, 60% of HCC patients were without hepatitis or cirrhosis (Fig. 8.3). These non-cirrhotic, hepatitis-free patients were found to be significantly older (70 vs. 55 years; $P = 0.001$), to be more often female (40.3 vs. 24.4%; $P = 0.01$), to have a larger tumor size (6.5 vs. 3.9 cm; $P = 0.004$), to have fewer liver lesions (median 1 vs. 3; $P = 0.22$), and to more frequently undergo surgical therapy (75.6 vs. 53.8%; $P = 0.01$) than the patients with cirrhosis or hepatitis. Furthermore, the non-cirrhotic,

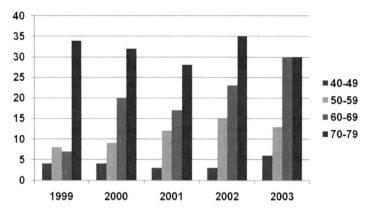

Fig. 8.3 Age-specific increase in incidence of HCC in the state of Kentucky. Y-axis is percent of patients in each of the age groups specified

non-hepatitis patients had a median AFP level of 16 vs. 320 in the group with hepatitis or cirrhosis ($P = 0.02$). We found that there was a similar increase in HCC incidence across all 5 regions of Kentucky. Whether this phenomenon is specific to Kentucky (and other regions of the Midwest) is not known; however, others have seen a similar rise in HCC without cirrhosis.

In a comparison of other studies that have presented the incidence of this variant non-cirrhotic HCC, the data from the University of Louisville demonstrate the single largest incidence rate. A recent report from Reichman demonstrated an incidence of 26%; however, it also noted a worse overall survival when compared to the cirrhotic population [7]. Similar high incidence (31%) was reported from Fong et al., without a difference in overall survival [8]. Both of these reports were from the United States, in New Jersey and New York, which has a higher incidence of Asian immigrants and thus probable higher incidence of hepatitis. Other reports have detailed the incidence of this variant HCC in Europe and Asia [9–11] to be much lower, most likely due to etiologic influences.

Fibrolamellar Carcinoma

Fibrolamellar carcinoma (FLC) was first described by Edmonson in 1956 [12]. It is a rare hepatic malignancy, comprising less than 1% of primary liver malignancies in a US population-based study [13]. The histologic appearance of FLC is distinctive, consisting of deeply eosinophilic malignant hepatocytes surrounded by thick fibrous bands arranged in a lamellar-like fashion [14]. Radiographically, the tumors are hyper-vascular and tend to be large, be calcified, and have a central scar [15], all distinct differences from conventional HCC (Table 8.2). Many consider it a variant of HCC, though the epidemiology, clinicopathologic factors, and prognosis differ widely from HCC.

FLC is largely tumors of youth and young adulthood. The median age of patients with FLC is on the order of 25 years [16–18], far younger than conventional HCC.

Table 8.2 Differences between fibrolamellar carcinoma and traditional HCC

Fibrolamellar		Traditional HCC	
Patient related	Young age	Patient related	Older age
	Lack fibrosis		Cirrhotic
	Better survival		Worse survival
Tumor related	Central scar	Tumor related	No scar
	Typically solitary		Often multifocal
	Higher resection rate		Lower resection rate

FLC is not associated with an underlying history of cirrhosis [19–21], and this fact may account for the differences in age distribution, given that a background of fibrosis is not common in younger populations. There also does not appear to be any connection with viral hepatitis, ethanol, or estrogen use, all factors commonly considered in association with conventional HCC [19].

There are conflicting data comparing the survival of patients with FLC with traditional HCC. Some authors have reported no survival benefit for FLC patients who have undergone resection (when compared to traditional HCC), although the number of cases was too small to draw firm conclusions [22]. These data are similar to that published by others, although the rate of resectability for patients with FLC might be higher [23]. In contrast to these data are reports demonstrating an improved survival for patients with FLC, including one report of a 56% 5-year survival for resected patients [24]. Further data suggesting a more favorable biologic behavior for FLC include high resectability rates and improved survival following resection [17, 19, 20, 23].

Like traditional HCC, FLC is prone to recurrence following resection. The most common site for recurrence appears to be in the liver remnant. Unlike traditional HCC, however, recurrent FLC might fare better following recurrence. Data demonstrate that patients with recurrent FLC survive longer than those patients with recurrent traditional HCC [25, 26]. Furthermore, patients with recurrent FLC might be amenable to re-resection, with data demonstrating a survival advantage to this aggressive approach [27]. FLC might have a higher risk for nodal metastasis upon presentation, and the rate of metastatic lymph nodes has been reported to be as high as 30% [28]. This raises the question of the role of routine portal lymphadenectomy at the time of initial hepatectomy.

Hereditary Hemochromatosis

Hereditary hemochromatosis (HH) is an autosomal recessive syndrome of iron overload. It is characterized by increased absorption of iron in the intestines with deposition in organs such as the heart, skin, pancreas, pituitary, and liver [29]. It is an under-recognized congenital condition caused by missense mutations at the HFE gene; some authors report HH is 10 times more common than cystic fibrosis [30], approximately 5 of 1000 patients of northern European descent having homozygosity for the *C282Y* mutation [31]. The end-stage results of HH-induced iron overload are diabetes, cirrhosis, and HCC, which are responsible for a reduced life expectancy from HH [32].

Patients with HH have a 20- to 200-fold increased risk of developing HCC [33–35]; in fact, primary liver carcinomas can account for up to 45% of deaths in HH patients [36]. Histologically, the overwhelming majority of these tumors are HCC and most occur in patients in their sixties. In a prospective longitudinal cohort study from Italy published in 2001, all cases of HCC in patients developed in those with cirrhotic livers [37]. However, there are approximately 10 case reports in the literature of HCC in patients (all male, all between 50 and 70 years of age) with HH and non-cirrhotic livers [38–40]. Vigilance in this group is warranted, as increased iron deposition alone may be a risk factor for development of HCC in the non-cirrhotic setting.

Aflatoxin

Aflatoxin B1 (AFB1) is a toxin produced by a fungus of the genus *Aspergillus.* It is found in Asia and sub-Saharan Africa where climate and food storage techniques allow the fungus to be a common contaminant of foods, especially grains, and release its toxin which is then ingested. As discussed previously, these endemic areas have high incidences of not only HCC but also viral hepatitis, specifically hepatitis B [41]. Therefore, aflatoxin may be more likely a potentiator of HCC rather than a director cause.

Non-alcoholic Fatty Liver Disease

Non-alcoholic fatty liver disease (NAFLD) is a spectrum of liver disease ranging from benign fatty infiltration of the liver to fulminate hepatic failure secondary to cirrhosis from non-alcoholic steatohepatitis (NASH). NASH, first described in 1980 [42], is defined by the histologic presence of findings associated with alcoholic liver disease in the absence of a history of alcohol consumption. The prevalence of NASH has been reported to be as high as 2% of the general population [43], making this one of the most common causes of non-viral liver disease. It is associated with obesity and diabetes mellitus and likely represents the hepatic manifestations of the metabolic syndrome.

Despite the prevalence of underlying liver disease, NASH-associated HCC has been rarely reported in the literature [44–46] beyond case reports. The connection can be difficult to establish because of regression of steatosis, inflammation, ballooning degeneration, and Mallory bodies is common once cirrhosis appears, and some HCCs in NASH patients occur in non-cirrhotic livers. There is no gender predominance in the literature; most cases occur in patients in their seventh decade.

Prospective studies linking NASH and HCC have been undertaken. They are limited by small numbers, highly selected subjects, and short-term follow-up [47]. The prodrome from the progression of fatty liver to NASH-associated cirrhosis can be quite pronounced, with estimates ranging from 10 to 16 years. As undiagnosed HCC may be somewhat indolent initially, it may be years after the onset of cirrhosis that a malignancy is diagnosed. Therefore, two decades of follow-up may be required to fully establish the relationship and true incidence.

References

1. Botha JF, Langnas AN (2006) Liver transplantation for hepatocellular carcinoma: an update. J Natl Compr Canc Netw 4:762–767.
2. El Serag HB, Davila JA, Petersen NJ et al (2003) The continuing increase in the incidence of hepatocellular carcinoma in the United States: an update. Ann Intern Med 139:817–823
3. Davila JA, Morgan RO, Shaib Y et al (2004) Hepatitis C infection and the increasing incidence of hepatocellular carcinoma: a population-based study. Gastroenterology 127:1372–1380
4. Martin RC, Loehle J, Scoggins CR et al (2007) Kentucky hepatoma: epidemiologic variant or same problem in a different region? Arch Surg 142:431–436.
5. Yancik R, Ries LA (2000) Aging and cancer in America. Demographic and epidemiologic perspectives. Hematol Oncol Clin North Am 14:17–23.
6. Muss HB (2001) Older age–not a barrier to cancer treatment. N Engl J Med 345:1127–1128
7. Reichman TW, Bahramipour P, Barone A et al (2005) Hepatitis status, child-pugh classification, and serum AFP levels predict survival in patients treated with transarterial embolization for unresectable hepatocellular carcinoma. J Gastrointest Surg 9 ;638–645
8. Fong Y, Sun RL, Jarnagin W et al (1999) An analysis of 412 cases of hepatocellular carcinoma at a Western center. Ann Surg 229 :790–799
9. Figueras J, Ramos E, Ibanez L et al (1999) Surgical treatment of hepatocellular carcinoma in cirrhotic and noncirrhotic patients. Transplant Proc 31:2455–2456
10. Torzilli G, Makuuchi M, Inoue K et al (1999) No-mortality liver resection for hepatocellular carcinoma in cirrhotic and noncirrhotic patients: is there a way? A prospective analysis of our approach. Arch Surg 134:984–992
11. Tsukioka G, Kakizaki S, Sohara N et al (2006) Hepatocellular carcinoma in extremely elderly patients: an analysis of clinical characteristics, prognosis and patient survival. World J Gastroenterol 12:48–53
12. Edmonson H (1956) Differential diagnosis of tumors and tumor-like lesion of liver in infancy and childhood. AMA J Dis Child 91:168–186
13. El-Serag HB, Davila JA (2004) Is fibrolamellar carcinoma different from hepatocellular carcinoma? A US population-based study. Hepatology 39:798–803
14. Craig JR, Peters RL, Edmondson HA et al (1980) Fibrolamellar carcinoma of the liver: a tumor of adolescents and young adults with distinctive clinico-pathologic features. Cancer 46:372–379
15. Ichikawa T, Federle MP, Grazioli L et al (1999) Fibrolamellar hepatocellular carcinoma: imaging and pathologic findings in 31 recent cases. Radiology 213:352–361
16. Pinna AD, Iwatsuki S, Lee RG et al (1997) Treatment of fibrolamellar hepatoma with subtotal hepatectomy or transplantation. Hepatology 26:877–883
17. Stipa F, Yoon SS, Liau KH et al (2006) Outcome of patients with fibrolamellar hepatocellular carcinoma. Cancer 106:1331–1338
18. Moreno-Luna LE, Arrieta O, Garcia-Leiva J et al (2005) Clinical and pathologic factors associated with survival in young adult patients with fibrolamellar hepatocarcinoma. BMC Cancer 5:142.

19. Okuda K (2002) Natural history of hepatocellular carcinoma including fibrolamellar and hepato-cholangiocarcinoma variants. J Gastroenterol Hepatol 17:401–405.
20. Hemming AW, Langer B, Sheiner P et al (1997) Aggressive surgical management of fibrolamellar hepatocellular carcinoma. J Gastrointest Surg 1:342–346
21. Patt YZ, Hassan MM, Lozano RD et al (2003) Phase II trial of systemic continuous fluorouracil and subcutaneous recombinant interferon Alfa-2b for treatment of hepatocellular carcinoma. J Clin Oncol 21:421–427
22. Vauthey JN, Klimstra D, Franceschi D et al (1995) Factors affecting long-term outcome after hepatic resection for hepatocellular carcinoma. Am J Surg 169:28–34.
23. Nagorney DM, Adson MA, Weiland LH et al (1985) Fibrolamellar hepatoma. Am J Surg 149:113–119
24. Soreide O, Czerniak A, Bradpiece H et al (1986) Characteristics of fibrolamellar hepatocellular carcinoma. A study of nine cases and a review of the literature. Am J Surg 151:518–523
25. Schlitt HJ, Ringe B, Rodeck B et al (1992) Bone marrow dysfunction after liver transplantation for fulminant non-A, non-B hepatitis. High risk for young patients. Transplantation 54:936–937
26. Busuttil RW, Farmer DG (1996) The surgical treatment of primary hepatobiliary malignancy. Liver Transpl Surg 2:114–130
27. Ichikawa T, Federle MP, Grazioli L et al (2000) Hepatocellular adenoma: multiphasic CT and histopathologic findings in 25 patients. Radiology 214:861–868
28. El-Gazzaz G, Wong W, El-Hadary MK et al (2000) Outcome of liver resection and transplantation for fibrolamellar hepatocellular carcinoma. Transpl Int 13(Suppl 1):S406–S409
29. Kohler HH, Hohler T, Kusel U et al (1999) Hepatocellular carcinoma in a patient with hereditary hemochromatosis and noncirrhotic liver. A case report. Pathol Res Pract 195:509–513
30. Merryweather-Clarke AT, Pointon JJ, Shearman JD et al. (1997) Global prevalence of putative haemochromatosis mutations. J Med Genet 34:275–278
31. Pietrangelo A (2004) Hereditary hemochromatosis–a new look at an old disease. N Engl J Med 350:2383–2397
32. Niederau C, Fischer R, Purschel A et al (1996) Long-term survival in patients with hereditary hemochromatosis. Gastroenterology 110:1107–1119
33. Niederau C, Fischer R, Sonnenberg A et al (1985) Survival and causes of death in cirrhotic and in noncirrhotic patients with primary hemochromatosis. N Engl J Med 313:1256–1262
34. Elmberg M, Hultcrantz R, Ekbom A et al (2003) Cancer risk in patients with hereditary hemochromatosis and in their first-degree relatives. Gastroenterology 125:1733–1741.
35. Hsing AW, McLaughlin JK, Olsen JH et al (1995) Cancer risk following primary hemochromatosis: a population-based cohort study in Denmark. Int J Cancer 60:160–162
36. Fargion S, Mandelli C, Piperno A et al (1992) Survival and prognostic factors in 212 Italian patients with genetic hemochromatosis. Hepatology 15:655–659
37. Fracanzani AL, Conte D, Fraquelli M et al (2001) Increased cancer risk in a cohort of 230 patients with hereditary hemochromatosis in comparison to matched control patients with non-iron-related chronic liver disease. Hepatology 33:647–651
38. von DS, Lersch C, Schulte-Frohlinde E et al (2006) Hepatocellular carcinoma associated with hereditary hemochromatosis occurring in non-cirrhotic liver. Z Gastroenterol 44:39–42
39. Sato K, Ueda Y, Ueno K et al (2005) Hepatocellular carcinoma and nonalcoholic steatohepatitis developing during long-term administration of valproic acid. Virchows Arch 447:996–999
40. Britto MR, Thomas LA, Balaratnam N et al (2000) Hepatocellular carcinoma arising in non-cirrhotic liver in genetic haemochromatosis. Scand J Gastroenterol 35:889–893
41. Gomaa AI, Khan SA, Toledano MB et al (2008) Hepatocellular carcinoma: epidemiology, risk factors and pathogenesis. World J Gastroenterol 14:4300–4308
42. Ludwig J, Viggiano TR, McGill DB et al (1980) Nonalcoholic steatohepatitis: Mayo Clinic experiences with a hitherto unnamed disease. Mayo Clin Proc 55:434–438

43. Bacon BR, Farahvash MJ, Janney CG et al (1994) Nonalcoholic steatohepatitis: an expanded clinical entity. Gastroenterology 107:1103–1109

44. Yoshioka Y, Hashimoto E, Yatsuji S et al (2004) Nonalcoholic steatohepatitis: cirrhosis, hepatocellular carcinoma, and burnt-out NASH. J Gastroenterol 39:1215–1218

45. Mori S, Yamasaki T, Sakaida I et al (2004) Hepatocellular carcinoma with nonalcoholic steatohepatitis. J Gastroenterol 39:391–396

46. Cuadrado A, Orive A, Garcia-Suarez C et al (2005) Non-alcoholic steatohepatitis (NASH) and hepatocellular carcinoma. Obes Surg 15:442–446

47. Bugianesi E (2007) Non-alcoholic steatohepatitis and cancer. Clin Liver Dis 11, 191–198

Chapter 9
Liver Resection for Hepatocellular Carcinoma

Daria Zorzi, Jean-Nicolas Vauthey, and Eddie K. Abdalla

Keywords Liver resection · Orthotopic liver transplantation · HCC surgical resection · Multinodular HCC · Child–Pugh (CP) classification · Metabolic assessment · Future liver remnant · HCC preoperative therapy · Fibrolamellar carcinoma (FLHCC)

Preoperative Assessment

The natural history of untreated HCC varies depending on the stage at presentation and the degree of underlying liver disease. However, even in patients with early stages, the prognosis is poor if the disease is left untreated [1, 2]. As primary medical therapy has failed to significantly improve survival, surgical resection and orthotopic liver transplantation (OLT) represent the only treatment options offering a prospect for cure with 5-year survival rates of up to 50% [3–5] and 70% [6, 7], respectively.

Unfortunately, only approximately 20–40% [8, 9] of patients are candidates for resection due to the burden of hepatic tumor, the presence of extrahepatic spread, or the extent of underlying liver disease. Despite this, liver resections are increasingly being performed due to better perioperative care, improved imaging, and advances in surgical technique.

OLT represents the only surgical option in patients with small HCC and impaired liver function. However, in view of the severe graft shortage and restricted indications for OLT, liver resection is considered the mainstay of therapy in patients with preserved hepatic function. At M.D. Anderson Cancer Center the criteria for resection in chronic liver disease are illustrated in Table 9.1.

J.-N. Vauthey (✉)
Department of Surgical Oncology, The University of Texas MD Anderson Cancer Center, Houston, TX, USA

K.M. McMasters, J.-N. Vauthey (eds.), *Hepatocellular Carcinoma*,
DOI 10.1007/978-1-60327-522-4_9, © Springer Science+Business Media, LLC 2011

Table 9.1 University of Texas M.D. Anderson Cancer Center criteria for resection in chronic liver disease

Resection	Criteria
Minor	Child–Pugh A
	Bilirubin $\leq$ 2 mg/dL
	Absence of ascites
	Platelets > 100.000/mm3
Major	Criteria for minor resection plus:
	Bilirubin $\leq$ 1 mg/dL
	Absence of portal hypertension
	Portal vein embolization for future liver remnant of < 40%

Patient Selection

Optimal outcomes after surgical resection for HCC – optimal postoperative morbidity and mortality as well as optimal long-term survival – are contingent upon proper identification of appropriate candidates for safe, complete resection. A systematic and careful assessment of the patient's general medical fitness, the tumor extent, the tumor stage, the underlying liver function, and the volume of the anticipated future liver remnant (FLR) is critical in ensuring proper patient selection.

Patient age should not be considered per se a contraindication for resection, since it has not been shown to be an independent predictor of increased operative risk. However, in elderly patients, comorbid illnesses are prevalent and hidden medical diseases are not uncommon. Recently it has been reported that the presence of comorbidities was one of the two independent factors predictive of postoperative mortality after extended hepatectomy. In general, patients with American Society of Anesthesiology (ASA) scores greater than 1 represent a population at greater risk for postoperative complications and death. The surgical risk becomes unacceptably high in some patients with congestive heart failure, severe chronic obstructive pulmonary disease, and chronic renal failure [10, 11].

Evaluation of Tumor Extent

The assessment of tumor extent is the essential step for determining resectability and the appropriate type of surgical resection. At M. D. Anderson Cancer Center each patient is first staged with a triple phase (early vascular or arterial phase, portal phase, and delayed phase) helical computed tomography (CT) of the thorax and the abdomen because of its superior resolution throughout the whole body and the excellent liver anatomy detail. The liver is studied using thin slices acquired during the unenhanced phase and during the arterial, portal, and late or equilibrium phase after contrast administration. Tumors, such as HCC, are hypervascular during the early arterial phase and hypovascular in late phase ("washout"). Magnetic resonance imaging (MRI) is the imaging modality of choice when contrast agents are contraindicated, better lesion characterization is needed, or the anatomic relationship between tumor and major vascular or biliary structures requires further delineation.

As mortality rates after partial hepatectomy have fallen, in recent years to almost zero, many centers worldwide have expanded eligibility criteria for resection. Now included are tumors once considered unresectable such as large HCCs, multinodular and bilobar HCCs, and HCCs with portal vein or hepatic vein involvement. Based on preoperative imaging, patients are considered for resection when all tumor nodules can be safely excised with negative margins and when the volume and function of the FLR is adequate. Formal contraindications for resection are the presence of extrahepatic disease, extensive tumor thrombus in the inferior vena cava, and involvement of the common hepatic artery and portal vein trunk. Extension to surrounding structures, such as the diaphragm, does not represent a contraindication if a margin negative resection can be attained.

Large Tumor Size

In western countries, because of the lack of effective HCC screening, up to 50% of cases of HCC are diagnosed at an advanced stage, and tumor diameters sometimes exceed 10 cm. Large HCCs are more aggressive tumors, as indicated by higher alpha-fetoprotein levels and higher incidences of tumor rupture, multiple tumors, and invasion of portal or hepatic veins. Despite the technical problems encountered with large tumors – such as problems with liver mobilization, access and control of the hepatic veins – liver resection for large HCCs has been shown to be safe. A recent study reported a 30-day mortality rate of 5% in 300 patients who underwent partial hepatectomy for HCCs larger than 10 cm [12]. The 5-year survival rate in patients with tumors larger than 10 cm is about 27% and can reach up to 73% [13]. Thus, since in these patients cadaveric OLT and radiofrequency ablation (RFA) are not indicated, surgical resection remains the only treatment of choice that may cure large HCCs (Fig. 9.1).

Multinodular Disease

Multinodular HCC may represent independent tumors derived from multiple loci of hepatocarcinogenesis or may be a manifestation of advanced disease with intrahepatic metastasis, an event associated with a poor prognosis. Multinodular HCC (>3 nodules or >1 nodule exceeding 3 cm in diameter) have been considered unsuitable for resection. Surgical resection for these patients often requires major resection because of substantial tumor volume. Ng et al. [14] reported the outcome after resection in a cohort of 380 patients with intermediate-stage HCC: the mortality rate was 2.4% with a 5-year survival rate of 39%. Some authors investigated the role of liver resection for bilobar HCC. In a series of 78 patients with bilobar HCC, Liu et al. [15] compared 15 patients treated with hepatectomy plus treatment of tumor nodules in the contralateral lobe (wedge resection in five patients,

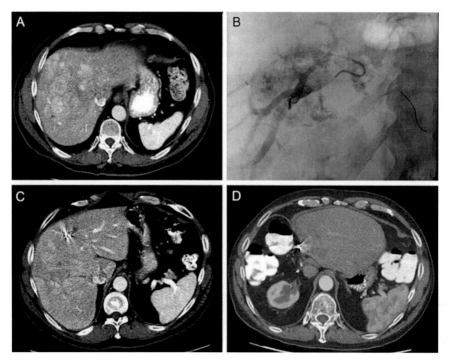

Fig. 9.1 A 59-year-old male patient had a 16 cm hepatocellular carcinoma in the right liver without evidence of extrahepatic disease. (**a**) Computed tomography revealed that the standardized FLR (sFLR) was 12%. (**b**) Right PVE was performed. (**c**) Four weeks after PVE, the sFLR was 21%. (**d**) The patient had no evidence of disease 5 years postresection (From [35], with permission)

alcohol injection in five, cryotherapy in two, and transarterial oily chemoembolization in two) with 63 patients who underwent nonsurgical therapy and showed that partial hepatectomy resulted in better survival outcomes. Hence, when liver function permits and clearance of all tumor nodules is possible, en bloc extended hepatectomy, multiple bilobar resections, or hepatectomy plus effective local ablative therapy for treatment of contralateral nodules should be considered for patients with bilobar HCC.

Major Portal or Hepatic Vein Involvement

HCCs with major portal or hepatic vein involvement represent a technical and onco-logic challenge. These tumors are aggressive and often multifocal, and surgery to remove them may be difficult. However, hepatic resection for such tumors seems justified because resection results in better survival rates than are achieved with nonsurgical treatment. A recent series focusing on 102 patients with major portal vein branches or hepatic vein involvement reported a 5-year survival rate of 23% in patients without cirrhosis, which still exceeded the historical survival rate in similar patients treated nonsurgically [16]. In a series of 23 patients with portal vein involvement who were treated with partial hepatectomy, Minagawa et al. [17] reported a median survival of 3.4 years and 1-, 3-, and 5-year survival rates of 82, 42, and 42%, respectively.

Recurrent HCC

Tumor recurrence represents the major drawback after curative liver resection and the most common cause of treatment failure. The cumulative 5-year recurrence rate is reported to be 70 to 100%. Recurrence in the liver remnant occurs in about 80–90% of cases as a result of vascular invasion leading to microsatellite tumors within the liver ("early recurrence") or second primaries in the remnant liver associated with field effect from hepatitis and cirrhosis ("late recurrence"). In the largest series, reresection rates have been reported between 10 and 31% and depend on the underlying liver status, pattern of recurrence, and extent of first resection with lower rates in series with high proportion of major resection during the first hepatectomy. Repeat hepatectomy has been proven to be a safe and worthwhile procedure with mortality and 5-year survival rates of 0–8% and 50–69%, respectively.

Evaluation of Hepatic Function

In western countries, the Child–Pugh (CP) classification (Table 9.2), which was originally designed to estimate the risk of cirrhotic patients undergoing portocaval shunt surgery for portal hypertension [18], has traditionally been used to evaluate the hepatic function. Usually only patients with Child–Pugh class A disease are considered good candidates for hepatectomy. However, Child–Pugh class is a crude measure and is prone to underestimate the surgical risk.

Table 9.2 Child–Pugh classification

Clinical and biochemical parameters	Points		
	1	2	3
Albumin (g/dL)	>3.5	2.8–3.5	<2.8
Bilirubin (mg/dL)	<2	2–3	>3
Prothrombin time			
Seconds prolonged	<4	4–6	>6
%	>60	40–60	<60
INR	<1.7	1.7–2.3	>2.3
Encephalopathy	Absent	Moderate (Stage I–II)	Severe (Stage III–IV)
Ascites	Absent	Moderate	Refractory

Total points: 5–6 points, Child–Pugh A; 7–9 points, Child–Pugh B; 10–15 points, Child–Pugh C

While no individual test accurately predicts liver function, the CP classification, combining different parameters, provides a rough estimation of the gross synthetic and detoxification capacity of the liver. In general, the risk of death after surgery increases with each CP class. Operative mortality rates for CP class A, B, and C patients undergoing abdominal operations are approximately 10, 30, and 82%, respectively [19], therefore liver resection is only considered in CP class A patients. Nevertheless, recent series of hepatectomy in CP class A patients have reported a wide range of perioperative mortality rates, from 0 to 16% [20–22].

Portal hypertension is present if the portal venous pressure is greater than 10 mmHg (the normal value ranges from 5 to 8 mmHg). Undiagnosed and latent portal hypertension in a cirrhotic patient undergoing liver resection puts the patient at risk of major complications, such as variceal bleeding, endotoxemia, and hepatic decompensation, in the postoperative period. In a prospective study in CP class A cirrhotic patients, Bruix et al. [23] showed that the hepatic venous pressure gradient (HVPG), a surrogate measurement of portal venous pressure, was the only predictor of hepatic decompensation following hepatic resection. Specifically, unresolved hepatic decompensation developed in 11 of 15 patients with an HVPG > 10 mmHg versus none of the patients with an HVPG < 10 ($P < 0.002$) suggesting that the CP classification may be somewhat inaccurate in assessing risk. Thus, in most patients with clinical or radiologic signs of portal hypertension, including splenomegaly, abdominal collaterals, thrombocytopenia (platelets <100,000/mm^3), or esophagogastric varices, resection is contraindicated.

Additionally, postoperative mortality has been shown to be almost sixfold higher in a cohort of 285 patients who underwent hepatectomy for HCC when there was histologic evidence of cirrhosis and active hepatitis versus cirrhosis alone [24]. Although the presence of hepatitis does not always correlate with serum transaminase levels [25, 26], increased complication and death rates have been reported in those patients with elevated liver function tests. Patients with aspartate aminotransferase level greater than 100 IU/L [27] or alanine aminotransferase level at least twice normal [28] are considered to be poor candidates for major hepatic resection. Bilirubin levels greater than 2 mg/dL contraindicate hepatic resection while patients with bilirubin levels between 1.1 and 2.0 mg/dL should be carefully selected and considered for only limited resection.

In eastern countries several hepatobiliary units have employed more sophisticated quantitative liver function tests, such as indocyanine green (ICG) clearance, galactose elimination capacity, and aminopyrine clearance, to evaluate the hepatic metabolic function and to predict the risk of postoperative liver failure. The most widely used and validated metabolic assessment is the ICG clearance test. Makuuchi et al. have incorporated the ICGR15 and two clinical features, i.e., bilirubin and ascites, into a treatment-selection algorithm (Fig. 9.2) [22]. In patients without ascites and bilirubin levels less than 1.0 mg/dL, ICGR15 is used to predict the number of liver segments that can be safely resected (ICGR15 <10%, extended hepatectomy and right hemihepatectomy are safe; ICGR15 10–19%, left hemihepatectomy and bisegmentectomy are safe; ICGR15 20–29%, only segmentectomies

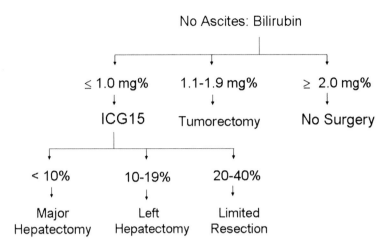

Fig. 9.2 Japanese algorithm for resection in cirrhosis (Adapted from [22] used with permission)

are safe; ICGR15 30–39%, only wedge resections are safe; ICGR15 ≥40%, only enucleations are safe). This algorithmic approach was prospectively validated in 107 patients; the 30-day mortality rate was zero, and there were no major complications [29].

Evaluation of Future Liver Remnant Volume

Computed tomography (CT) can now provide an accurate, reproducible method for preoperatively measuring the volume of the future liver remnant (FLR). The FLR is measured directly by three-dimensional CT volumetry, and the total liver volume is calculated using a mathematical formula that relies on the linear correlation between liver size and body surface area (BSA). The ratio of the CT measure FLR volume/calculated total liver volume (TLV) is defined as the standardized FLR and it provides the percent of TLV remaining after resection [30]. The formula used to estimate TLV based on BSA was recently evaluated in a meta-analysis and recommended as one of the least biased and most precise formulas for the estimation of the total liver volume in adults [31] (Fig. 9.3).

Although there is a general consensus that the extent of resection that is safe is mainly limited by the function, attention has also focused on the FLR volume after major hepatectomy. In general, a FLR of 20% is considered the minimum safe volume needed following extended hepatic resection in patients with normal underlying liver, while an FLR of 40% is required in patients with chronic liver disease (cirrhosis or hepatitis) [32, 33] (Fig. 9.4). Current suggested indications for PVE in normal, injured, and cirrhotic liver are presented in Fig. 9.5.

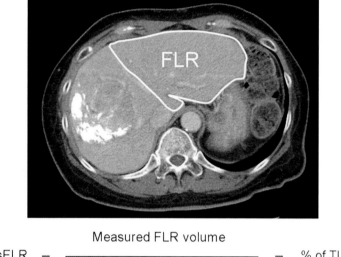

$$sFLR \ = \ \frac{\text{Measured FLR volume}}{\text{TLV} = -794 + 1267 \times \text{BSA}} \ = \ \% \text{ of TLV}$$

Fig. 9.3 Method of systemic preoperative liver volume calculation using three-dimensional CT volumetry. CT outline of the segments included in the measurement of future liver remnant (FLR) volume for a planned extended right hepatectomy (white outline = FLR). (**a**) The FLR is measured directly by three-dimensional CT volumetry, and the total liver volume (TLV) is calculated using a mathematical formula that relies on the linear correlation between liver size and body surface area (BSA). The ratio of the CT measure FLR volume/calculated total liver volume (TLV) is defined as the standardized FLR (sFLR) and it provides the percent of TLV remaining after resection

Preoperative Therapy

Transarterial Chemoembolization (TACE) and Portal Vein Embolization (PVE)

In patients who are otherwise candidates for hepatic resection, an inadequate FLR volume – ≤20 or <40% of the estimated TLV in patients with normal or cirrhotic liver, respectively – may be the only obstacle to curative resection. Three-dimensional CT volumetry and calculation of the FLR allows the planning of hepatic resection to be individualized for each patient. Portal vein embolization (PVE) can be performed to prime the growth of the anticipated FLR, thereby making a major or extended hepatectomy possible.

PVE is safe with less than a 5% complication rate, causes little periportal reaction, and generates durable portal vein occlusion especially when used in combination with coils. PVE has been shown to increase both the size of the FLR as well as the percentage of indocyanine green (ICG) excretion and bile volume flow in the remnant liver. In addition, in patients with chronic liver disease PVE has also been reported to decrease the incidence of postoperative complications, intensive care unit stay, and the total hospital stay after major hepatic resection. Thus, the

A   B

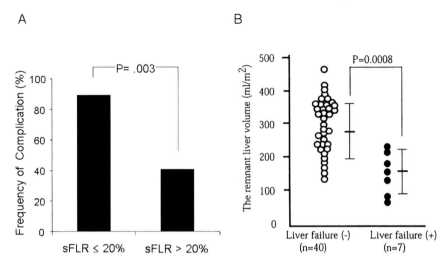

Fig. 9.4 Standardized calculation of future liver remnant (FLR) volume accurately predicts the likelihood of postoperative complications after hepatic resection in normal liver (**a**) and in chronic liver disease (**b**). (**a**) Complication rate stratified by standardized future liver remnant (% FLR) volume in relation to FLR in normal liver; 90% of patients with a % FLR of 20% or less had complications; 39% of patients with a % FLR of greater than 20% had complications ($P = 0.003$) [33]. (**b**) A comparison of FLR volume of patients who died of liver failure and those without liver failure after surgery in chronic liver disease. Remnant liver volume in patients who died of liver failure was significantly smaller than that in patients who did not die of liver failure ($P = 0.0008$) and it was never more than 250 mL/m^2 (From [33], used with permission)

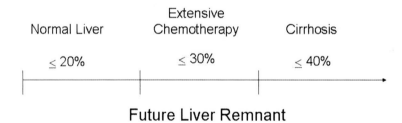

Fig. 9.5 Indications for portal vein embolization (PVE). There is a consensus that in patients treated with aggressive preoperative chemotherapy, the remnant liver volume should be at least 30% of the total liver volume to avoid a high risk of complications following hepatic resection. BMI, body mass index (From [34], used with permission)

selective use of PVE may enable safe and potentially curative extended hepatec-tomy in a subset of patients with advanced hepatobiliary malignancies who would otherwise have been marginal candidates for resection.

Palavecino et al. [35] reported on 54 patients who underwent major hepatic resec-tion for HCC with or without PVE before resection. This study demonstrates that PVE before major hepatectomy for HCC is associated with decreased perioperative mortality. The overall and disease-free survival rates were similar between patients

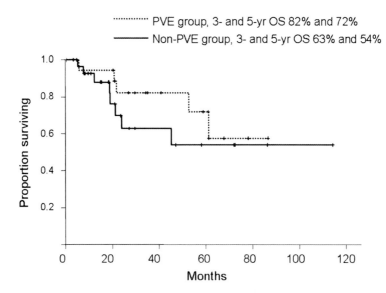

Fig. 9.6 Overall survival after major hepatectomy in patients with and without preoperative portal vein embolization (PVE), excluding postoperative deaths ($P = 0.35$) (From [35], used with permission)

who underwent major hepatectomy with and without PVE (Fig. 9.6). Thus, PVE increases the safety of major hepatectomy in patients with HCC without compromising long-term oncologic outcomes.

Because the main blood supply for HCC is the hepatic artery and PVE results in increased hepatic arterial flow, concerns have been raised about the potential for accelerated tumor growth after PVE [36, 37]. To avoid this possibility, TACE has been proposed as a complementary procedure to PVE in patients with HCC (Fig. 9.7). TACE eliminates the arterial blood supply to the tumor and embolizes potential arteriovenous shunts resulting from cirrhosis and/or HCC that attenuate the effects of PVE. In addition, 60–80% complete necrosis of tumor can be achieved by the combination of TACE and PVE [38, 39]. Our results support a study by Ogata et al. [38] in which patients who underwent TACE before PVE had improved disease-free survival and increased FLR hypertrophy than patients who underwent PVE alone [35] (Fig. 9.8). Our current recommendation for those patients with bilobar HCC and tumor nodules in the FLR is to perform TACE before PVE to avoid tumor growth in the FLR after PVE.

Chemotherapy

Sorafenib is an oral multikinase inhibitor, which exerts an antiangiogenic effect by targeting vascular endothelial growth factor receptors (VEGFRs)

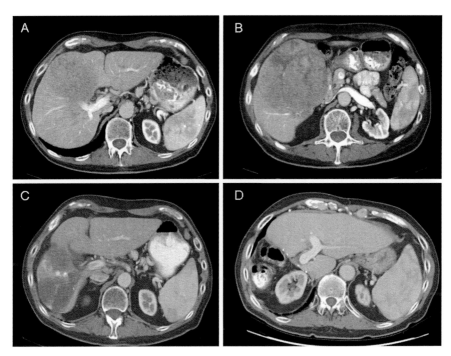

Fig. 9.7 Sequential transartherial chemoembolization (TACE) and portal vein embolization (PVE) in cirrhotic liver. A 74-year-old male patient HCV genotype 2b with a 12.5 hepatocellular carcinoma involving the right liver with periportal fibrosis and focal bridging. (**a, b**) Future liver remnant (FLR) volume of segments 1, 2, 3, and 4 equal to 27%. Computed tomography following TACE and right PVE shows hypertrophy of the FLR (47%) (**c**). Right hepatectomy was performed. The specimen indicated complete pathologic response with no residual tumor. The patient had no evidence of disease 53 months postresection (**d**)

and platelet-derived growth factor receptor (PDGFR). Recently, a randomized, placebo-controlled phase III trial of sorafenib reported an improvement in median overall survival along with increased time to progression and disease control rate in advanced HCC [40]. There is no evidence that sorafenib has a role as a neoadjuvant agent in downstaging patients to render them resectable because the response rate to sorafenib is only 3%.

In contrast the PIAF treatment regimen (platinum, interferon, adriamycin, and 5 FU) allows a selected group of patients with normal liver and HCC confined to the liver to become eligible for aggressive surgical techniques [41, 42] (Fig. 9.9). Using the PIAF regimen in patients with preserved liver function Lau et al. found 18% major tumor response rate (more than 50% reduction in tumor size). Furthermore, 10% percent of the entire cohort, who presented with tumors that were considered unresectable, underwent subsequent complete resection after chemotherapy; 53% of the resected patients were alive 3 years after hepatic resection [43].

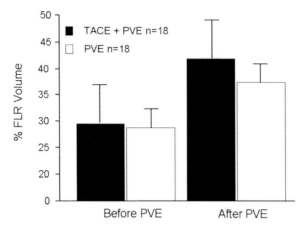

Fig. 9.8 Sequential arterial and portal vein embolization. Patients who underwent transartherial chemoembolization (TACE) before portal vein embolization (PVE) had increased future liver remnant (FLR) hypertrophy than patients who underwent PVE alone ($P = 0.13$) (From [36], used with permission)

Surgical Technique

In patients with HCC, the goal of the surgical approach is to optimize the oncologic resection (negative margin) while sparing the noncancerous hepatic parenchyma. Advances in anesthetic and surgical techniques, as well as a thorough understanding of the liver anatomy and tumor biology, have contributed dramatically to the safety and effectiveness of liver resection for HCC. Modern surgical principles include anatomic resection, the use of vascular inflow occlusion, and low central venous pressure anesthesia. New surgical approaches such as the anterior approach and liver hanging maneuver have been developed along with the use of more effective instruments for parenchymal transection.

For a safe liver resection, both the bilateral subcostal incision, with or without superior/midline extension to the xiphoid (hockey-stick incision), and the J-type incision are valid options. At M.D. Anderson Cancer Center the modified Makuuchi J-incision where the vertical midline portion converges with the horizontal limb at the level of the umbilicus. Our modification aims to spare the nerves supplying the skin and the rectus muscle, thus reducing skin numbness, muscle atrophy, and post-operative pain [44]. After mobilization of the liver, intraoperative ultrasound (IOUS) is systematically performed to confirm the extent of disease, review the intrahepatic portal and hepatic vein anatomy, and define the parenchymal transection plane. IOUS identifies new nodules in 15–30% of patients with HCC [45, 46], although only about 25% of these new nodules are malignant. The classic description of HCC by IOUS is a mosaic pattern with posterior enhancement and lateral shadowing. In nodules that lack specific findings of HCC, malignancy is found in 24–30% of

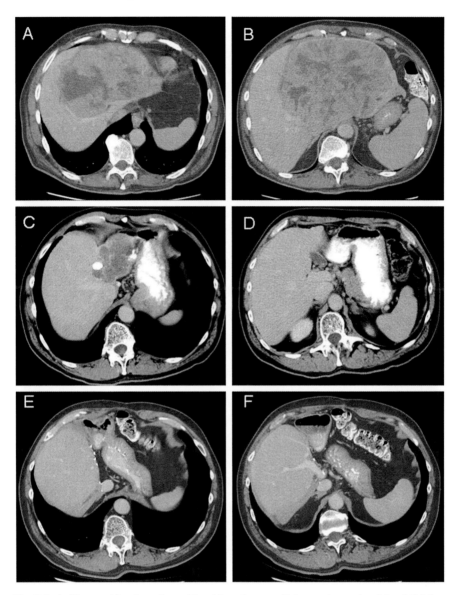

Fig. 9.9 A 60-year-old male patient with a 15 cm hepatocellular carcinoma involving left lobe, right anterior sector and abutting the right hepatic vein. (**a, b**) Computed tomography following six cycles of chemotherapy with PIAF (platinum, interferon, adriamycin, and 5 FU), three cycles of capecitabine + interferon, and transarterial chemoembolization (TACE) revealed response of the tumor. (**c, d**) Extended left hepatectomy with caudate and vena cava resection was performed. The patient had no evidence of disease 4 years postresection (**e, f**)

hypoechoic nodules and 0–18% of hyperechoic nodules [45, 46]. IOUS may therefore decrease recurrence through the identification of unrecognized multifocal HCC.
In addition, IOUS is considered an essential aid for guidance of resection [47] and
has proven useful in obtaining a margin negative resection [48] (see Chapter 10).

Anatomic Resection

HCC has a high propensity to invade the portal and hepatic veins; thus, the spread
of HCC is essentially through the bloodstream – first via the portal vein to cause
intrahepatic metastasis, a primary mechanism of intrahepatic recurrence, and later
to extrahepatic organs such as the lungs, bone, and adrenal glands. These two forms
of spread, vascular invasion and intrahepatic metastasis, are among the risk factors
that most strongly influence the postoperative prognosis. On this basis, Makuuchi
et al. introduced the concept of anatomic resection – segmentectomy and subsegmentectomy – which involves systematic removal of a hepatic segment confined
by tumor-bearing portal tributaries that might contain portal metastases or daughter
micronodules.

The theoretical advantage of anatomic over nonanatomic resection has been
demonstrated in two large series in which anatomic resection was found to be an
independent factor for both overall and disease-free survival [49, 50]. Therefore,
segment-oriented anatomical resection should be proposed for any HCC, whenever
technically and functionally possible. The width of a negative resection margin has
also been investigated. A study predating the reports on anatomic resection showed
that the rate of postoperative recurrence of HCC was not related to the width of the
resection margin but rather to microvascular invasion or the presence of microsatel-
lites [51], further supporting the superior value of the anatomic approach. As the
margin size has not been found to be an independent predictor of recurrence across
multiple studies, functional liver should not be sacrificed in an attempt to obtain a
wide margin [51–54].

Resection of Large Right Liver Tumors

Surgical resection of a large right lobe tumor represents one of the most challenging situations. With the conventional technique for hepatectomy, mobilization of the
right lobe from the retroperitoneum and anterior surface of the IVC may be challenging because of the tumor volume and adhesion to the diaphragm and may result
in injury to the right hepatic vein or the venous branches between the IVC and the
posterior aspect of the right lobe.

To overcome these problems, the anterior approach has been proposed [55]. With
this approach, after hilar control of the vascular inflow is achieved, the parenchyma
is transected from the anterior surface of the liver down to the anterior surface of
the IVC, without prior mobilization of the right lobe. After control is achieved of
all venous tributaries to the IVC, including the right hepatic vein, the right lobe
is detached from the diaphragm. In a retrospective comparative analysis, Liu et al.
demonstrated that the anterior approach for large right lobe HCCs resulted in less

intraoperative blood loss, lower transfusion requirements, a lower in-hospital death rate, and significantly better overall and disease-free survival compared to the conventional approach to right or extended right hepatectomy [56]. More recently in a prospective randomized controlled study, Liu et al. confirmed findings of the previous study, demonstrating improved operative and survival outcomes of the anterior approach technique compared to the conventional approach [57]. With the anterior approach, it may be difficult to control bleeding in the deeper parenchymal plane. Because of this, in 2001, Belghiti et al. proposed a new technique of hanging the liver after lifting it with a tape passed between the anterior surface of the IVC and the liver parenchyma ("liver-hanging maneuver") [58]. To allow for passage of the tape, the space between the right and middle hepatic veins is initially dissected for 2 cm downward. The dissection of the anterior plane of the IVC begins with placement of a long vascular clamp posterior to the caudate lobe on the left side of the right inferior hepatic vein, if present (Fig. 9.10). Then the clamp is gently pushed cranially in the middle plane of the IVC to allow a blind dissection. When the clamp appears between the right and middle hepatic veins, the tape is seized and

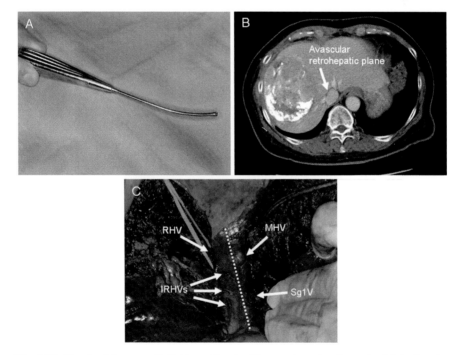

Fig. 9.10 Hanging Maneuver. Pediatric suction (grafting suction tube, 4-mm tip, 9.5 in. length; Cardinal Health/V Mueller Products) is used to explore the space of Couinaud and to perform the liver hanging maneuver (**a**). Avascular retrohepatic plane between right and middle hepatic veins (*arrow*) (**b**). Intraoperative view after removal of the specimen. Avascular retrohepatic plane is shown with a *dot line* (**c**). Right hepatic vein (RHV), middle hepatic vein (MHV), inferior right heparic veins (IHRVs), segment 1 vein (Sg1V)

passed around the hepatic parenchyma. The parenchymal dissection is facilitated by upward traction on the tape, which allows the surgeon to follow a direct plane and facilitates exposure and hemostasis of the posterior parenchymal plane in front of the IVC.

Prevention and Control of Bleeding

Many studies have shown that intraoperative blood loss and transfusion requirements are independent predictors of major morbidity and death from surgery. Blood transfusion can add to the risk of coagulopathy as well as exert immunosuppressive effects. Given this, efforts to minimize blood loss become critical. Techniques of temporary vascular occlusion such as portal triad clamping and total vascular exclusion (TVE) have been used to reduce bleeding from the cut edge of the liver.

In a prospective randomized study, portal triad clamping, otherwise known as the Pringle maneuver, has been shown to significantly reduce blood loss resulting in improved postoperative liver function [59]. Further, the authors suggested that the reduction in blood loss offset the potential adverse effects of ischemia–reperfusion-induced hepatocellular injury. In a different randomized trial, Belghiti et al. demonstrated that intermittent Pringle maneuver – 15 min of inflow occlusion followed by 5 min of liver revascularization – is safer than continuous inflow occlusion in patients with chronic liver disease and should be considered, in this population, the technique of choice [60]. While Pringle maneuvers exceeding 4 h have been reported, Wei et al. found that inflow occlusion time exceeding 80 min was associated with a higher mortality rate [11]. Total vascular exclusion (TVE), a technique which involves the Pringle maneuver as well as clamping of the supra- and infra-hepatic vena cava, has not been shown to be more effective in decreasing blood loss when compared to portal triad clamping alone, while associated with increased morbidity [61]. Indications for TVE are limited to those cases with tumor involvement of the cavo-hepatic junction [62].

The drawback of hepatic pedicle clamping is that it does not prevent back bleeding from the hepatic veins. In fact, one of the most important factors related to intraoperative blood loss is pressure within the inferior vena cava (IVC). In a prospective study examining blood loss and IVC pressure, there was a direct linear correlation between mean caval pressure and blood loss [63]. As hepatic vein pressure directly reflects the caval pressure, the maintenance of a low central venous pressure is an effective technique to reduce back bleeding from the hepatic veins [64, 65]. At our institution, all patients who undergo hepatic resection have maintenance of a low central venous pressure (<5 cm H_2O), with a minimal acceptable urine output of 0.5 mL/kg/h, until the parenchymal transection is completed. Infusions and transfusions are minimized, and transient hypotension that can occur with hepatic mobilization is treated with vasopressor support (usually phenylephrine). When the parenchymal transection is complete and hemostasis achieved, patients are rendered euvolemic with crystalloid and/or albumin infusions.

Several different parenchymal dissection techniques have been developed to minimize blood loss and expedite hepatic resection. Advances in instrumentation, such as development of the ultrasonic aspirator, the jet cutter, the argon beam coagulator, and saline-linked cautery, have all been purported to improve surgical technique. The ultrasonic dissector is a handheld device that destroys hepatocytes by cavitation based on water content and aspirates the liquefied tissue. Vessels and biliary ducts, which contain less water, are preserved allowing for a clear delineation of these structures within the transection plane. Saline-linked cautery (SLC) uses a metal probe to deliver radiofrequency energy conducted through a slow infusion of saline. At our institution, we recently combined saline-linked cautery with ultrasonic dissection in a standardized fashion (Fig. 9.11). This combination allows a clear delineation of the vascular and biliary anatomy within the transection plane, resulting in a significant decrease in total operative time, blood loss, and need for suture control of intraparenchymal vessels. The primary surgeon dissects the hepatic parenchyma from the patient's left side utilizing the ultrasonic dissector while the second surgeon operates the SLC from the patient's right side. Vessels of 3 mm or smaller are coagulated and divided using the SLC device, while those of 3–5 mm in diameter are controlled with titanium clips and divided sharply. Larger vessels and portal triads are sutured with 3-0 silk ties in continuity and divided sharply. This two-surgeon technique resulted in a significant decrease in blood loss and total operative time [66]. The combined technique using the ultrasonic dissector and the SLC has recently been validated by two different groups. Takatsuki

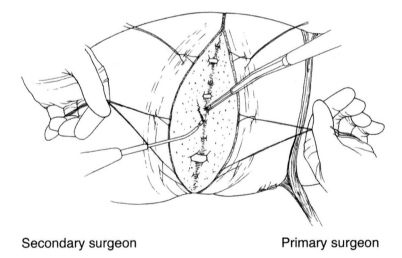

Secondary surgeon   Primary surgeon

Fig. 9.11 Two-surgeon technique for hepatic parenchymal transection. Using the ultrasonic dissection device, the primary surgeon directs the dissection from the patient's left side. Simultaneously, the secondary surgeon operates the saline-linked cautery device from the patient's right side. Traction on 4-0 polypropylene stay sutures is used to expose the deepening transection plane (From [66], used with permission)

et al. [67] analyzed outcomes in living donor hepatectomy. The authors found a statistically significant lower level of blood loss and donors complications when the two-surgeon technique was used. In a randomized controlled trial, El Moghazy et al. [68] demonstrated a lower blood loss and a faster parenchymal transection time in the group randomized to ultrasonic dissector and saline-linked cautery compared to ultrasonic dissector and bipolar cautery in living donor hepatectomy. This is of utmost importance since a faster parenchymal phase may reduce the time of the Pringle maneuver and of ischemic injury of the liver. In addition a recent study reported the level of intraoperative blood loss during resection of HCC to be an independent predictor of overall survival, disease-specific survival, and disease-free survival [69], hence a decreased intraoperative blood loss during HCC resection using the two-surgeon technique may improve oncologic outcome.

Drainage

Drains have not been shown to be beneficial after hepatic resection for HCC. In a meta-analysis of three randomized controlled trials, the incidence of postoperative biloma was approximately 5% and either equal or even higher in drained patients compared with not drained patients [70]. In one of these trials, which only included patients with chronic liver disease, drainage after resection was an independent predictor of postoperative complications [71]. Drains also failed to detect significant postoperative complications such as bile leak and hemorrhage that needed surgical or radiologic interventions.

Outcome After Resection

Morbidity and Mortality

Improvements in patient selection and surgical technique have resulted in a remarkable decrease in perioperative mortality rates. A large, multicenter review from the 1970s by Foster and Berman reported a perioperative mortality of 21% for major hepatectomy and 58% for patients with cirrhosis [72]. Currently, the mortality rate is approximately 5% with some centers approaching close to zero mortality [22, 29, 73]. Refinements are multifactorial and include surgical technique, anesthesia management, perioperative care, and the establishment of high-volume referral centers specializing in hepatobiliary surgery.

Morbidity rates range from 25 to 50% in recent large series [4, 5, 9–11]. In addition to complications associated with all major surgery, posthepatectomy specific complications include right pleural effusion, subphrenic abscess, bleeding, biliary leak/fistula, ascites, and hepatic insufficiency. Blood loss and the need for transfusion have clearly been shown to increase morbidity and mortality [74, 75]. In a review of extended hepatectomies for HCC, multivariate analysis identified the Pringle maneuver and blood transfusion as risk factors for morbidity with comorbid illness and blood transfusion as independent risk factors for death [11]. The risk of morbidity with Pringle maneuver was primarily for minor complications such as ascites/effusion and mainly in those patients with clamping time exceeding 80 min.

Long-Term Outcome

During the past two to three decades, survival after hepatic resection has markedly improved over earlier results, likely due to early diagnosis in high-risk patients screened with AFP and ultrasound, improved patient selection, and surgical management. Large series have reported 30–50% 5-year overall survival rates following curative resection [69, 76–78].

The main cause of treatment failure is tumor recurrence. Indeed, cumulative 5-year recurrence rates of 70–100% have been reported after hepatic resection. Recurrence occurs in the liver remnant in about 80–90% [78, 79] of cases, as a result of vascular invasion leading to microsatellite tumors within the liver, i.e., intrahepatic metastases (early recurrence), or second primaries in the remnant liver associated with field effect from hepatitis and cirrhosis (late recurrence).

Though surgical resection of intrahepatic tumor recurrence is a demanding procedure because of reduced hepatic parenchyma and a more hostile environment, repeat hepatectomy has been proven to be safe and worthwhile [80–85]. About 10–31% of the patients with intrahepatic recurrence can be treated with a second hepatectomy. Utilizing the same selection criteria as for primary resection, three clinicopathologic variables were found to be independent prognostic factors: absence of portal invasion at the second resection, single HCC at the primary hepatectomy, and a disease-free interval of at least 1 year after the primary hepatectomy [86]. In a series of 67 patients, the overall 5-year survival after a repeat hepatectomy was 56% – a rate comparable to those reported in many series of initial resection [85]. Aggressive nonsurgical treatment with ethanol injection, radiofrequency ablation, and transarterial chemoembolization may yield favorable results in patients not suitable for repeat resection.

The prognosis after potentially curative therapy depends on tumor-related factors and underlying liver disease. Thus, clinical and pathologic predictors of survival have been extensively investigated. For example, in a stepwise analysis approach on 5,800 patients, the Liver Cancer Study Group of Japan established portal involvement as the predominant prognostic factor, followed by number of tumor nodules, AFP level, tumor size, cirrhosis, age, and surgical curability (as defined by resection margin, stage, and absence of remaining macroscopic tumor) [87].

Resection Prior to Liver Transplantation

For those patients whose poor underlying liver function and tumor number or location preclude traditional hepatic resection, total hepatectomy with orthotopic liver transplantation (OLT) has been advocated. Initial series of OLT for HCC reported poor results, with tumor recurrence in up to 75% of patients. Bismuth et al. were the first to show that in the early era of liver transplantation, the surgical strategy for the treatment of hepatocellular carcinoma in cirrhosis had followed a misconception in selecting patients suffering from advanced, unresectable cancers as transplant candidates [88]. Currently, those patients suffering from HCC and cirrhosis with three or less tumor nodules up to 3 cm in maximum diameter or a single tumor not exceeding 5 cm and no signs of vascular invasion are considered for transplantation (Milano criteria) [6]. OLT based on these Milan criteria have been shown to provide very good disease-free survival, so that it is considered to be the optimal treatment of small HCC, especially in patients with underlying chronic liver disease [7, 89]. The evidence that OLT should be the preferred treatment choice for these patients has increased the demand resulting in longer waiting list in the face of a relative shortage of available donors. During long waiting times, some patients suffer progression of disease such that they can never benefit from OLT. Bridge treatments to halt or delay tumor progression during the waiting period for OLT include also liver resection [90–94]. Poon et al. noted that 80% of patients who recur after primary resection for HCC remain eligible for OLT [90]. Thus a new strategy was proposed for patients with preserved liver function and HCC: hepatic resection prior to "salvage" or secondary OLT. The major drawbacks of this concept of primary liver resection prior to transplantation could be the increase technical difficulty during OLT procedure and the risk of impaired posttransplant survival. Belghiti et al. showed that in selected patients with cirrhosis and resectable HCC perioperative and postoperative course of OLT following liver resection did not differ in terms of operative time, blood loss, morbidity and mortality compared to upfront OLT. Also, long-term survival after liver resection prior to OLT was not different compared to upfront OLT [95].

Fibrolamellar Variant of HCC

Fibrolamellar carcinoma (FLHCC) is a distinct clinical variant of HCC. This hepatic tumor usually occurs in young patients, most commonly within the second and third decades of life with no gender predominance. There seems to be a preponderance of FLHCC in American Caucasians, with few cases reported in Asian populations. The incidence of FLHCC has been reported at 6–23% of western patients with HCC. Pathologically, FLHCC typically consists of well-circumscribed, large solitary lesions with a central scar. Unlike classic HCC, cirrhosis is not a common component of the hepatic disease in patients with FLHCC. In addition, hepatitis infection is uncommon and serum alpha-fetoprotein levels are usually within normal limits. Abdominal computed tomography (CT) and magnetic resonance imaging (MRI) often demonstrate a heterogeneous mass with a central scar that is similar to those seen in cases of focal nodular hyperplasia (FNH). Central calcifications within the mass have been used to distinguish FLHCC from FNH, but this is not specific.

Conflicting data exist regarding whether patients with fibrolamellar carcinoma have a better survival when compared to patients with classic HCC. In a series published from Memorial Sloan-Kettering Cancer Center, resected patients with FLHCC did not have an improved long-term survival compared to classic HCC, although there were too few patients with FLHCC to make meaningful conclusions [96]. These survival data were similar to those published by Nagorney et al. [97] who found no survival advantage for FLHCC over classic HCC without cirrhosis. They noted, however, a higher resection rate for patients with FLHCC. In contrast, Soreide et al. reported a 56% 5-year survival and a 58% resectability rate for patients with FLHCC [98]. In a large review of the literature, Okuda noted a 95% resectability rate and improved survival for patients with FLHCC as compared to HCC patients [99]. Tumor stage has a profound influence on survival as demonstrated by Hemming et al., with stage II FLHCC patients experiencing extended survival times as compared to patients with stage III disease [100]. Ringe et al. observed the number of hepatic lesions and the presence of nodal disease to be significant variables in predicting survival in resected patients [101]. Survival times are longer in patients with recurrences of FLHCC following resection when compared to recurrences of classic HCC. In addition, patients with recurrent FLHCC following resection have been reported to have prolonged survival following re-excision of a local recurrence. Unlike HCC, patients with FLHCC are more likely to have solitary tumors, thus potentially increasing the resection rate. The rate of metastases, both nodal and distant, has been reported up to 30% at the time of diagnosis. Indeed, the rate of lymph node positivity is quite high in FLHCC, raising the question of en bloc lymphadenectomy at the time of the primary surgery. To date, no one has reported data to adequately answer this question. Patients with unresectable metastatic FLHCC have been reported to have a median survival of 14 months, double that for matched-for-stage HCC patients.

Controversy exists as to whether resection or transplantation for FLHCC provides superior survival. One study from the UK noted a 3-year survival of 100% for patients treated with major liver resection versus 76% 3-year survival following hepatic transplantation for FLHCC ($P < 0.025$) [102]. These data are similar to data published from Pittsburgh. Pinna et al. [103] documented superior survival for FLHCC patients treated with resection as compared to transplanted patients. Additionally, the survival gap at 5 years was 44%, with 75% of resected patients alive versus 36% of transplant recipients. Further evidence of the apparent superiority of hepatic resection compared to transplantation in patients with FLHCC came from Germany, where resected patients had a median survival of 44.5 months versus 28.5 months for transplantation. In a review of the literature on transplantation for HCC, Neuhaus et al. concluded that transplantation is not appropriate for FLHCC without cirrhosis [104].

The potential neoadjuvant role for continuous infusion fluorouracil and subcutaneous interferon alpha-2b has been suggested based on a phase II trial conducted at the M.D. Anderson Cancer Center [105]. There was a 62.5% response rate following chemotherapy seen in patients with FLHCC as compared to a 14% response rate in patients with HCC. This suggests that in patients with advanced stage FLHCC, downstaging with chemotherapy should be considered to increase the resectability rate, although further trials are necessary.

References

1. Nagasue N, Yukaya H, Hamada T, Hirose S, Kanashima R, Inokuchi K (1984) The natural history of hepatocellular carcinoma. A study of 100 untreated cases. Cancer 54:1461–1465
2. Barbara L, Benzi G, Gaiani S et al (1992) Natural history of small untreated hepatocellular carcinoma in cirrhosis: a multivariate analysis of prognostic factors of tumor growth rate and patient survival. Hepatology 16:132–137
3. Shuto T, Hirohashi K, Kubo S et al (1998) Changes and results of surgical strategies for hepatocellular carcinoma: results of a 15-year study on 452 consecutive patients. Surg Today 28:1124–1129
4. Zhou XD, Tang ZY, Yang BH et al (2001) Experience of 1000 patients who underwent hepatectomy for small hepatocellular carcinoma. Cancer 91:1479–1486
5. Takenaka K, Kawahara N, Yamamoto K et al (1996) Results of 280 liver resections for hepatocellular carcinoma. Arch Surg 131:71–76
6. Mazzaferro V, Regalia E, Doci R et al (1996) Liver transplantation for the treatment of small hepatocellular carcinomas in patients with cirrhosis. N Engl J Med 334:693–699
7. Llovet JM, Bruix J, Fuster J et al (1998) Liver transplantation for small hepatocellular carcinoma: the tumor-node-metastasis classification does not have prognostic power. Hepatology 27:1572–1577
8. Cance WG, Stewart AK, Menck HR (2000) The National Cancer Data Base Report on treatment patterns for hepatocellular carcinomas: improved survival of surgically resected patients, 1985–1996. Cancer 88:912–920
9. Fong Y, Sun RL, Jarnagin W, Blumgart LH (1999) An analysis of 412 cases of hepatocellular carcinoma at a Western center. Ann Surg 229:790–799
10. Belghiti J, Hiramatsu K, Benoist S, Massault P, Sauvanet A, Farges O (2000) Seven hundred forty-seven hepatectomies in the 1990s: an update to evaluate the actual risk of liver resection. J Am Coll Surg 191:38–46
11. Wei AC, Tung-Ping Poon R, Fan ST, Wong J (2003) Risk factors for perioperative morbidity and mortality after extended hepatectomy for hepatocellular carcinoma. Br J Surg 90:33–41
12. Pawlik TM, Poon RT, Abdalla EK et al (2005) Critical appraisal of the clinical and pathologic predictors of survival after resection of large hepatocellular carcinoma. Arch Surg 140:450–457
13. Kosuge T, Makuuchi M, Takayama T, Yamamoto J, Shimada K, Yamasaki S (1993) Long-term results after resection of hepatocellular carcinoma: experience of 480 cases. Hepatogastroenterology 40:328–332
14. Ng KK, Vauthey JN, Pawlik TM et al (2005) Is hepatic resection for large or multinodular hepatocellular carcinoma justified? Results from a multi-institutional database. Ann Surg Oncol 12:364–373
15. Liu CL, Fan ST, Lo CM, Ng IO, Poon RT, Wong J (2003) Hepatic resection for bilobar hepatocellular carcinoma: is it justified? Arch Surg 138:100–104
16. Pawlik TM, Poon RT, Abdalla EK et al (2005) Hepatectomy for hepatocellular carcinoma with major portal or hepatic vein invasion: results of a multicenter study. Surgery 137: 403–410
17. Minagawa M, Makuuchi M, Takayama T, Ohtomo K (2001) Selection criteria for hepatectomy in patients with hepatocellular carcinoma and portal vein tumor thrombus. Ann Surg 233:379–384
18. Pugh RN, Murray-Lyon IM, Dawson JL, Pietroni MC, Williams R (1973) Transection of the oesophagus for bleeding oesophageal varices. Br J Surg 60:646–649
19. Mansour A, Watson W, Shayani V, Pickleman J (1997) Abdominal operations in patients with cirrhosis: still a major surgical challenge. Surgery 122:730–735
20. Teh SH, Christein J, Donohue J et al (2005) Hepatic resection of hepatocellular carcinoma in patients with cirrhosis: model of end-stage liver disease (MELD) score predicts perioperative mortality. J Gastrointest Surg 9:1207–1215

21. Belghiti J, Regimbeau JM, Durand F et al (2002) Resection of hepatocellular carcinoma: a European experience on 328 cases. Hepatogastroenterology 49:41–46
22. Makuuchi M, Kosuge T, Takayama T, et al (1993) Surgery for small liver cancers. Semin Surg Oncol 9:298–304
23. Bruix J, Castells A, Bosch J et al (1996) Surgical resection of hepatocellular carcinoma in cirrhotic patients: prognostic value of preoperative portal pressure. Gastroenterology 111:1018–1122
24. Eguchi H, Umeshita K, Sakon M et al (2000) Presence of active hepatitis associated with liver cirrhosis is a risk factor for mortality caused by posthepatectomy liver failure. Dig Dis Sci 45:1383–1388
25. Haber MM, West AB, Haber AD, Reuben A (1995) Relationship of aminotransferases to liver histological status in chronic hepatitis C. Am J Gastroenterol 90:1250–1257
26. Healey CJ, Chapman RW, Fleming KA (1995) Liver histology in hepatitis C infection: a comparison between patients with persistently normal or abnormal transaminases. Gut 37:274–278
27. Poon RT, Fan ST, Lo CM, Liu CL, Ng IO, Wong J (2000) Long-term prognosis after resection of hepatocellular carcinoma associated with hepatitis B-related cirrhosis. J Clin Oncol 18:1094–1101
28. Noun R, Jagot P, Farges O, Sauvanet A, Belghiti J (1997) High preoperative serum alanine transferase levels: effect on the risk of liver resection in Child grade A cirrhotic patients. World J Surg 21:390–394
29. Torzilli G, Makuuchi M, Inoue K et al (1999) No-mortality liver resection for hepatocellular carcinoma in cirrhotic and noncirrhotic patients: is there a way? A prospective analysis of our approach. Arch Surg 134:984–992
30. Vauthey JN, Abdalla EK, Doherty DA et al (2002) Body surface area and body weight predict total liver volume in Western adults. Liver Transpl 8:233–240
31. Johnson TN, Tucker GT, Tanner MS, Rostami-Hodjegan A (2005) Changes in liver volume from birth to adulthood: A meta-analysis. Liver Transpl 11:1481–1493
32. Shirabe K, Shimada M, Gion T et al (1999) Postoperative liver failure after major hepatic resection for hepatocellular carcinoma in the modern era with special reference to remnant liver volume. J Am Coll Surg 188:304–309
33. Ribero D, Abdalla EK, Madoff DC, Donadon M, Loyer EM, Vauthey JN (2007) Portal vein embolization before major hepatectomy and its effects on regeneration, resectability and outcome. Br J Surg 94:1386–1394
34. Zorzi D, Laurent A, Pawlik TM, Lauwers GY, Vauthey JN, Abdalla EK (2007) Chemotherapy-associated hepatotoxicity and surgery for colorectal liver metastases. Br J Surg 94:274–286
35. Palavecino M, Chun YS, Madoff DC et al (2009) Major hepatic resection for hepatocellular carcinoma with or without portal vein embolization: Perioperative outcome and survival. Surgery 145:399–405
36. Kokudo N, Tada K, Seki M et al (2001) Proliferative activity of intrahepatic colorectal metastases after preoperative hemihepatic portal vein embolization. Hepatology 34:67–72
37. Nagino M, Nimura Y, Kamiya J, Kanai M, Hayakawa N, Yamamoto H (1998) Immediate increase in arterial blood flow in embolized hepatic segments after portal vein embolization: CT demonstration. AJR Am J Roentgenol 171:1037–1039
38. Ogata S, Belghiti J, Farges O, Varma D, Sibert A, Vilgrain V (2006) Sequential arterial and portal vein embolizations before right hepatectomy in patients with cirrhosis and hepatocellular carcinoma. Br J Surg 93:1091–1098
39. Aoki T, Imamura H, Hasegawa K et al (2004) Sequential preoperative arterial and portal venous embolizations in patients with hepatocellular carcinoma. Arch Surg 2004;139(7):766–774
40. Llovet JM, Ricci S, Mazzaferro V et al (2008) Sorafenib in advanced hepatocellular carcinoma. N Engl J Med 359:378–390

41. Leung TW, Patt YZ, Lau WY et al (1999) Complete pathological remission is possible with systemic combination chemotherapy for inoperable hepatocellular carcinoma. Clin Cancer Res 5:1676–1681
42. Zorzi D, Abdalla EK, Pawlik TM, Brown TD, Vauthey JN (2006) Subtotal hepatectomy following neoadjuvant chemotherapy for a previously unresectable hepatocellular carcinoma. J Hepatobiliary Pancreat Surg 13:347–350
43. Lau WY, Leung TW, Lai BS et al (2001) Preoperative systemic chemoimmunotherapy and sequential resection for unresectable hepatocellular carcinoma. Ann Surg 233:236–241
44. Chang SB, Palavecino M, Wray CJ, Kishi Y, Pisters PW, Vauthey JN (2010) Modified Makuuchi incision for foregut procedures. Arch Surg 145:281–284
45. Kokudo N, Bandai Y, Imanishi H et al (1996) Management of new hepatic nodules detected by intraoperative ultrasonography during hepatic resection for hepatocellular carcinoma. Surgery 119:634–640
46. Takigawa Y, Sugawara Y, Yamamoto J et al (2001) New lesions detected by intraoperative ultrasound during liver resection for hepatocellular carcinoma. Ultrasound Med Biol 27:151–156
47. Torzilli G, Makuuchi M (2003) Intraoperative ultrasonography in liver cancer. Surg Oncol Clin N Am 12:91–103
48. Lau WY, Leung KL, Lee TW, Li AK (1993) Ultrasonography during liver resection for hepatocellular carcinoma. Br J Surg 80:493–494
49. Hasegawa K, Kokudo N, Imamura H, et al (2005) Prognostic impact of anatomic resection for hepatocellular carcinoma. Ann Surg 242:252–259
50. Regimbeau JM, Kianmanesh R, Farges O, Dondero F, Sauvanet A, Belghiti J (2002) Extent of liver resection influences the outcome in patients with cirrhosis and small hepatocellular carcinoma. Surgery 131:311–317
51. Poon RT, Fan ST, Ng IO, Wong J (2000) Significance of resection margin in hepatectomy for hepatocellular carcinoma: a critical reappraisal. Ann Surg 231:544–551
52. Jwo SC, Chiu JH, Chau GY, Loong CC, Lui WY (1992) Risk factors linked to tumor recurrence of human hepatocellular carcinoma after hepatic resection. Hepatology 16:1367–1371
53. Yamamoto J, Kosuge T, Takayama T et al (1996) Recurrence of hepatocellular carcinoma after surgery. Br J Surg 83:1219–1222
54. Cha CH, Ruo L, Fong Y et al (2003) Resection of hepatocellular carcinoma in patients otherwise eligible for transplantation. Ann Surg 238: 315–321
55. Ozawa K (1990) Hepatic function and liver resection. J Gastroenterol Hepatol 5:296–309
56. Liu CL, Fan ST, Lo CM, Tung-Ping Poon R, Wong J (2000) Anterior approach for major right hepatic resection for large hepatocellular carcinoma. Ann Surg 232:25–31
57. Liu CL, Fan ST, Cheung ST, Lo CM, Ng IO, Wong J (2006) Anterior approach versus conventional approach right hepatic resection for large hepatocellular carcinoma: a prospective randomized controlled study. Ann Surg 244:194–203
58. Belghiti J, Guevara OA, Noun R, Saldinger PF, Kianmanesh R (2001) Liver hanging maneuver: a safe approach to right hepatectomy without liver mobilization. J Am Coll Surg 193:109–111
59. Man K, Fan ST, Ng IO, Lo CM, Liu CL, Wong J (1997) Prospective evaluation of Pringle maneuver in hepatectomy for liver tumors by a randomized study. Ann Surg 226:04–11
60. Belghiti J, Noun R, Malafosse R et al (1999) Continuous versus intermittent portal triad clamping for liver resection: a controlled study. Ann Surg 229:369–375
61. Belghiti J, Noun R, Zante E, Ballet T, Sauvanet A (1996) Portal triad clamping or hepatic vascular exclusion for major liver resection. A controlled study. Ann Surg 224:155–161
62. Torzilli G, Makuuchi M, Midorikawa Y et al (2001) Liver resection without total vascular exclusion: hazardous or beneficial? An analysis of our experience. Ann Surg 233: 167–175
63. Johnson M, Mannar R, Wu AV (1998) Correlation between blood loss and inferior vena caval pressure during liver resection. Br J Surg 85:188–190

64. Rees M, Plant G, Wells J, Bygrave S (1996) One hundred and fifty hepatic resections: evolution of technique towards bloodless surgery. Br J Surg 83:1526–1529
65. Cunningham JD, Fong Y, Shriver C, Melendez J, Marx WL, Blumgart LH (1994) One hundred consecutive hepatic resections. Blood loss, transfusion, and operative technique. Arch Surg 129:1050–1056
66. Aloia TA, Zorzi D, Abdalla EK, Vauthey JN (2005) Two-surgeon technique for hepatic parenchymal transection of the noncirrhotic liver using saline-linked cautery and ultrasonic dissection. Ann Surg 242:172–177
67. Takatsuki M, Eguchi S, Yamanouchi K et al (2009) Two-surgeon technique using saline-linked electric cautery and ultrasonic surgical aspirator in living donor hepatectomy: its safety and efficacy. Am J Surg 197, e25–e27
68. El Moghazy WM, Hedaya MS, Kaido T, Egawa H, Uemoto S, Takada Y (2009) Two different methods for donor hepatic transection: cavitron ultrasonic surgical aspirator with bipolar cautery versus cavitron ultrasonic surgical aspirator with radiofrequency coagulator-A randomized controlled trial. Liver Transpl 15:102–105
69. Katz SC, Shia J, Liau KH et al (2009) Operative blood loss independently predicts recurrence and survival after resection of hepatocellular carcinoma. Ann Surg 249:617–623
70. Petrowsky H, Demartines N, Rousson V, Clavien PA (2004) Evidence-based value of prophylactic drainage in gastrointestinal surgery: a systematic review and meta-analyses. Ann Surg 240:1074–1084
71. Liu CL, Fan ST, Lo CM et al (2004) Abdominal drainage after hepatic resection is contraindicated in patients with chronic liver diseases. Ann Surg. 239:194–201
72. Foster JH, Berman MM (1977) Solid Liver Tumors.W. B. Saunders, Philadelphia
73. Jaeck D, Bachellier P, Oussoultzoglou E, Weber JC, Wolf P (2004) Surg.ical resection of hepatocellular carcinoma. Post-operative outcome and long-term results in Europe: an overview. Liver Transpl 10(2 Suppl 1):S58–S63
74. Makuuchi M, Takayama T, Gunven P, Kosuge T, Yamazaki S, Hasegawa H (1989) Restrictive versus liberal blood transfusion policy for hepatectomies in cirrhotic patients. World J Surg. 13:644–648
75. Shimada M, Takenaka K, Fujiwara Y et al (1998) Risk factors linked to postoperative morbidity in patients with hepatocellular carcinoma. Br J Surg. 85:195–198
76. Bismuth H, Majno P, Adam R (1999) Hepatocellular carcinoma: from ethanol injection to liver transplantation. Acta Gastroenterologica Belgica 62:330–341
77. Capussotti L, Borgonovo G, Bouzari H, Smadja C, Grange D, Franco D (1994) Results of major hepatectomy for large primary liver cancer in patients with cirrhosis. Br J Surg. 81:427–431
78. Belghiti J, Panis Y, Farges O, Benhamou JP, Fekete F (1991) Intrahepatic recurrence after resection of hepatocellular carcinoma complicating cirrhosis. Ann Surg. 214:114–117
79. Nagasue N, Kohno H, Chang YC et al (1993) Liver resection for hepatocellular carcinoma. Results of 229 consecutive patients during 11 years. Ann Surg. 217:375–384
80. Suenaga M, Sugiura H, Kokuba Y, Uehara S, Kurumiya T (1994) Repeated hepatic resection for recurrent hepatocellular carcinoma in eighteen cases. Surg.ery 115:452–457
81. Kakazu T, Makuuchi M, Kawasaki S et al (1993) Repeat hepatic resection for recurrent hepatocellular carcinoma. Hepatogastroenterology 40:337–341
82. Matsuda Y, Ito T, Oguchi Y, Nakajima K, Izukura T (1993) Rationale of surg.ical management for recurrent hepatocellular carcinoma. Ann Surg. 217:28–34
83. Shimada M, Takenaka K, Taguchi K et al (1998) Prognostic factors after repeat hepatectomy for recurrent hepatocellular carcinoma. Ann Surg. 227:80–85
84. Arii S, Monden K, Niwano M et al (1998) Results of surg.ical treatment for recurrent hepatocellular carcinoma; comparison of outcome among patients with multicentric carcinogenesis, intrahepatic metastasis, and extrahepatic recurrence. J Hepatobiliary Pancreat Surg. 5:86–92

85. Minagawa M, Makuuchi M, Takayama T, Kokudo N (2003) Selection criteria for repeat hepatectomy in patients with recurrent hepatocellular carcinoma. Ann Surg. 238:703–710

86. Shimada K, Sakamoto Y, Esaki M et al (2007) Analysis of prognostic factors affecting survival after initial recurrence and treatment efficacy for recurrence in patients undergoing potentially curative hepatectomy for hepatocellular carcinoma. Ann Surg. Oncol 14:2337–2347

87. The Liver Cancer Study Group of Japan (1994) Predictive factors for long-term prognosis after partial hepatectomy for patients with hepatocellular carcinoma in Japan. Cancer 74:2772–2780

88. Bismuth H, Chiche L, Adam R, Castaing D, Diamond T, Dennison A (1993) Liver resection versus transplantation for hepatocellular carcinoma in cirrhotic patients. Ann Surg. 218: 145–151

89. Jonas S, Herrmann M, Rayes N et al (2001) Survival after liver transplantation for hepatocellular carcinoma in cirrhosis according to the underlying liver disease. Transplant Proc 33:3444–3445

90. Poon RT, Fan ST, Lo CM, Liu CL, Wong J (2002) Long-term survival and pattern of recurrence after resection of small hepatocellular carcinoma in patients with preserved liver function: implications for a strategy of salvage transplantation. Ann Surg. 235:373–382

91. Fisher RA, Maroney TP, Fulcher AS et al (2002) Hepatocellular carcinoma: strategy for optimizing surg.ical resection, transplantation and palliation. Clin Transplant 16 (Suppl 7):52–58

92. Majno PE, Sarasin FP, Mentha G, Hadengue A (2000) Primary liver resection and salvage transplantation or primary liver transplantation in patients with single, small hepatocellular carcinoma and preserved liver function: an outcome-oriented decision analysis. Hepatology 31:899–906

93. Otto G, Heuschen U, Hofmann WJ, Krumm G, Hinz U, Herfarth C (1998) Survival and recurrence after liver transplantation versus liver resection for hepatocellular carcinoma: a retrospective analysis. Ann Surg. 227:424–432

94. Yamamoto J, Iwatsuki S, Kosuge T et al (1999) Should hepatomas be treated with hepatic resection or transplantation? Cancer 86:1151–1158

95. Belghiti J, Cortes A, Abdalla EK et al (2003) Resection prior to liver transplantation for hepatocellular carcinoma. Ann Surg. 238:885–892

96. Vauthey JN, Klimstra D, Franceschi D et al (1995) Factors affecting long-term outcome after hepatic resection for hepatocellular carcinoma. Am J Surg. 169:28–34

97. Nagorney DM, Adson MA, Weiland LH, Knight CD, Jr., Smalley SR, Zinsmeister AR (1985) Fibrolamellar hepatoma. Am J Surg. 149,:113–119

98. Soreide O, Czerniak A, Bradpiece H, Bloom S, Blumgart L (1986). Characteristics of fibrolamellar hepatocellular carcinoma. A study of nine cases and a review of the literature. Am J Surg. 151:518–523

99. Okuda K (2002) Natural history of hepatocellular carcinoma including fibrolamellar and hepato-cholangiocarcinoma variants. J Gastroenterol Hepatol 17:401–405

100. Hemming AW, Langer B, Sheiner P, Greig PD, Taylor BR (1997) Aggressive surg.ical management of fibrolamellar hepatocellular carcinoma. J Gastrointest Surg. 1:342–346

101. Ringe B, Wittekind C, Weimann A, Tusch G, Pichlmayr R (1992) Results of hepatic resection and transplantation for fibrolamellar carcinoma. Surg. Gynecol Obstet 175:299–305

102. El-Gazzaz G, Wong W, El-Hadary MK et al (2000) Outcome of liver resection and transplantation for fibrolamellar hepatocellular carcinoma. Transpl Int 13 (Suppl 1):S406–S409

103. Pinna AD, Iwatsuki S, Lee RG et al (1997) Treatment of fibrolamellar hepatoma with subtotal hepatectomy or transplantation. Hepatology 26(4):877–883

104. Neuhaus P, Jonas S, Bechstein WO (2000) Hepatoma of the liver–resection or transplantation? Langenbecks Arch Surg. 385:171–178

105. Patt YZ, Hassan MM, Lozano RD et al (2003) Phase II trial of systemic continuous flurorouracil and subcutaneous recombinant interferon Alfa-2b for treatment of hepatocellular carcinoma. J Clin Oncol 21:421–427

Chapter 10
Ultrasound-Guided Liver Resection for Hepatocellular Carcinoma

Guido Torzilli

Keywords Hepatic surgery · Ultrasound-guided percutaneous therapies · Liver resection · Contrast-enhanced Ultrasonography performed intraoperatively

Introduction

Hepatic surgery performed without a parenchyma-sparing policy carries relevant risks for patients' survival due to the not negligible occurrence of postoperative liver failure. In particular, the coexistence of liver cirrhosis in most cases of hepatocellular carcinoma (HCC) has a considerable adverse effect on the surgical results. As a matter of fact, recent series are still associated with mortality rates above 5%, which is not negligible [1]. For this reason and for the broadening of ultrasound-guided percutaneous therapies [2], the role of surgical treatment of HCC as the first-choice treatment is now reserved only for patients with normal bilirubin level, no signs of portal hypertension, and moreover carriers of single small HCC [3]. Imaging techniques also have been introduced as aids for surgeons in performing liver resection. In fact, since the early 1980s, intraoperative ultrasonography (IOUS) has been used to guide hepatic surgery in patients with liver cirrhosis [4]. Now, liver resections can be carried out with no mortality, even if cirrhosis is associated, combining the needs for oncological radicality and liver parenchyma sparing. This goal is mainly achievable because of IOUS [5, 6]. Recently, the demonstration of the feasibility and efficacy of contrast-enhanced ultrasonography performed intraoperatively (CE-IOUS) has further stressed the relevance of IOUS guidance during liver surgery [7, 8]. In this chapter, technical aspects of IOUS and the impact of this tool during surgery for HCC for both staging and resection guidance are discussed.

G. Torzilli (✉)
Department of Surgery, Istituto Clinico Humanitas IRCCS, University of Milan, School of Medicine, Milan, Italy

K.M. McMasters, J.-N. Vauthey (eds.), *Hepatocellular Carcinoma*,
DOI 10.1007/978-1-60327-522-4_10, © Springer Science+Business Media, LLC 2011

Technical Aspects

For a proper IOUS, high-frequency echoprobes (7.5–10 MHz) are necessary and should have a flat shape to allow their management in deep and narrow spaces. For this purpose, T-shaped probes, interdigital probes, and microconvex probes are available. Main factors for probe selection are its volume, its stability, and the wideness of the ultrasonographic scanning window: the best probe should be small, thin in width, and short in transverse length, stable, and with a wide ultrasonographic scanning window. In this sense the microconvex probe represents the best compromise among all these requirements. Indeed, the T-shaped probe is more stable but has a lower ratio between lateral length and ultrasonographic scanning window than the microconvex one. Linear transducers with enlarged scanning windows are also available now: in the future this solution may combine stability with larger scanning windows (Fig. 10.1).

For CEIOUS, we use a convex 3–6 MHz frequency and 1.88–3.76 MHz harmonic frequency transducer from Aloka (Aloka Co., Tokyo, Japan). Once CEIOUS is needed, 4.8 mL sulphur-hexafluoride microbubbles (SonoVue®, Bracco Imaging, Italy) is injected intravenously through a peripheral vein by the anesthesiologist. For HCC, CEIOUS is used for characterizing the new lesions eventually detected

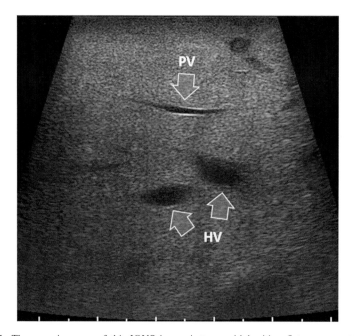

Fig. 10.1 The scanning area of this IOUS image is trapezoidal with a flat upper part that represents the contact area between the probe and the liver and a scanning window which enlarges as it gets deeper. It is also evident, how at IOUS, the portal vein (PV) and the hepatic vein (HV) have different thicknesses of their walls: in particular the wall of the portal branch is thicker, as commonly happens

at IOUS [7]: the rationale is to check the vascular pattern during contrast enhancement of each new lesion. Because in the case of HCC it is very important to identify the arterial vascularization, which lasts from 20–30 sec, each nodule has to be carefully evaluated and this demands multiple injections in the presence of multiple nodules. This may no longer be a necessity once the new hepato-specific contrast agents become commercially available for clinical use (for the moment available only in Japan): indeed, behaving as the hepato-specific contrast medium used in magnetic resonance does, they could provide new criteria for nodule differentiation. Furthermore, the contrast enhancement remains visible from several minutes to even hours after injection, thus CEIOUS should gain that panoramicity and reduce the need for reinjections. These features make their use extremely promising and begin further scenarios for the application of CEIOUS in patients who undergo surgery for HCC.

Ultrasound Liver Anatomy

A background of perfect knowledge of the liver anatomy surgically and ultrasonographically is needed in order to perform IOUS properly. For surgical anatomy, Brisbane Terminology is considered here [9]. After entering into the abdominal cavity, liver mobilization dividing the round and falciform ligaments, and division of eventual adhesions to free the antero-superior and inferior surfaces of the liver are the steps that should precede the liver exploration with IOUS. Of course, adhesions with other organs or structures should not be divided in the event there is the possibility that they are expressions of tumor infiltration: in this eventuality, IOUS could be helpful for ruling out or confirming the tumor invasion and then changing the surgical strategy accordingly.

By pulling the round ligament, the liver surface is widely exposed and following the portal branches and the hepatic veins, the liver can be studied in its entirety. The probe should be managed using enough pressure to ensure good contact with the liver surface but not to compress the intrahepatic vascular structures and in particular the hepatic vein. The three main hepatic veins are readily identified at their junction with the inferior vena cava (IVC) positioning the probe at this level and tilting it upward once the confluence of the hepatic veins into the IVC is recognized. Then gently withdrawing the probe, the hepatic vein paths can be traced into the liver. Hepatic veins appear as echofree zones into the liver parenchyma with the vessel wall which appears as a thin hyperechogenic line (Fig. 10.1): hepatic vein wall thickness can be larger in the cirrhotic liver and its lumen thinner in function of the hard stiffness of the organ.

The portal vein branches can be followed first positioning the probe horizontally above the segment 4 inferior to visualize the first-order bifurcation and then first-, second-, and third-order portal branches can be followed with the probe. Because of the existence of the Glisson's capsule, the portal pedicles, which run together with the arteries and the bile ducts, have thicker vessel walls compared with the hepatic vein and for this reason they appear at IOUS as echofree zones surrounded by a thicker hyperechogenic layer (Fig. 10.1); furthermore, other parallel thinner vascular structures are visible, namely the arteries and bile ducts of the Glissonian triad. However, in principle, distinction between hepatic veins and portal branches should be based not only on their appearance but mainly on their anatomy: indeed in the cirrhotic liver, as already mentioned, the vessel wall of the hepatic vein could be thicker and not immediately differentiable from a peripheral portal branch. Following the portal pedicles at the sectional, segmental, and subsegmental levels and positioning it in relation to the hepatic vein it is possible to precisely define the location of the IOUS target in terms of sections and segments.

The appearance of bile ducts at IOUS is worthwhile mentioning because of their peculiarity. Indeed, normally they result as thin echofree zones in the Glissonian triad. Once dilated they appear more evidently as echofree zones and with a serpiginous path pattern. The element that is difficult to recognize in the IOUS study of the bile ducts is their segmental anatomy. Indeed, bifurcation of sectional and segmental ducts is closer to the hilum compared with the portal branches and for that it is possible with one scan to visualize more than a segmental bile duct. If this fact is not considered it could be more difficult to address which part of the liver is not well drained. Conversely, if recognized, IOUS could allow the exact definition of the bile duct anatomy both in normal and pathological conditions.

Indications

The use of IOUS in liver resections can be schematically divided into three principal phases: the liver exploration for the staging of the disease, the planning of the surgical strategy, and the guidance of the surgical maneuvers.

Liver Exploration

The hard and irregular surface of a cirrhotic liver makes the detection of small nodules by palpation difficult; IOUS allows the detection of new lesions in around 30% of cases [10]. However, most of the nodules detected by IOUS in the cirrhotic liver are not really tumors: in this way, IOUS introduces the risk of overestimating the tumor stage. Indeed, except for those nodules with mosaic ultrasonographic pattern (Fig. 10.2a) that are malignant in 84% of cases, only 24–30% of hypoechogenic (dark) nodules (Fig. 10.2b), and 0–18% of those hyperechogenic (bright) (Fig. 10.2c) are neoplasm [10, 11]. To overcome this problem even biopsy seems inadequate. The only nodule that can be easily differentiated intraoperatively from a HCC or liver metastases is the small hemangioma which is often discovered primarily at IOUS; it has a typical ultrasonographic pattern, and moreover when compressed changes its size and appearance. Therefore, the problem of the differentiation of the lesions depicted at IOUS exploration becomes crucial. Further

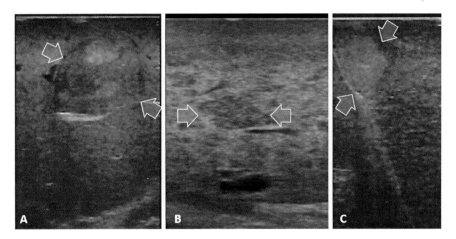

Fig. 10.2 (**a**) A mosaic pattern lesion at IOUS (*arrows*); (**b**) a hypoechogenic lesion at IOUS (*arrows*); (**c**) a hyperechogenic lesion at IOUS (*arrows*)

improvement in differential diagnosis of liver nodules with IOUS may be expected with the introduction and diffusion of the intraoperative use of the last-generation contrast agents.

Contrast-Enhanced Intraoperative Ultrasonography

More recently the introduction of CE-IOUS has set the rate for modified operative decision making on 30–40% of cases [7, 8]. Tumor vascularity as a criterion for differentiating the regenerative or dysplastic nodules from the HCC correlates well with the histological evidence of a progressive increase in unpaired arteries from dysplastic to neoplastic nodules in a cirrhotic liver [12]. Certainly, the pattern of vascular enhancement is insufficient for differentiating malignant from nonmalignant nodules in a cirrhotic liver with 100% specificity. However, CE-US provides differential diagnosis of FLL with a 95% specificity rate [13]; of course, it must be considered that this last rate referred to another type of lesion when compared to the CEIOUS target. Indeed, the intraoperative exploration takes advantage of the higher resolution of the ultrasonography done in direct contact with the liver. Therefore, the need for differentiating nodules detected at IOUS is mostly focused on lesions smaller than 1 cm: for these nodules the vascularity as the criterion for differential diagnosis is less specific. However, some improvements compared with conventional IOUS could be expected. For this reason, in the early 1990s attempts were made to use CE-IOUS with carbon dioxide as the contrast material for IOUS, however, the need for arterial catheterization made this technique too invasive [14].

In our preliminary experience CE-IOUS provided remarkable findings, either by adding information on nodular vascularity in patients with HCC, or by detecting nodules that were not visible at IOUS, in patients with colorectal cancer liver mctastascs [8]. Focusing attention on patients operated on for HCC specificity of CEIOUS is around 69% [7]. This value is probably not that high especially when compared with that reported for CE-US [13]. However, as we mentioned before, the small size of the lesions targeted for CEIOUS study could explain this discrepancy: for these tiny nodules the neovascularity as criterion for differentiation between malignant and benign lesions has limits independent from the method we use for studying them. Therefore, CEIOUS can be helpful in a certain percentage of nodules but not in all: in this perspective the rate of 69% of specificity is encouraging as it means that we can provide proper information with this new technique in seven out of ten lesions we detect at the time of laparotomy. For the remaining three, even histology may be lacking as we know that there is no common agreement among Western and Eastern pathologists on the definition of early HCC and dysplastic lesions [12, 15]. A new perspective in this sense will certainly be provided by a more extensive use of the new contrast agent, at the moment only clinically available in Japan [16]. This agent, having a Kupffer phase adds a further criterion for differentiating those nodules detected at IOUS, and for disclosing others eventually missed at IOUS; in this sense this new contrast agent mimics the contrast agents used with magnetic resonance.

In practice, at CEIOUS we can follow in real-time the enhancement of the liver parenchyma with vessels appearing hyperechogenic instead of the echofree pattern at the unenhanced US. Any lesion with a pathological behavior appearing as hypoechogenic with or without inner vessels and with or without an arterial phase in which it is enhanced prior to the remaining liver parenchyma is removed (Fig. 10.3). Those lesions that disappear once the contrast enhances the liver are not considered neoplastic, and thus are not removed.

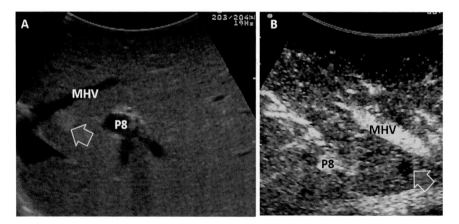

Fig. 10.3 (**a**) At IOUS a small hyperechogenic nodule is found (*arrows*) close to the middle hepatic vein (MHV) and the segment 8 main portal branch (P8); (**b**) at CE-IOUS, the black hole (*arrows*) of that nodule in the late phase is evident showing a pathological pattern

Planning of the Surgical Strategy

IOUS exploration of the liver could have a great impact on the surgical strategy; however, more recently the impact of IOUS on operative decision making, when compared with those of preoperative imaging techniques, is reported to be just around 4–7% [17, 18]. The problem of the impact of IOUS on the operative decision making depends on two main factors: the surgical policy of each specific team and the type of tumor. Indeed, the relatively low rates reported [17, 18] are also partially motivated by the surgeon's surgical policy: in fact, because a considerable number of patients undergo major hepatectomies, new nodules detected by IOUS in the same hemiliver would not have modified the surgical strategy. Recently, it has been shown how major hepatectomies are carried out in the minority of patients [5, 6] just because of the extensive use of the IOUS guidance for achieving parenchymal-sparing resections, so that detection of new nodules is more suitable for changing the surgical strategy. IOUS allows an accurate three-dimensional reconstruction of the relationship among the tumor, the portal branches, and hepatic veins; this is a fundamental step in the definition of the proper surgical strategy. Indeed, surgical decision making should be obtained having portal branches and hepatic veins as landmarks to reduce the risk of major morbidity and mortality.

Definition of the tumor–vessels relationship is relevant for planning the type of resection, and based on that, specific and original operations can be performed [5, 6]. IOUS easily allows the surgeon to recognize if an HCC is separated by some normal parenchyma from the vessel, if it is in contact with the vessel without invading its wall (Fig. 10.4), or conversely if the HCC is invading the vessel wall, is determining the proximal bile duct dilation, or if it is associated with a tumor thrombus.

Extension of the hepatectomy is always considered for the parenchyma fed by infiltrated portal branch at IOUS [5]: vein Glissonian triad invasion is considered in the presence of portal or biliary tumor thrombus, in the absence of vessel wall visualization, or in the case of HCC in contact with the Glissonian triad with proximal bile duct dilation. Inversely, in the case of infiltration of a hepatic vein, an extension of the resection to the whole liver parenchyma theoretically drained by this vein is considered only if one of the following ultrasonographic signs is missing:

- Presence of accessory hepatic veins at IOUS
- Color-Doppler IOUS showing hepatopetal blood flow in the feeding portal branch once the hepatic vein is clamped [7] by means of encirclement more simply by vein compression at its extrahepatic route using the fingertip as described later
- Communicating veins connecting adjacent hepatic veins (Fig. 10.5)

Adopting these criteria we have been able to minimize the rate of major hepatectomy and to devise new procedures. One of them is the Systematic Extended Right Posterior Sectionectomy (SERPS) as an alternative to right hemihepatectomy [19]. Another new procedure that can be accomplished adopting the aforementioned criteria is the so-called minimesohepatectomy [20]. This last represents an alternative to the conventional mesohepatectomy in the case of tumors invading the middle

Fig. 10.4 This patient was a
carrier of a HCC in contact
(*arrows*) with the right
hepatic vein (RHV), which
maintains intact its wall
represented by an
hyperechogenic layer. P6–7
= portal branch to segments 6
and 7

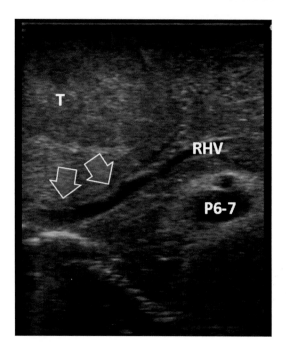

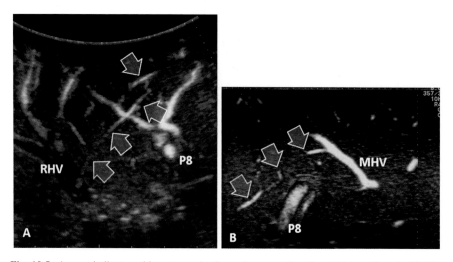

Fig. 10.5 *Arrows* indicate a thin communicating vein connecting the right hepatic vein (RHV)
(**a**) with the middle hepatic vein (MHV) (**b**). This vein has been disclosed compressing the RHV
(**a**): the latter has no flow (*color*) inside whereas flow directed from RHV to MHV (*red color* means
upward, towards the probe, direction of the flow) is shown in the communicating vein (**a,b**), and
flow directed toward the inferior vena cava (*blue color* means downward, opposite to the probe,
direction of the flow) is shown inside the MHV (**b**). P8 = portal branch to segment 8

hepatic vein at its caval confluence, and consists in a limited resection including the tract of the invaded vein without its reconstruction.

Resection Guidance

Systematic Segmentectomy

In a cirrhotic patient, the liver volume to be resected must be determined with particular care with the purpose of associating surgical radicality and noncancerous liver parenchyma sparing. Liver function tests and liver volumetry on CT scans help in this decision. Tumor dissemination from the main lesion through the portal branches cannot be detected with certainty by the pre- and intraoperative imaging modalities [21]. Consequently, some authors consider that the resected specimen should comprise at least the portal area, which includes the lesion [21]. This last is impossible to be correctly identified without the aid of IOUS, especially in a cirrhotic liver where there are generally wide variations and abnormalities in the distributions of the portal branches. For this purpose systematic segmentectomy was devised in the early 1980s [4], and we have recent alternatives to this approach.

Compression of the Portal Branch

Initially used for tumors located in the left hemiliver [22], recently we have successfully extended the application of this technique to any segmental location [23], and even to a sectional portion of the liver [24]. Once the feeding portal branch has been identified at IOUS, it is compressed using the IOUS probe at one side of the liver and the finger at the opposite side (Fig. 10.6a–c): in this way it is possible to induce a transient ischemia of the portion of the liver distal to the compression site. This portion can be marked with the electrocautery, the compression released, and the resection carried out. This technique is simple, fast, noninvasive, and reversible: the possibility to modify the site of compression and then the resection volume allows us

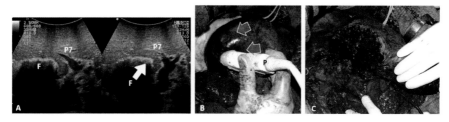

Fig. 10.6 (a) The portal branch to segment 7 (P7) is visualized at IOUS on the left and the surgeon's finger is positioned (F), and P7 is compressed on the right (*arrow*); (b) the hepatic ischemic area generated by compression with the surgeon's finger and probe (P), which corresponds to the area to be resected is well evident on the liver surface (*arrows*); (c) the cut surface at the end of the segment 7 segmentectomy

to size the resection in the function of the tumor features and the status of the background liver. Furthermore, the compression can be used in a countercompression perspective [23, 24], borrowing the philosophy proposed by Takayama et al. of defining the adjacent segmental margins to disclose those of the targeted segment which was applied by the author for segment 1 resection using the portal branch puncture technique [25]. Indeed for segments such as 8 and 4 superior for which the direct compression of the feeding portal branch could be infeasible, compressing the adjacent segmental branch allows the definition of their segmental margins [23]. Similarly, this technique can be applied to disclose the margin of the right anterior section of the liver by compressing the Glissonian pedicles to the right posterior section and to the left hemiliver, respectively [24]. For this last it avoids the need of portal pedicle dissection or blunt encirclement resulting in a simpler, safer, and equally anatomical procedure [26–28].

Hooking of the Portal Branch

The segmental portal branches to segment 4 are generally divided in two groups, those for the superior and those for the inferior portion, but the most common branching pattern can be recognized in just half the cases [29]. These branches rather than being punctured, under IOUS guidance can be approached dissecting the umbilical portion: once exposed the vessel can be encircled with a suture and pulled under IOUS control to verify if it is the branch to segment 4 inferior or not. Then the proper portal branch can be ligated and divided and the discolored area that will appear on the liver surface should correspond to the segment 4 inferior which can be marked with the electrocautery to proceed with the liver dissection; this is a peculiar application of the so-called hooking technique [30]. Furthermore, the subsegment 4 superior could be resected just clamping the portal branch to the subsegment 4 inferior, as it is identified with the just-described hooking technique; the discolored subsegment 4 inferior caudally, the plan at IOUS which includes the middle hepatic vein laterally, and that marked by the falciform ligament medially, delimit the area to be resected.

Limited Resection

The anatomical versus nonanatomical surgical approach for HCC is still a controversial issue [21, 31–36], inasmuch as there are no really randomized studies comparing the two different operations. However, recent reports seem to confirm adequacy in terms of oncological radicality of limited resections for HCC once IOUS is extensively used [5, 6, 31, 36]. The IOUS-guided limited resection is simpler than the systematic segmentectomy because there is no need for identifying the area of the liver fed by the portal branch to be ligated, although nowadays, with the compression technique, there could be no more need for puncturing the portal branches or dissecting the pedicles. Indeed, for limited resection, once the tumor is identified, the surgeon under IOUS control can mark with the electrocautery the border of the lesion and that of the area to be removed on the surface of the liver. To carry out this maneuver the flat and thin tip of the electrocautery is positioned between the probe and the liver surface: this maneuver results in a shadow at the IOUS image which runs deeply just below the electrocautery. In this way it is possible to define the position of the electrocautery with the tumor edge and consequently to mark with the electrocautery itself the nodule profile on the liver surface and select the safer edge for the incision. Furthermore, the adequacy of the marked edge can be checked with IOUS as the air trapped between the probe and the irregular surface of the demarcation line drawn with the electrocautery on the liver surface can be visualized at IOUS.

Another way to draw precisely on the liver surface with the aid of IOUS the tumor edge is carried out using the fingertips. With the probe positioned on the liver surface the surgeon's fingertip pushes on the opposite side and its profile is visualized at IOUS: as a consequence the relation between the fingertip and the tumor edge can be precisely estimated and the resection area can be marked on the liver surface.

The main target to be obtained once the resection area is drawn on the liver surface is that of achieving at the end of the dissection the flattest and most regular cut surface.

Liver Parenchyma Dissection

The main advantage provided by the resection guidance accomplished with the aid of IOUS is the modification of the traditional way to dissect the liver tissue, which was done on vertical planes to avoid tumor exposure on the cut surface. IOUS allows to follow in real-time the dissection plane, to put it constantly in relation to the tumor edge, and then to modify its direction when needed. This is because it is possible to visualize on the IOUS image the dissection plane which appears as an echogenic line due to the entrapment of air bubbles and clots between the faced cut surfaces (Fig. 10.7). If the dissection plane is not clearly visible, it can be better visualized inserting a gauze or a specifically devised silicon gauze between the faced cut surfaces. These techniques allow the surgeon to keep the proper dissection plane: an early recognition of a wrong dissection plane permits to modify it properly, and to avoid a possible tumor exposure. In this way it is possible to carry out a rounded trajectory of the dissection plane around the tumor avoiding its exposure, and allowing to spare important vascular structures; this results in more conservative but radical treatments and in a lower rate of major hepatectomies.

The artifacts which allow to show the dissection plan at IOUS could sometimes mask structures such as portal branches that should be ligated or conversely respected. For this reason, to better visualize the targeted point where the portal branch should be divided, the so-called hooking technique has been devised [30]. When the Glissonian sheath is exposed and skeletonized, it is encircled with a stitch, which is visualized by IOUS as an echogenic spot with a posterior shadow. Then under sonographic control, the stitch, hooking the exposed vessel, is gently pulled up, which stretches the portal branch slightly and the traction point is shown clearly by IOUS. If the exposed portal branch is not clearly visible because it has collapsed, the portal triad is unclamped to enable it to fill with blood and then it is better

Fig. 10.7 The dissection line (DL) can be well visualized (*arrows*) at IOUS, and it runs towards the tumor (T)

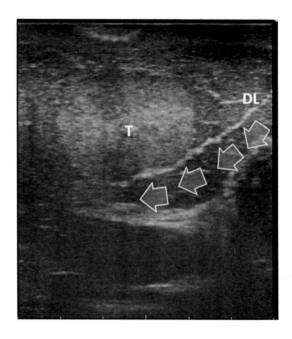

visualized by IOUS. If the target site is correct, the portal branch is ligated and divided and segmentectomy is completed under IOUS guidance; conversely, if the exposed vessel was not the targeted one, it is spared and useless sacrifice of further liver parenchyma is avoided.

A practical example in which the hooking technique is used is during ventral or dorsal subsegmentectomy of segment 8. The portal trunk to this segment may show bifurcation in its dorsal branch and ventral trunk just close to the origin of the portal vessel to segment 5. In this situation, there is the risk of ligating and dividing the portal branch of segment 5 instead of the planned subsegmental branch of segment 8 and then, necrosis of segment 5 may occur. The hooking technique under IOUS control enables the identification of the branch, which was encircled, and then the surgeon can decide with certainty whether to ligate it. This technique is also useful in the case of tumor thrombus in major portal branches. In this situation, once the portal branch is skeletonized, it is encircled with a stitch and, under IOUS control, the stitch is gently pulled up; this traction stretches the portal branch slightly and the traction point is shown clearly by IOUS (Fig. 10.8). If the traction point is not at the level of the tumor thrombus it is possible to ligate the portal branch and proceed with the liver resection being sure that the thrombus will not migrate because of surgical manipulation.

During liver dissection the backflow bleeding from the hepatic veins is an important source of blood loss, and it is one of the most important factors in determining the short- and long-term outcome for the patient. Therefore, limiting the backflow bleeding from the hepatic veins is a priority in liver resections. An ultrasound-guided technique for backflow bleeding control from the right hepatic vein (RHV)

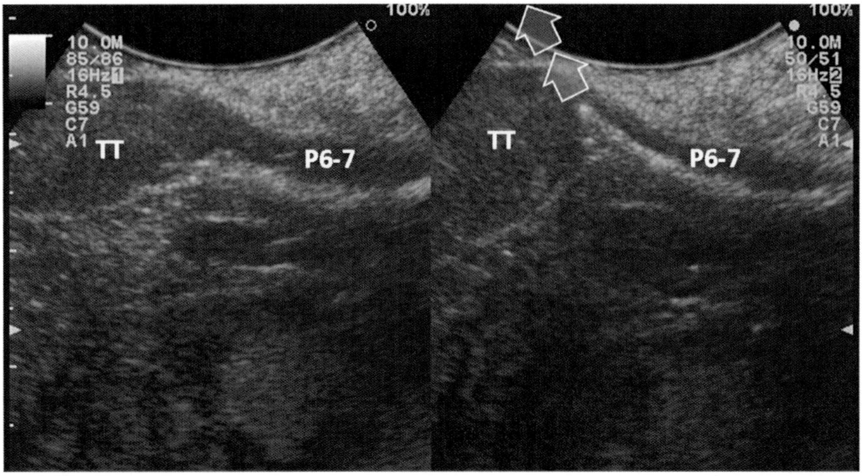

Fig. 10.8 On the left, the portal branch to segments 5 and 8 (P5–8) is occupied by a tumor thrombus (TT) approaching its origin; at this level P5–8 is encircled. On the right, traction is applied (*arrows*) pulling up the stitch and at IOUS the level of the traction does not involve the tumor thrombus; therefore, P5–8 can be safely ligated at that level. P6–7: portal branch to segments 6 and 7

during right-sided liver resection has been recently described [37]. The technique is very simple and is now applied to every hepatic vein. Once the hepatocaval confluence is exposed anteriorly, dissection proceeds until the right surface of the extrahepatic RHV is exposed in case the RHV has to be controlled, the left surface of the extrahepatic left hepatic vein (LHV) for the LHV itself, and the right-anterior surface of the middle hepatic vein (MHV) for the MHV itself. The surgeon's fingertips compress the vessel at the exposed side, and the effectiveness of finger compression is checked by IOUS, and color-Doppler.

Postresectional Control

There are two possibilities given by IOUS after nodule removal: one is the "water bath" technique which consists in the real-time control of the proper resection of the targeted nodule verifying its complete inclusion in the specimen just removed from the liver [38]; the second is done checking the cut surface refilled with saline to avoid the artifacts generated by the residual air bubbles and clots.

Major Hepatectomy

In those patients in which major resections are needed with removal of at least three adjacent segments, IOUS allows us to better achieve the proper dissection plane, which should run along the hepatic vein to be fully anatomic. Color-Doppler is a useful aid in these patients because it helps verify the preserved vascular supply of the liver to be spared, before ligation of the vessels skeletonized at the hepatic hilum. Furthermore, color-Doppler IOUS allows the proper positioning of the remaining liver till the in- and outflow are proper in terms of velocity and waveform [39].

Conclusions

IOUS still remains the best method for staging liver involvement by the tumor, and it has been discussed how new improvements are expected by adding the CEIOUS with the aim of ameliorating the specificity of ultrasound exploration. IOUS is certainly the best method for the surgeon to understand the liver anatomy and the relations between tumors and intrahepatic vessels. This information is crucial for planning the resection and in this sense IOUS probably has the most important role guiding the surgeon's hand in real-time during the liver parenchyma dissection. The aforementioned methods for performing an IOUS-guided resection guarantee whenever possible both anatomical and limited resection with a radical intent: this has consequences for the effectiveness of the surgical treatment as well as for its safety. Indeed, this kind of surgery allows radical surgical treatment of HCC without mortality. Procedures that are not IOUS-guided lead to dangerous and useless major resection or incomplete operations. Inversely, IOUS tumor-vessel classification and the related surgical policy have proven that in selected patients it is possible to get close to the tumor burden without increasing the risk of incomplete removal and, consequently, of local recurrence [5, 6]. In practice this evidence means that with IOUS guidance it is possible to perform conservative but radical hepatectomies also in complex presentations, and then to enlarge the surgical indications. With this approach the rate of major hepatectomies has been limited to up to 8% in patients with tumors involving one or more hepatic veins close to their caval confluence, without performing any vascular reconstruction [6]. These results not only underline how IOUS guidance allows otherwise infeasible operations but, just because this approach reduces the rate of major hepatectomies, there can be discussion of the real need for interventions such as preoperative portal vein embolization which are adopted to secure the patient from liver failure after major removal of liver parenchyma.

Nowadays, it can be affirmed that liver resection is an imaging-guided procedure and as with every interventional imaging-guided procedure, its features are the highest therapeutic efficacy combined with minimal invasiveness. With IOUS aid it is nowadays possible to carry out surgical procedures comparatively safely, oncologically radical, and conservative for the liver function. Mostly because of that, surgery can still be considered the treatment of choice for most liver tumors. For this purpose, IOUS should be a familiar instrument for hepatic surgeons. The American College of Surgeons has recently recognized the need for surgeons with specific training in US, and similarly a School for Surgical Ultrasonography has been started in Europe; meanwhile dedicated monographs have been published almost simultaneously in America and in Europe [40, 41]. The way for a wider diffusion of ultrasound in the surgeon's practice has been definitely opened.

References

1. Liu CL, Fan ST, Lo CM, Wong Y, Ng IO, Lam CM, Poon RT, Wong J (2004) Abdominal drainage after hepatic resection is contraindicated in patients with chronic liver diseases. Ann Surg 239:194–201

2. Livraghi T, Giorgio A, Marin G et al (1995) Hepatocellular carcinoma and cirrhosis in 746 patients: long-term results of percutaneous ethanol injection. Radiology 197:101–108

3. Bruix J, Sherman M (2005) Practice Guidelines Committee, American Association for the Study of Liver Diseases. Management of hepatocellular carcinoma. Hepatology 42: 1208–1236

4. Makuuchi M, Yamazaki S, Hasegawa H et al (1980) Ultrasonically guided liver surgery. Jpn J Ultrasonics in Med 7:45–49

5. Torzilli G, Montorsi M, Donadon M et al (2005) "Radical but conservative" is the main goal for ultrasonography-guided liver resection: prospective validation of this approach. J Am Coll Surg 201:517–528

6. Torzilli G, Montorsi M, Del Fabbro D, Palmisano A, Donadon M, Makuuchi M (2006) Ultrasonographically guided surgical approach to liver tumors involving the hepatic veins close to the caval confluence. Br J Surg 93:1238–246

7. Torzilli G, Palmisano A, Del Fabbro D et al (2007) Contrast-enhanced intraoperative ultra-sonography during surgery for hepatocellular carcinoma in liver cirrhosis: is it useful or useless? A prospective cohort study of our experience. Ann Surg Oncol 14:1347–1355

8. Torzilli G, Del Fabbro D, Olivari N, Calliada F, Montorsi M, Makuuchi M (2004) Contrast-enhanced ultrasonography during liver surgery. Br J Surg 91:1165–1167

9. Terminology Committee of the International Hepato-Pancreato-Biliary Association (2000) The Brisbane 2000 Terminology of Liver Anatomy and Resections. HPB 2:333–339

10. Kokudo N, Bandai Y, Imanishi H et al (1996) Management of new hepatic nodules detected by intraoperative ultrasonography during hepatic resection for hepatocellular carcinoma. Surgery 119:634–640

11. Takigawa Y, Sugawara Y, Yamamoto J et al (2001) New lesions detected by intraopera-tive ultrasound during liver resection for hepatocellular carcinoma. Ultrasound Med Biol 27: 151–156

12. Roncalli M, Roz E, Coggi G et al (1999) The vascular profile of regenerative and dysplas-tic nodules of the cirrhotic liver: implications for diagnosis and classification. Hepatology 30:1174–1178

13. Quaia E, Calliada F, Bertolotto M et al (2004) Characterization of focal liver lesions with contrast-specific US modes and a sulfur hexafluoride-filled microbubble contrast agent: diagnostic performance and confidence. Radiology 232:420–430

14. Takada T, Yasuda H, Uchiyama K, Hasegawa H, Shikata J (1990) Contrast-enhanced intraoperative ultrasonography of small hepatocellular carcinoma. Surgery 107: 528–532

15. Kojiro M (2004) Focus on dysplastic nodules and early hepatocellular carcinoma: an Eastern point of view. Liver Transpl 10(2 Suppl 1):3–8

16. Hatanaka K, Kudo M, Minami Y et al (2008) Differential diagnosis of hepatic tumors: value of contrast-enhanced harmonic sonography using the newly developed contrast agent, Sonazoid. Intervirology 51(Suppl 1):61–69

17. Jarnagin WR, Bach AM, Winston CB et al (2001) What is the yield of intraoperative ultrasonography during partial hepatectomy for malignant disease? J Am Coll Surg 192: 577–583

18. Cerwenka H, Raith J, Bacher H et al (2003) Is intraoperative ultrasonography dur-ing partial hepatectomy still necessary in the age of magnetic resonance imaging? Hepatogastroenterology 50:1539–1541

19. Torzilli G, Donadon M, Marconi M et al (2008) Systematic extended right posterior sectionectomy: a safe and effective alternative to right hepatectomy. Ann Surg 247:603–611

20. Torzilli G, Palmisano A, Procopio F, Botea F, Del Fabbro D, Montorsi M (2010) A new systematic small for size resection for liver tumors invading the middle hepatic vein at its caval confluence: the mini-mesohepatectomy. Ann Surg 251:33–39

21. Hasegawa K, Kokudo N, Imamura H et al (2005) Prognostic impact of anatomic resection for hepatocellular carcinoma. Ann Surg 242:252–259

22. Torzilli G, Makuuchi M (2004) Ultrasound-guided finger compression in liver subsegmentectomy for hepatocellular carcinoma. Surg Endosc 18:136–139

23. Torzilli G, Procopio F, Cimino M, Del Fabbro D, Palmisano A, Donadon M, Montorsi M (2010) Anatomical segmental and subsegmental resection of the liver for hepatocellular carcinoma: a new approach by means of ultrasound-guided vessel compression. Ann Surg 251:229–235

24. Torzilli G, Procopio F, Palmisano A, Cimino M, Del Fabbro D, Donadon M, Montorsi M (2009) New technique for defining the right anterior section intraoperatively using ultrasound-guided finger counter-compression. J Am Coll Surg. 209(2):e8–11

25. Takayama T, Makuuchi M, Watanabe K, Kosuge T, Takayasu K, Yamazaki S, Hasegawa H (1991) A new method for mapping hepatic subsegment: counterstaining identification technique. Surgery 109:226–229

26. Takasaki K, Kobayashi S, Tanaka S, Saito A, Yamamoto M, Hanyu F (1990) Highly anatomically systematized hepatic resection with Glissonean sheath code transection at the hepatic hilus. Int Surg 75:73–77

27. Launois B, Jamieson GG (1992) The posterior intrahepatic approach for hepatectomy or removal of segments of the liver. Surg Gynec Obstet 174:155–158

28. Strasberg S, Linehan DC, Hawkins WG (2008) Isolation of right main and right sectional portal pedicles for liver resection without hepatotomy or inflow occlusion. J Am Coll Surg 206:390–396

29. Onishi H, Kawarada Y, Das BC et al (2000) Surgical anatomy of the medial segment (S4) of the liver with special reference to bile ducts and vessels. Hepatogastroenterology 47: 143–150

30. Torzilli G, Takayama T, Hui AM, Kubota K, Harihara Y, Makuuchi M (1999) A new technical aspect of ultrasound-guided liver surgery. Am J Surg 178:341–343

31. Kaibori M, Matsui Y, Hijikawa T, Uchida Y, Kwon AH, Kamiyama Y (2006) Comparison of limited and anatomic hepatic resection for hepatocellular carcinoma with hepatitis C. Surgery, 139(3):385–394

32. Kobayashi A, Miyagawa S, Miwa S, Nakata T (2008) Prognostic impact of anatomical resection on early and late intrahepatic recurrence in patients with hepatocellular carcinoma. J Hepatobiliary Pancreat Surg 15:515–521

33. Eguchi S, Kanematsu T, Arii S et al (2008) Comparison of the outcomes between an anatomical subsegmentectomy and a non-anatomical minor hepatectomy for single hepatocellular carcinomas based on a Japanese nationwide survey. Surgery 143:469–475

34. Cho YB, Lee KU, Lee HW et al (2007) Anatomic versus non-anatomic resection for small single hepatocellular carcinomas. Hepatogastroenterology, 54(78):1766–1769

35. Wakai T, Shirai Y, Sakata J, Kaneko K, Cruz PV, Akazawa K, Hatakeyama K (2007) Anatomic resection independently improves long-term survival in patients with T1-T2 hepatocellular carcinoma. Ann Surg Oncol 14:1356–1365

36. Tanaka K, Shimada H, Matsumoto C, Matsuo K, Nagano Y, Endo I, Togo S (2008) Anatomic versus limited nonanatomic resection for solitary hepatocellular carcinoma. Surgery 143: 607–615

37. Torzilli G, Donadon M, Palmisano A et al (2007) Back-flow bleeding control during resection of right-sided liver tumors by means of ultrasound-guided finger compression of the right hepatic vein at its caval confluence. Hepatogastroenterology 54:1364–1367

38. Makuuchi M (1987) Abdominal intraoperative utrasonography. Igaku-Shoin, Tokyo-New York

39. Ogata S, Kianmanesh R, Belghiti J (2005) Doppler assessment after right hepatectomy confirms the need to fix the remnant left liver in the anatomical position. Br J Surg 92:592–595
40. Machi J, Staren ED (2004) Ultrasound for surgeons, 2nd edn Lippincott-Williams & Wilkins, Philadelphia
41. Torzilli G, Olivari N, Livraghi T, Di Candio G (1997) Ecografia in chirurgia: modalità diagnostiche e terapeutiche. Poletto Editore, Milano

Chapter 11
Portal Vein Embolization Prior to Resection

David C. Madoff and Rony Avritscher

Keywords Portal vein embolization · Hepatic resection · Liver regeneration · Preoperative PVE · Indications and contraindications for PVE · FLR volume

With improvements in perioperative care, major hepatic resections are increasingly being performed for primary and metastatic hepatobiliary neoplasia. Although fatal hepatic failure and major technical complications are now rare after resection, impaired synthetic function, fluid retention, and cholestasis still contribute to prolonged recovery time and extended hospital stay [1, 2]. Although there are many potential contributing causes for perioperative hepatic failure, volume of the future liver remnant (FLR) constitutes one of the most important risk factors. Patients considered at "high risk" for perioperative failure are those with chronic liver disease in whom more than 60% of the functional liver mass will be removed or those with normal underlying liver who undergo resection of more than 80% of their functional liver mass [2–5].

Preoperative portal vein embolization (PVE) is a procedure used to reduce the risk of extensive surgery in patients with small remnant livers [5–15]. PVE redirects portal blood flow to the intended future liver remnant in an attempt to initiate hypertrophy of the non-embolized segments and has been shown to improve the functional reserve of the FLR before surgery. In appropriately selected patients, PVE has also been shown to reduce perioperative morbidity and allow for safe, potentially curative hepatectomy for patients previously considered ineligible for resection based on anticipated small remnant livers [5–16]. For this reason, PVE is now performed at many comprehensive hepatobiliary centers worldwide prior to major hepatectomy.

The clinical use of PVE is based on laboratory investigations first reported by Rous and Larimore [17] in 1920. In their experiments, Rous and Larimore observed the effects of segmental portal venous occlusion in rabbits and found hypertrophy (i.e., enlargement) of the hepatic segments with patent portal veins and atrophy

D.C. Madoff (✉)
Interventional Radiology Section, Division of Diagnostic Imaging, The University of Texas MD Anderson Cancer Center, Houston, TX, USA

K.M. McMasters, J.-N. Vauthey (eds.), *Hepatocellular Carcinoma*,
DOI 10.1007/978-1-60327-522-4_11, © Springer Science+Business Media, LLC 2011

(i.e., shrinkage) of the hepatic segments with ligated portal veins. Clinical researchers subsequently reported their results showing that portal vein or bile duct occlusion resulting from tumor invasion or ligation leads to atrophy of the liver to be resected (i.e., ipsilateral liver) and hypertrophy of liver to remain in situ after resection (i.e., contralateral liver) [18–20]. In the 1980s, Kinoshita and colleagues [21] first described the use of PVE to limit the extension of segmental portal tumor thrombi from hepatocellular carcinoma (HCC) for which transcatheter arterial embolization (TAE) was ineffective. In 1990, Makuuchi and colleagues [10] were first to report on the use of PVE solely as a method to prepare the contralateral liver for major hepatectomy in 14 patients with hilar biliary tract cancer.

Since publication of these seminal articles, many investigators have stressed the importance of PVE in their multidisciplinary management of patients with HCC, cholangiocarcinoma, and liver metastases. Given this, extensive research efforts into the mechanisms of liver regeneration, indications and contraindications for PVE, methods of measuring the FLR before and after PVE, technical aspects of PVE, and potential surgical strategies are ongoing and in continual evolution. This chapter reviews the current indications for and technical aspects of PVE before hepatic resection, with an emphasis on strategies to improve outcomes.

Mechanisms of Liver Regeneration

The liver's ability to regenerate after injury or resection has long been known with the earliest reference being from classical Greek literature, in Hesiod's *Theogony* (750–700 B.C.) [22]. However, the human liver's regenerative capacity was not scientifically documented until 1890 [23].

Despite its sizeable metabolic burden, the liver is basically an inactive organ in terms of hepatocyte replication, with only 0.0012–0.01% of hepatocytes undergoing mitosis at any time [22, 24, 25]. However, this low rate of cell turnover in healthy liver can be altered by substantial toxic damage or surgical resection, which stimulates sudden, massive hepatocyte proliferation resulting in recovery of the functional liver mass within 2 weeks after the loss of up to two-thirds of the liver. This regenerative response is usually mediated by the proliferation of surviving hepatocytes within the acinar architecture of the remnant liver. After resection, this response results in hypertrophy of the remnant liver rather than restoration of the resected segments, a phenomenon that is appropriately termed "compensatory hyperplasia" rather than true "regeneration" [25]. The term "hypertrophy" actually means an increase in cell size and may be misleading because the primary mechanism of volume restitution after liver resection or embolization is more precisely termed "hyperplasia," or increase in cell number [26–28]. However, studies also suggest that both hypertrophy and hyperplasia aid in restoring functional hepatic volume [29–31]. Thus, the term "hypertrophy" after PVE or resection will be used throughout this chapter since this is the term used throughout the published literature.

Most information about the molecular and cellular events during liver regeneration comes from studies of partial hepatectomy in animal models [22, 32]. In short, the events that occur in hepatocytes result from growth factor stimulation in response to injury. In regenerating liver, hepatocyte growth factor (HGF), transforming growth factor-α (TGF-α), and epidermal growth factor (EGF) are important stimuli for hepatocyte replication. HGF is the most potent mitogen for hepatocyte replication, and in combination with other mitogenic growth factors, such as TGF-α and EGF, it can induce the production of cytokines, including tumor necrosis factor-α and interleukin-6, and activate immediate response genes that ready the hepatocytes for cell cycle progression and regeneration. Insulin is synergistic with HGF, resulting in slower regeneration rates seen in patients with diabetes [33, 34]. The extrahepatic factors are transported primarily from the gut to the liver via the portal vein and not from the hepatic artery and are directed [9, 23, 35, 36].

Rate of Liver Regeneration

Hepatocyte regeneration occurs soon after partial hepatectomy, PVE, or liver injury. Shortly after the stimulus, hepatocytes leave the dormant stage of the cell cycle and undergo mitosis, with an initial peak of DNA synthesis occurring in the parenchymal cells (e.g., hepatocytes and biliary epithelial cells) at 24 and 40 h after resection in rat and mouse models, respectively [37]. In both species, non-parenchymal cells exhibit a first peak of proliferation about 12 h after the parenchymal cells [38]. In large animal models of regeneration after partial hepatectomy, DNA synthesis peaks later, at 72–96 h in canines [39] and 7–10 days in primates [40]. Notably, the extent of hepatocyte proliferation is directly proportional to the extent of insult (i.e., a small liver injury will result in a mitotic reaction limited to only a small area, but any insult greater than 10% will lead to proliferation of cells all over the liver) [41]. When more than half of the liver is resected, a second, less distinct rise of hepatocyte mitoses is observed. In rat and mouse models, this second rise is observed at 3–5 days; in larger-sized animals, this second rise occurs over the course of many days. Studies performed in other injury models have hinted that comparable timelines for regeneration and cellular signaling are implicated in the regenerative response. For example, examination of the regenerative response after PVE in swine showed induction of hepatocyte proliferation at 2–7 days [42]. Replication peaked at 7 days, taking place in roughly 14% of hepatocytes, and then decreased to baseline levels by day 12, a process similar to what is observed with PVE clinically. When contrasted with replication after resection, the peak replication after PVE is delayed about 3–4 days, implying that the stimulus of removing hepatocytes is superior to the stimulus of apoptosis seen with PVE [26].

Also critical to the understanding of liver regeneration is the observation that diseased (i.e., cirrhotic) liver has a reduced regenerative capacity when compared to healthy liver [26]. This may be the result of the diminished capacity of hepatocytes to react to hepatotropic factors or due to parenchymal damage such as fibrosis that leads to slower portal blood flow velocities [43]. Lee and colleagues [26] assessed rats with normal or chemically induced cirrhotic livers and showed that the weight of normal livers increased after 24 h, tripled after 7 days, and reached a plateau between 7 and 14 days, whereas the regeneration rate of the cirrhotic livers was delayed and of a lesser degree. Findings in clinical studies have been similar. Non-cirrhotic livers in humans regenerate quickest, at rates of 12–21 cm^3/day at 2 weeks, 11 cm^3/day at 4 weeks, and 6 cm^3/day at 32 days after PVE [34, 44]. The regeneration rates are slower (9 cm^3/day at 2 weeks) in patients with cirrhotic livers, with equivalent rates found in diabetics [34, 45]. Kawarada et al. [46] reported that dogs subjected to a 70% hepatectomy combined with a pancreatectomy had delayed recovery of hepatic function and more limited regenerative capacity than dogs that underwent hepatectomy alone. The reduction in hepatic regeneration was proportional to the extent of the pancreatectomy.

Steatosis also appears to impair liver regeneration in animal models but regeneration may still occur after PVE [47]. Currently, however, the severity of clinically significant steatosis is unknown. In laboratory animals, exposure to a high-fat diet impairs liver regeneration after partial hepatectomy and is also associated with increased hepatocellular injury (i.e., necrosis with severe steatosis [48] and apoptosis with mild steatosis [49]). Thus, a high-fat diet not only may limit liver regeneration but may also increase the risk for hepatic injury and result in delayed functional recovery after major hepatectomy [50].

Pathophysiology of Preoperative PVE

Makuuchi and colleagues [10] published the first experience using preoperative PVE to induce left liver hypertrophy prior to right hepatectomy. Their rationale for performing PVE in this situation was to lessen the sudden increase in portal pressure at resection that can result in hepatocellular damage to the FLR, to dissociate portal pressure-induced hepatocellular injury from the direct trauma to the FLR during physical handling of the liver at the time of surgery, and to improve overall tolerance to major resection by increasing hepatic mass before resection in order to reduce the risk of postresection metabolic changes.

The justification for using PVE has also been based on data showing that increases in FLR volume are associated with improved function as verified by increases in biliary excretion [51, 52] and in technetium-99m-galactosyl human serum albumin uptake [53] and by significant improvements in the postoperative liver function tests after PVE compared with no PVE [3].

After PVE, changes in liver function tests are generally small and short-lived. When transaminase levels rise, they typically reach their zenith at levels less than three times baseline 1–3 days after PVE and return to baseline within 10 days, regardless of the embolic agent used [10, 11, 34, 45, 54–56]. Minor alterations in total serum bilirubin concentration and white blood cell count may be seen after PVE, and prothrombin time is rarely affected.

Unlike arterial embolization, the postembolization syndrome is not associated with PVE [9]. This relative lack of symptomatology results from the histopathological basis of PVE; it produces no distortion of the hepatic anatomy, leads to negligible inflammation except for immediately around the embolized vein, and little, if any, parenchymal or tumor necrosis [10, 57]. Animal studies demonstrated that hepatocytes undergo apoptosis and not necrosis after portal venous occlusion [42, 58], which accounts for the relative lack of systemic symptoms after PVE.

Portal blood flow to the non-embolized hepatic segments measured by Doppler sonography increases significantly and then falls to near-baseline values after 11 days. The resultant hypertrophy rates correlate with the portal blood flow rates [9, 43].

FLR Volume Measurement and Predicting Function After PVE

Computed tomography (CT) with volumetry is an important tool to predict liver function after resection of the tumor-bearing liver, and several methods have been offered [14, 59, 60]. However, CT volumetry must be employed within the context of the patient's underlying liver function and should not be used as a "stand-alone" value upon which resection will be solely based.

Three-dimensional CT volumetric measurements are obtained by demarcating the hepatic segmental contours and calculating the volumes from the surface measurements from each sequential image. Multiphasic contrast-enhanced CT must be performed to best delineate the vascular landmarks of the segments [60]. This technique makes it possible to easily obtain an accurate and reproducible FLR volume that can be calculated within minutes of imaging and with a margin of error <5% [61, 62]. The FLR can then be standardized to the total liver volume (TLV) to determine the %TLV that will need to remain after resection.

Although measurement of the TLV is possible with CT, direct TLV measurements may not be appropriate for surgical planning for many reasons. First, in patients with considerable tumor burden, the TLV is changed, and attempts to deduct tumor volume from the TLV require additional time to calculate, especially when multiple tumors are present, and this may lead to additive mathematical errors in volume calculation (TLV minus tumor volume) [7, 63]. Furthermore, this approach does not account for the actual functional liver mass when chronic liver disease, vascular obstruction, or biliary dilatation is present within the liver to be resected. Patients with cirrhosis frequently have enlarged or shrunken livers such that the measured TLV may not be useful as an index to which FLR volume is standardized, leading various researchers to advocate clinical algorithms in which functional tests (e.g., indocyanine green retention at 15 min (ICGR15) are evaluated in combination with the planned extent of resection [64].

A straightforward, precise, and reproducible technique (Fig. 11.1) standardizes liver remnant size to individual patient size to account for the fact that large patients

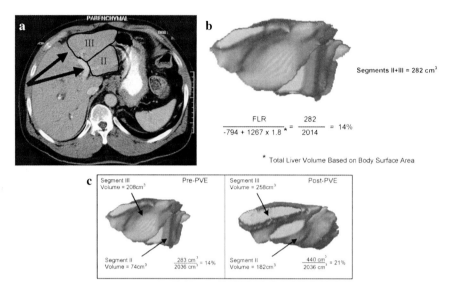

Fig. 11.1 Hypertrophy of the future liver remnant after portal vein embolization as determined by three-dimensional reconstruction of computed tomography images. (**a**) Three-dimensional volumetric measurements are determined by outlining the hepatic segmental contours and then calculating the volumes from the surface measurements of each slice. (**b**) The formula for calculating total liver volume is based on the patient's body surface area. (Modified from [22], used with permission.) (**c**) Before embolization, the volume of segments 2 and 3 was 283 cm^3 or 14% of the total liver volume (2,036 cm^3). After embolization, the volume of segments 2 and 3 was 440 cm^3 or 21% of the total liver volume (a degree of hypertrophy of 7%) (Modified from [3], used with permission)

require larger liver remnants than do smaller patients. CT is used to directly quantify the FLR, which is by definition disease free. The total estimated liver volume (TELV) is calculated by the formula (TELV = −794.41 + 1,267.28 × BSA) derived from the close association between liver size and patient size based on body weight and body surface area (BSA) [3, 14, 65]. The FLR/TELV ratio is subsequently calculated to give a volumetric estimate of FLR function. From this method of calculation, termed "standardized FLR measurement," a correlation between the anticipated liver remnant and the operative outcome has been recognized [3]. This formula was recently appraised in a meta-analysis evaluating 12 different formulas and was found to be one of the least biased and most accurate for TELV estimation [66]. At our institution, CT scans are routinely performed before PVE and approximately 3–4 weeks after PVE to assess the degree of FLR hypertrophy. We have recently found that in addition to the FLR/TELV measurement, the degree of hypertrophy (DH) (i.e., [FLR/TELV after PVE] − [FLR/TELV before PVE]) is also a predictor of postoperative course. If a patient has a DH <5% after PVE, they are at increased risk for postoperative complications [67].

Shirabe and colleagues [2] also realized the significance of standardizing liver volume to BSA and showed that no patient with underlying liver disease who had a standardized liver volume of more than 285 mL/m^2 BSA died of liver failure after liver resection. Given analogous data from a different study, the guideline for utilizing PVE in patients with cirrhotic livers has been set at a standardized FLR volume <40% [7].

Developments in nuclear imaging technology are currently being designed to quantify both anatomical and functional differences in liver volume. Technetium-99m-labeled diethylenetriamine pentaacetic acid-galactosyl-human serum albumin binds specifically to asialoglycoprotein receptors on hepatocyte cell membranes. Agent distribution is monitored in real time with single-photon emission scintigraphy and has been shown to correlate with ICGR15 [68]. Another technique, axial image reconstruction, can be used to estimate the differential functions of the right and left liver. However, neither technique is as of yet sufficiently accurate in assessing segmental or bisegmental function during the planning for extended hepatectomy.

Indications and Contraindications for PVE

General Indications

To determine whether a particular patient will benefit from PVE, several factors must be considered [15]. The first is whether or not there is underlying liver disease as this will have a profound impact on the liver remnant volume needed for adequate function. Patient size also must be considered as larger patients require larger liver remnants. Next, the extent and complexity of the planned resection and the likelihood that associated non-hepatic surgery will be performed at the time of liver resection must be considered. These three factors are considered in the setting of the patient's age and comorbidities (e.g., diabetes) that may affect hypertrophy and perioperative outcome. Thus, after all of these factors have been evaluated and the patient remains a candidate for resection, appropriate liver CT volumetry is performed so that the standardized FLR volume expressed as a percentage of the estimated TLV can be used to determine the need for PVE.

As mentioned above, a normal liver has a superior regenerative capacity than a cirrhotic liver, functions more efficiently, and tolerates injury better. Patients with normal underlying liver can survive resection of up to 90% of the liver, but in cirrhotic patients, survival after resection beyond 60% of the functional parenchyma is unlikely [5]. Furthermore, complications of the poorly functioning remnant liver (e.g., ascites and wound breakdown from poor protein synthesis) and fatal postoperative liver failure are more common after resection in patients with cirrhosis than in those without cirrhosis. With regard to liver volume, there is a limit to how small a liver can remain after resection. If too little liver remains after resection, immediate postresection hepatic failure leads to multisystem organ failure and death. If a marginal volume of liver remains, cirrhotic or not, the lack of reserve often leads to a cascade of complications, prolonged hospital and intensive care unit stays, and slow recovery or slowly progressive liver failure over weeks to months with eventual death [1–3].

Normal Underlying Liver

In patients with a normal underlying liver, the indications for PVE have evolved with the greater precision of liver CT volumetric measurements and the use of standardized liver volumes. Although extensive resections are now achieved with a very low risk of death from liver failure, small-for-patient-size normal liver remnants are still associated with an increased number of complications and slower postoperative recovery [3]. An FLR/TELV of more than 20% is associated with a fourfold reduction in complications compared with an FLR/TELV of 20% or less [5]. This finding was corroborated in a retrospective series that revealed that residual liver volume, not resected volume, more accurately predicts postoperative course [4].

It is also crucial to recognize and individualize the indication for PVE with regard to the standardized 20% cutoff for liver volume as there is considerable intrahepatic segmental variability. Liver volume analysis revealed that the lateral left liver (segments 2 and 3) contributes less than 20% of the TLV in more than 75% of patients in the absence of compensatory hypertrophy. Further, the left liver (segments 2, 3, and 4) contributes 20% or less of the TLV in more than 10% of patients [69]. Therefore, an FLR/TELV of less than 20% can be expected in most patients who do not develop compensatory hypertrophy from tumor growth and require an extended right hepatectomy. In these patients, RPVE extended to segment 4 is indicated. However, left PVE is rarely needed; Nagino and colleagues [12] showed that an extended left hepatectomy with caudate lobectomy results in resection of only 67% of the liver, leaving an FLR of 33%, the same residual volume after right hepatectomy in a normal liver. Volumetric analysis of normal livers also confirms the consistently large volume of the posterior right liver (segments 6 and 7) [70].

Recently, Farges et al. [71] showed that RPVE performed before right hepatectomy in patients with an otherwise normal liver showed no clinical benefit, and they concluded that in this setting, PVE may be unnecessary (except in the small subset of patients whose left liver is <20% of the TLV). Failure to follow these well-established guidelines may result in overuse of PVE.

Underlying Liver Disease

Although major resection can be performed safely in some cirrhotic patients, extended hepatectomy is seldom an option. In contrast to patients with normal liver, those with cirrhosis with marginal liver remnant volumes are at an increased risk for both postoperative complications and death from liver failure [2]. However, in carefully selected patients with cirrhosis with preserved liver function (Child's Class A) and normal ICGR15 (<10%), major hepatectomy can be performed safely and

PVE is indicated when the FLR volume is <40% of the TLV [7]. This guideline is supported by the finding that when liver volume is standardized to BSA, standardized FLR volume predicts death from liver failure after hepatectomy in chronic liver disease [2].

These studies were validated by the only prospective study that assessed the use of PVE prior to right hepatectomy. This study, reported by Farges and colleagues [71], showed that patients with chronic liver disease who did not have PVE before right hepatectomy had more complications and longer intensive care unit and hospital stays than those with chronic liver disease who underwent PVE before right hepatectomy. This guideline has been expanded to include patients in whom the liver is compromised by prolonged biliary obstruction who need extended hepatectomy [3, 9, 10, 34].

Highly selected patients with advanced liver disease might be able to undergo safe resection. Specifically, in patients with cirrhosis with a moderately abnormal ICGR15 (10–20%) but with preserved liver function, sequential chemoembolization and PVE has been advocated [72]. Recent studies have shown that this strategy leads to increased atrophy of the embolized liver and greater hypertrophy of the FLR than PVE alone. Furthermore, the combined use of chemoembolization with PVE may become the definitive treatment for patients initially considered to be candidates for resection whose disease ultimately becomes unresectable as their treatment progresses.

At M.D. Anderson Cancer Center, portal pressures are now measured routinely before and after PVE in patients with chronic liver disease because of the lack of reliability of assessment of hepatic fibrosis by core needle biopsy [73]. Patients with overt portal hypertension (splenomegaly, low platelets, imaging evidence of varices) are not candidates for major hepatectomy and therefore are not candidates for PVE. Mild portal hypertension, however, is not a contraindication to PVE followed by hepatectomy, provided liver function test results are otherwise normal (Child–Pugh A+). However, because "liver disease" is a continuum, the specific indications for PVE in patients with chronic liver disease remain to be precisely defined and will require an individualized approach. However, it is anticipated that refined criteria will be developed with the accumulation of additional experience with the standardized measurement of FLR.

High-Dose Chemotherapy

Retrospective data suggest an increased risk of surgical complications in patients after preoperative systemic or regional chemotherapy [74, 75], but no definite guidelines for a minimal FLR have been established. Patients with steatosis have an increased incidence of complications after resection, but the potential benefit and selection criteria for PVE in these patients are currently unknown [76]. Furthermore, knowledge of a patient's specific chemotherapeutic regimen is essential as patients may develop hepatic injuries such as steatohepatitis and sinusoidal dilatation from oxaliplatin and irinotecan-based fluoropyrimidine chemotherapy regimens, with an increased 90-day mortality rate after resection [77]. Thus, some investigators have advocated larger buffer zones (i.e., a larger FLR than required for normal underlying liver) when performing extended resection in selected patients who have received preoperative chemotherapy. Although such patients have been less well studied than patients with normal liver, PVE may be indicated when the FLR is ≤ 30% of the TLV [75, 78].

One issue that has been raised is whether maintaining patients on chemotherapy will have an impact on hepatic hypertrophy, especially in the setting of colorectal liver metastases. Recent articles have shown that systemic chemotherapy administered during the period between PVE and resection does not seem to affect FLR hypertrophy or outcome [79–81]. Further, no differences in regeneration rates after PVE were found in patients receiving chemotherapy with or without prior administration of the anti-vascular endothelial growth factor (VEGF) agent, bevacizumab [82].

General Contraindications

Contraindications to PVE include an inadequate FLR volume based on the criteria discussed above, extensive tumor invasion of the portal vein to be resected as portal flow is already diverted and may preclude safe catheter manipulation and optimal delivery of embolic material, disease progression that leads to overall unresectability and overt clinical portal hypertension [15, 59]. Relative contraindications to PVE include tumor extension to the FLR (PVE may still be performed if part of aggressive therapy involving multistage hepatectomy or thermal ablation of the lesions within the FLR), biliary dilatation in the FLR (if the biliary tree is obstructed, drainage is recommended), mild portal hypertension, uncorrectable coagulopathy, and renal insufficiency. The presence of an ipsilateral tumor may preclude safe transhepatic access if the tumor burden is great, but this is also unlikely, as there is no evidence that tumor spread occurs during PVE. If access to an adequate portal vein branch for PVE is not possible, the contralateral approach can be considered.

Technical Considerations for PVE

Standard Approaches

PVE is performed to redirect portal blood flow toward the anticipated FLR (i.e., hepatic segments that will remain after surgery). To ensure that sufficient hypertrophy occurs, embolization of portal vein branches should be as complete as possible so that recanalization of the occluded portal system does not occur. Therefore, the entire portal system to be resected must be occluded to avoid the development of intrahepatic portal collaterals that may limit regeneration [83].

PVE can be performed by any of three standard approaches: the transhepatic contralateral (i.e., portal access via the FLR), the transhepatic ipsilateral (i.e., portal access via the liver to be resected), and the intraoperative transileocolic venous approach. These approaches are chosen based on operator preference, type of hepatic resection planned, extent of embolization (e.g., right PVE [RPVE] with or without extension to segment 4), and type of embolic agent used.

The transileocolic venous approach was the original approach for performing preoperative PVE. This technique is performed during laparotomy by direct cannulation of the ileocolic vein and advancement of a balloon catheter into the portal venous system for embolization [10]. For years, this was the preferred approach for many Asian surgeons. Conventional teaching is that this approach is performed when an interventional radiology suite is not available, when a percutaneous approach is not considered feasible, or when additional treatment is needed during the same surgical exploration [60, 84]. The disadvantages of this method are the need for general anesthesia and laparotomy, with their inherent risks, and the inferior imaging equipment often (but not always) available in the operating room compared with the state-of-the-art imaging equipment available in most modern interventional radiology suites. However, as more minimally invasive techniques have become favored and the equipment used (e.g., imaging equipment, catheter systems, embolic agents) has become more sophisticated, the reasons mentioned above for using this technique apply in very limited situations such that the transileocolic venous approach is being used less often.

The transhepatic contralateral approach was initially developed by Kinoshita and colleagues [21] to slow the progression of tumor thrombus within the portal system (Fig. 11.2). However, this approach was later adapted for preoperative PVE. With this technique, a branch of the left lateral portal system (i.e., either a segment 2 or 3 branch) is accessed, and the catheter is advanced under imaging guidance into the

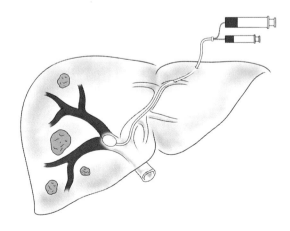

Fig. 11.2 Schematic representation of the contralateral approach. An occlusion balloon catheter is placed from the left lobe into right portal branch, with delivery of the embolic agent in the antegrade direction

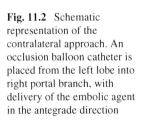

right portal venous system for embolization [54]. The advantage of this approach, albeit minor, is that catheterization of the desired right portal vein branches is more direct via the left system than via the right, making the procedure technically easier. However, the technique's major disadvantage is the potential risk of damage to the FLR parenchyma and the left portal vein. A multicenter European study was published in 2005 that included 188 patients who underwent contralateral PVE and it reported 24 (12.8%) adverse events including migration of embolic material to the FLR in 10 patients (5.3%), occlusion of a major portal branch requiring intervention in three patients (1.6%), bleeding in five patients (2.7%: 1 hemobilia, 1 hemoperitoneum, 1 rupture of gallbladder metastases, 2 subcapsular hematomas), and transient liver failure in six patients (3.2%) [85]. These adverse events may compromise the FLRs integrity and may make the planned resection more difficult or even impossible. Furthermore, embolization of segment 4, if needed, may prove difficult given the anatomical considerations related to catheter placement and the choice of embolic agent [15].

The transhepatic ipsilateral approach was first described by Nagino and colleagues [86] in the mid-1990s (Fig. 11.3) and it is now advocated by additional investigators [87–90]. For this approach, a peripheral portal vein in the liver to be resected is accessed through which embolic material is subsequently administered. Since Nagino's ipsilateral technique required the use of specially designed catheters that are unavailable outside of Japan, modifications of their technique were developed. At M.D. Anderson Cancer Center, standard angiographic catheters are utilized for combined particulate infusion and coil deployment [59, 87, 88] (Fig. 11.4). When right heptatectomy is planned, RPVE is performed (Fig. 11.5), and when extended right hepatectomy is planned, RPVE is extended to include the segment 4 portal veins (RPVE + 4) (Fig. 11.6). Ipsilateral RPVE ± 4 is performed through a 5- or 6-French sheath that is placed within a distal right portal vein branch. When RPVE + 4 is needed, embolization of segment 4 is done first so as to reduce the need to maneuver catheters through segments that have already been embolized. A 3-French microcatheter is then advanced coaxially through an

a   b

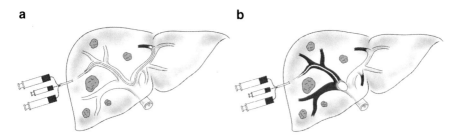

Fig. 11.3 Schematic representation of the ipsilateral approach for RPVE and segment 4 as described by Nagino et al. (13). Different portions of the balloon catheter are used for antegrade embolization of segment 4 veins (**a**) and for retrograde delivery of the embolic agent into the right portal system (**b**)

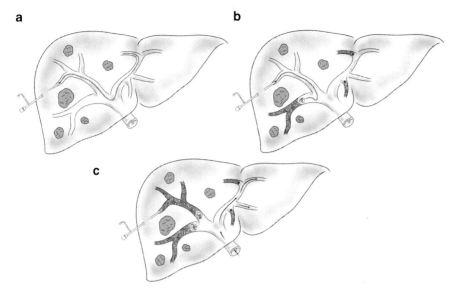

Fig. 11.4 Schematic representation shows modification of the ipsilateral technique for RPVE extended to segment 4. (**a**) Placement of a 6-French vascular sheath into the right portal branch. An angled 5-French catheter is placed into the left portal system with coaxial placement of a micro-catheter into a segment 4 branch. Particulate embolization is performed followed by placement of coils until all the branches are occluded. (**b**) After segment 4 embolization is completely occluded, a 5-French reverse-curve catheter is used for RPVE. (**c**) After embolization of the right and segment 4 portal veins are complete, the access tract is embolized with coils to prevent subcapsular hemorrhage

angled 5-French catheter into the portal vein branches supplying segment 4 so that particulate embolics and coils can then be delivered. Once complete occlusion of the segment 4 embolization is achieved, a 5-French reverse-curve catheter may be needed to embolize the portal veins supplying segments 5 through 8 (i.e., right liver). After complete occlusion of the right portal venous system, the access tract is embolized with coils and/or gelfoam to diminish the risk of perihepatic bleeding at the access site.

A distinct advantage of the ipsilateral approach is that the FLR is not instrumented. However, while disadvantages do exist, they are minor. Catheterization and embolization of the right portal vein branches may be slightly more difficult due to the severe angulations between right portal branches; however, this is rarely a problem when reverse-curve catheters are used. Another potential disadvantage is that some embolic material could be displaced upon catheter removal, leading to nontarget embolization, although this has not occurred in our experience with more than 200 RPVEs, most of which included extension to segment 4 branches. Similarly, in our experience, ipsilateral access has not been an issue in patients with large liver tumors.

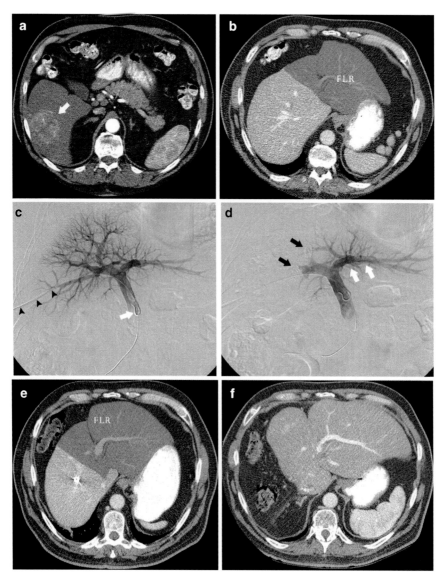

Fig. 11.5 A 72-year-old man with history of hepatitis B, cirrhosis, and hepatocellular carcinoma HCC, who had transhepatic ipsilateral RPVE with particles and coils prior to right hepatectomy. (**a**) Contrast-enhanced CT scan of the liver shows a hypervascular mass in the right hepatic lobe consistent with HCC (*arrow*). (**b**) Contrast-enhanced CT scan of the liver shows small left liver (FLR/TELV of 35%) with underlying cirrhosis (FLR is *shaded area*). (**c**) Anteroposterior flush portogram shows a 6-French vascular sheath (*arrowheads*) in a right portal vein branch and a 5-French flush catheter (*arrow*) in the main portal vein. (**d**) Postprocedure anteroposterior flush portogram shows occlusion of the portal vein branches to segments 5–8 (*black arrows*) with continued patency of the vein supplying the left lobe (segments 2–4) (*white arrows*). (**e**) Contrast-enhanced CT scan of the liver performed 1 month after RPVE shows hypertrophy of the left liver (FLR/TELV of 45%) (FLR is *shaded area*). (**f**) Contrast-enhanced CT scan of the liver performed after successful right hepatectomy shows hypertrophy of the liver remnant

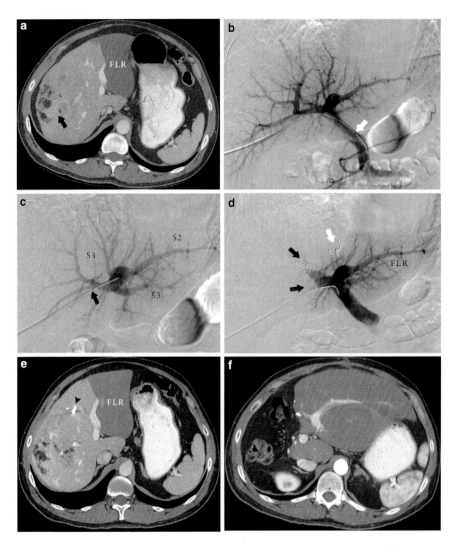

Fig. 11.6 A 45-year-old man with history of non-alcoholic steatohepatitis and HCC who had transhepatic ipsilateral RPVE extended to segment 4 with particles and coils prior to extended right hepatectomy. (**a**) Contrast-enhanced CT scan of the liver shows a heterogeneous mass in the right hepatic lobe consistent with HCC (*black arrow*) and small left lateral liver (*shaded area*) with FLR/TELV of 27%. (**b**) Anterior-posterior flush portogram from the ipsilateral approach shows a 6-French vascular sheath in a right portal vein branch and a 5-French flush catheter (*arrow*) in the main portal vein. (**c**) Selective left portogram with a 5-French catheter in the left portal vein (*arrow*) shows the veins that supply segments 2 (s2), 3 (s3), and 4 (s4). (**d**) Postprocedure portogram shows complete occlusion (with particles and coils) of the portal vein branches to segments 4–8 (*arrows*) with continued patency of the veins supplying the left lateral lobe (segments 2 and 3) (*shaded area*). (**e**) Contrast-enhanced CT scan performed 4 weeks after PVE shows hypertrophy of the left lateral liver (FLR/TELV now 39%, a degree of hypertrophy of 12%) with rounded margins (*shaded area*). Coil within segment 4 (*arrowhead*) is seen. (**f**) Contrast-enhanced CT scan of the liver performed after successful extended right hepatectomy shows hypertrophy of the liver remnant

Additional PVE Approaches

PVE Followed by Bland Transarterial Embolization

Other approaches have been used for PVE. The thought of combining PVE and TAE for complete portal venous and hepatic arterial occlusion has been reported in patients with biliary tract cancer and colorectal metastases who had inadequate hypertrophy after PVE alone [91, 92]. Nagino and colleagues [91] described a patient that required an extended left hepatectomy but the FLR volume (i.e., right posterior liver) did not increase 51 days after PVE. After TAE, the FLR volume increased from 485 cm^3 before PVE to 685 cm^3 after PVE, an addition of 215 cm^3. Another patient required a right hepatectomy, but no significant volume change was seen after PVE (pre-PVE: 643 cm^3 and post-PVE: 649 cm^3). After TAE, the left liver volume enlarged to 789 cm^3, an increase of 140 cm^3. Both patients underwent successful and uneventful resection after the staged procedures. However, there are potential drawbacks. As both arterial and portal systems are deprived of blood, the potential for hepatic infarction exists such that only half the target segments were treated with TAE, superselectively. While this approach was effective, the disadvantage is that two separate procedures are needed, performed at different times, leading to considerably longer waiting periods. During these waiting periods, tumor progression could occur to the degree that the tumors become unresectable.

Sequential Arterial Embolization and PVE

In 2004, Aoki and colleagues [72] described their experience with the use of sequential transcatheter arterial chemoembolization followed within 2 weeks by PVE in 17 patients with HCC (Fig. 11.7). Their justification for this approach was as follows: (1) The livers of most patients with HCC are compromised by underlying liver disease such that the liver's regenerative capability after hepatic resection is weakened, making it hard to predict if adequate FLR hypertrophy can be achieved after PVE. (2) Since most HCCs are hypervascular and supplied largely by arterial blood flow, termination of portal flow induces compensatory augmentation in arterial blood flow (i.e., "arterialization of the liver") in the embolized segments that may lead to rapid tumor progression after PVE. (3) Arterioportal shunts often found in cirrhotic livers and HCC may limit the effects of PVE. To this end, sequential chemoembolization and PVE were used to prevent tumor progression during the time between the PVE and planned hepatectomy and to strengthen the effect of PVE by embolizing arterioportal shunts with chemoembolization. As a result, the researchers found that the combined procedures were safe, induced sufficient FLR hypertrophy within 2 weeks, and caused no worsening of the basal hepatic functional reserve or increase in tumor progression. Importantly, when the explanted livers were evaluated, tumor necrosis was profound but without substantial injury to the non-cancerous liver, and they therefore encourage the aggressive application of this treatment strategy in patients with large HCC and chronically injured livers.

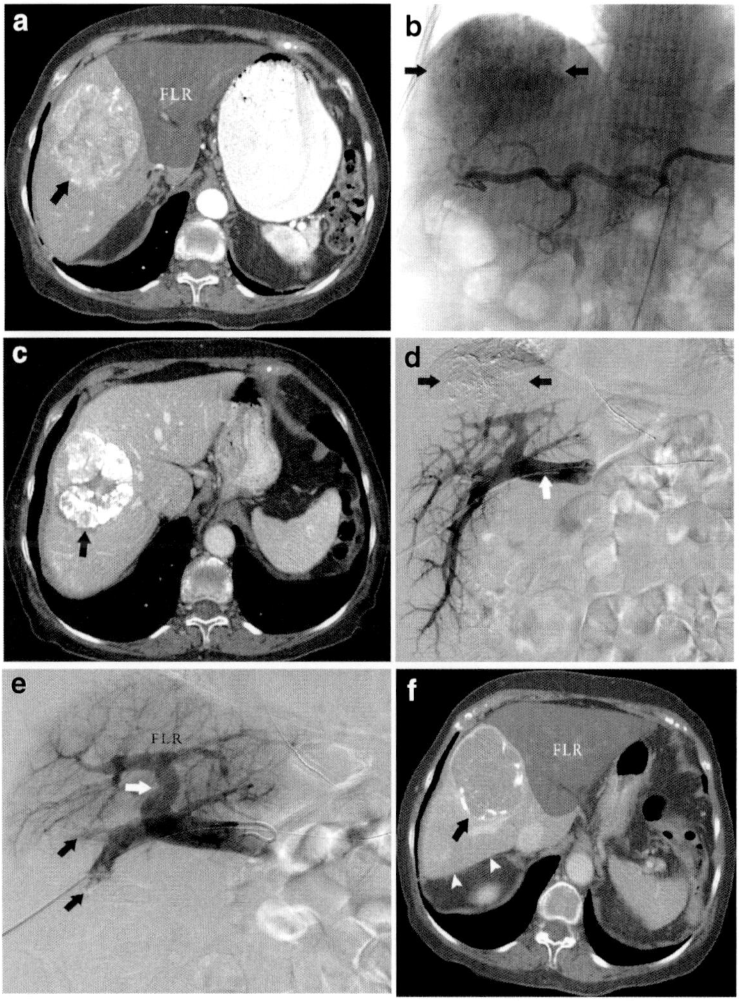

Fig. 11.7 A 71-year-old man with history of liver steatosis, fibrosis, and HCC, who underwent sequential transcatheter arterial chemoembolization followed 1 month later by RPVE prior to a right hepatectomy. (**a**) A single image from pre-PVE contrast-enhanced CT scan shows a large hypervascular mass in the right hepatic lobe (*arrow*) and a small left liver (*shaded area*) with a FLR/TELV of 27%. (**b**) Celiac arteriogram performed during chemoembolization shows a hypervascular mass with iodized oil uptake in the right hepatic lobe (*arrows*). (**c**) Contrast-enhanced CT shows iodized oil uptake in the HCC (*arrow*). (**d**) Anterior-posterior flush portogram from the ipsilateral approach shows a 6-French vascular sheath in a right portal vein branch and a 5-French flush catheter (*white arrows*) in the main portal vein. Persistent iodized oil uptake in the right hepatic mass is seen (*black arrows*). (**e**) Postembolization portogram shows complete occlusion of all branches to right portal vein (*black arrows*). The left portal vein remains patent (*white arrow*). (**f**) Contrast-enhanced CT scan of the liver after RPVE shows complete necrosis of the right liver mass (*black arrow*), hypertrophy of the left liver (*shaded area*), and massive atrophy of the right liver (*arrowheads*). The FLR/TELV increased to 56%. The patient underwent uncomplicated right hepatectomy

More recently, a French group reported on the use of PVE in 36 patients with HCC and chronic liver disease prior to right hepatectomy [93]. In their study, 18 patients underwent chemoembolization followed 3–4 weeks later by PVE and the remaining 18 patients underwent PVE alone. Although PVE was well tolerated in all patients, the mean increase in percentage FLR volume was significantly higher for patients in the combined chemoembolization and PVE group than those who underwent PVE alone ($P = 0.022$). The incidence of complete tumor necrosis (83%:15/18 vs. 6%: 1/18; P <0.001) and 5-year disease-free survival rate (37% vs. 19%; $P = 0.041$) were also significantly greater in patients who underwent chemoembolization and PVE. Given the risks of hepatic infarction, the authors recommended that the two procedures should be separated by at least 3 weeks to reduce procedure-related morbidity. However, similar to Nagino's TAE/PVE approach, the downside of the combined approach is that two separate procedures and an increased waiting times are required.

PVE with Transjugular Access

In 2003, a pilot study of performing PVE by means of the transjugular route was described [94]. This technique was tried because of the vast experience gained during the preceding decade with transjugular intrahepatic portosystemic shunts (TIPS). Under sonographic guidance, the right internal jugular vein was accessed, and then with fluoroscopy, a right or left portal branch was punctured from a right, middle, or left hepatic vein. A catheter was placed near the portal bifurcation and used to perform right PVE with a mixture of n-butyl-2-cyanoacrylate (NBCA) and iodized oil. All 15 procedures were technically successful without any serious complications. FLR hypertrophy was deemed sufficient and right hepatectomy was performed in 12 (80%) patients. While this approach appears safe and effective, the series was small, and further studies will be needed before this approach becomes widespread. For RPVE in patients with cirrhosis, this may be an attractive alternative; however, the technical feasibility of RPVE extended to segment 4 has not yet been explored.

Extent of Embolization

The optimal extent of PVE is presently a subject of much debate. Currently, several groups who utilize PVE to prepare patients for extended right hepatectomy occlude only branches of the right portal vein and leave the segment 4 portal veins patent even though segment 4 will be resected [11, 71, 95]. While FLR hypertrophy does occur, full diversion of portal flow to segments 2, 3 $\pm$ 1 ensures the maximal stimulus for FLR hypertrophy [12, 13]. Further, incomplete embolization of the liver to be resected will also lead to segment 4 hypertrophy. Segment 4 hypertrophy is undesirable for an extended right hepatectomy due to increased morbidity associated with a larger area of intraoperative parenchymal transection across this hypertrophic segment [12]. Nagino and colleagues [13] first showed that a greater left lateral bisegment hypertrophy occurs after RPVE + 4 (50% increase in FLR volume) than after only RPVE (31% increase, $P<0.0005$) [34]. Recent studies have corroborated Nagino's findings and without any increase in PVE-associated complications [96]. Because segment 4 embolization has shown to be of benefit, the ipsilateral approach for RPVE + 4 has been further refined and this has led to improved FLR hypertrophy and operative outcomes [88]. Lastly, left PVE is rarely needed due to consistently large volumes of the right posterior liver (i.e., segments 6/7) [12, 69, 70].

Another potential benefit of RPVE + 4, from an oncological standpoint, is that the entire tumor-bearing liver is systematically embolized (i.e., RPVE for right hepatectomy and RPVE + 4 for extended right hepatectomy) to reduce the risk of tumor growth that may result from increased portal blood flow and hepatotrophic factors. A recent M.D. Anderson study evaluated 112 patients where the entire tumor-bearing liver was systematically embolized and found no increase in the median tumor size during the waiting period [67]. However, tumor growth within the non-embolized liver has been discussed upon analysis of a very limited number of patients with primary and secondary liver tumors after RPVE alone (although no comparison to pre-PVE tumor growth rate was made so the true effect of PVE on tumor growth could not be proven) [97, 98]. Furthermore, liver hypertrophy occurs quickly in patients with normal liver, and thus resection can be undertaken in most patients with multiple colorectal metastases within 3–4 weeks of PVE.

Embolic Agents

Many embolic materials have been used for PVE, with no remarkable differences reported in the degree or rate of hypertrophy. These agents include, but are not limited to, fibrin glue, n-butyl cyanoacrylate (NBCA) mixed with ethiodized oil, gelatin sponge, thrombin, metallic coils, spherical and non-spherical microparticles (e.g., PVA particles and tris-acryl gelatin microspheres), and absolute alcohol. Choosing a particular embolic agent is at the operator's discretion, and the decision is based on the extent of the embolization and surgery, their preference for a particular catheter and approach, and their experience with a specific agent.

In the early experiences with PVE, gelatin sponge was widely used as an embolic agent. However, portal recanalization was frequently observed 2 weeks after the procedure [10, 21, 54] and when compared with other embolic agents, gelatin sponge seemed less efficient at 4 weeks in terms of hypertrophy. Also, fibrin glue combined with ethiodized oil is a commonly used mixture for PVE. This mixture usually induces <75% portal occlusion at 2 weeks and <25% portal occlusion at 4 weeks [10, 54].

Some authors prefer NBCA mixed with ethiodized oil because the mixture leads to fast, reliable hypertrophy and minimizes the delay between PVE and definitive resection. NBCA ensures portal vein occlusion that persists beyond 4 weeks. Since polymerization time can be modulated by varying the lipiodol volume added to the NBCA, distal and proximal branches can be aggressively embolized. Typically,

NBCA is mixed with lipiodol at a ratio of 1.1 to 1.3. Because it is a liquid, NBCA can be quickly delivered throughout the entire right portal system, which greatly decreases procedure time. In terms of effectiveness, de Baere and colleagues [54] reported that NBCA embolization led to a 90% increase in liver volume after 30 days and Denys and colleagues [99] found it helpful in inducing hypertrophy in patients with underlying cirrhosis or advanced fibrosis. However, there are a few drawbacks of NBCA embolization. For instance, the NBCA injections have to be precise because of the increased risk of non-target embolization, thus requiring a highly experienced operator. In addition, NBCA induces an inflammatory process that may make hepatectomy more difficult [54]. NBCA can be difficult to use in patients with reduced hepatopetal flow, as is commonly seen in patients with chronic hepatic disease. These altered flow dynamics have been associated with increased risk of procedural complications [85].

Lastly, while this agent may be straightforward when the anatomy is favorable (e.g., the anterior and posterior sector portal veins originating from a right portal vein), this agent may not be the best alternative in situations where variant anatomy is present or when multiple segment 4 veins are to be embolized (i.e., multiple microcatheters are needed leading to considerable expense; increased risk of non-target embolization to the FLR).

Absolute ethanol is another effective embolic agent for PVE. Osagawara and colleagues [100] demonstrated near doubling of the left liver volume within 4 weeks for patients with chronic hepatic disease and HCC who underwent PVE with this agent. Unfortunately, the most pronounced changes in liver function tests of all PVE embolic agents and poor patient tolerance are seen with absolute ethanol.

Recently, the use of particulate agents for PVE had been proposed [40, 54, 59, 101]. In the first clinical report in a single patient, no recanalization of the right portal vein was observed 5 weeks after PVE with PVA particles alone [101]. Later, Madoff and colleagues [87, 88] showed that a combination of particles (e.g., polyvinyl alcohol particles (PVA) and tris-acryl gelatin microspheres) and coils is safe and effective for PVE. Particles are safe, cause little periportal reaction, and generate durable portal vein occlusion, especially when used in combination with coils [59, 88]. In 2003, results from the first 26 patients who had PVE with non-spherical PVA particles ranging in size from 300 to 1000 μm and coils were reported; the mean FLR/TELV increased 7.8% (pre-PVE FLR/TELV, 17.6%; post-PVE FLR/TELV, 25.4%), and the mean absolute FLR increase was 47% [87]. The subsequent development of spherical particulate embolics has led to even further refinements in technique for PVE by using a stepwise infusion of very small (100–300 μm) tris-acryl microspheres followed by larger spheres (up to 700 μm) [88]. This type of distal embolization is thought to limit development of collateral circulation that may potentially reduce hypertrophy due to the improved targeting of distal portal vein branches (i.e., non-spherical particles tend to clump and therefore do not always reach the targeted size vessel). Metallic coils are then used proximally to block venous inflow and further reduce the possibility of recanalization. This approach was used for RPVE + 4 and led to an absolute increase in FLR volume of 69.0%, an FLR/TELV increase of 9.7%, and a subsequent resection rate of 86% that was a significant improvement over their previously reported method.

Complications of PVE

As with all transhepatic procedures, complications include subcapsular hematoma, hemoperitoneum, hemobilia, pseudoaneurysm, arteriovenous fistula, arterioportal shunts, portal vein thrombosis, transient liver failure, pneumothorax, and sepsis [85, 102]. Kodama and colleagues [102] compared the complication rate between the ipsilateral and contralateral approaches in 47 patients, who underwent PVE. They found that in 11 patients who underwent contralateral PVE, 2 (18.1%) experienced complications, and in 36 patients who underwent ipsilateral PVE, 5 (13.9%) experienced complications. This difference was not statistically significant. The rate of technical complications associated with percutaneous PVE using either approach was 14.9%. The patients in the study developed the following complications: two pneumothoraces, two subcapsular hematomas, one inadvertent arterial puncture, one pseudoaneurysm (in a patient who also had a subcapsular hematoma), one hemobilia, and one portal vein thrombosis. Complications more specific to percutaneous PVE included portal vein thrombosis and portal hypertension resulting in esophageal variceal hemorrhage. However, the authors emphasized that given the potential for injury to the FLR when using the contralateral approach, the ipsilateral approach should be tried first.

Di Stefano and colleagues [85] conducted a study of 188 patients who underwent PVE using the contralateral approach. They reported that only one patient experienced a major complication (complete portal vein thrombosis) directly related to the contralateral approach that precluded the planned surgical resection. Two other patients experienced inadvertent migration of embolic material into the FLR requiring intervention; one needed a portoportal graft during hepatic resection because of portal vein thrombosis. On CT imaging, another 10 patients were found to have embolic material in non-targeted portal venous branches.

Ribero and colleagues [67] recently studied 112 patients who underwent PVE with the ipsilateral approach. In this study, only one patient had non-targeted embolization to the FLR. However, the overall complication rate was 8.9%, which was not substantially different than the rate reported by Di Stefano and colleagues. If one takes into account the fact that Di Stefano and colleagues considered clinically occult incidental CT findings in their complication rate, the studies reported remarkably similar numbers. Further, the study by Ribero and colleagues found no difference in the complication rate whether right PVE was extended to segment 4 or not.

Outcomes Following PVE and Hepatectomy for HCC

In patients who developed HCC in the setting of chronic liver disease (e.g., chronic hepatitis, fibrosis, or cirrhosis), the increase in non-embolized liver volumes after PVE varies (range, 28–46%), and hypertrophy after PVE may take more than 4 weeks because of slower regeneration rates [45]. The degree of parenchymal fibrosis is thought to limit regeneration, possibly as a result of reduced portal blood flow

[75]. However, a study by Denys and colleagues [99], in which 40 patients with HCC in the setting of advanced liver fibrosis and cirrhosis, found that only two factors significantly affected hypertrophy: a lower degree of fibrosis, as indicated by a Knodell histological score [103] of <F4, and a pre-PVE lower functional liver ratio as defined by the ratio between the left liver (i.e., FLR) and the total liver volume minus tumor volume. Factors that did not correlate with improved hypertrophy included age, sex, history of diabetes, and prior chemoembolization. In addition, numerous studies have been performed that evaluated liver regeneration and the degree of hypertrophy after preoperative PVE in patients with and without underlying liver disease (Table 11.1) [104–106].

Rates of hepatectomy after PVE in patients with HCC are reported to be approximately 70%; series that report a very high rate of hepatectomy after PVE (over 90%) are either very small (<15 patients) or include patients who underwent less extensive PVE (e.g., embolization of only the right anterior or right posterior sector). Furthermore, in patients with HCC and chronic liver disease, hepatectomy outcomes, including the number and severity of complications and the incidence of postoperative liver failure and death, are better with PVE than without [26, 45, 71, 75, 107, 108]. Good outcomes following major hepatectomy after PVE in patients with HCC are regularly reported. In 2000, Azoulay and colleagues [75] reported long-term outcomes after resection of three or more liver segments for

Table 11.1 Future liver remnant (FLR) hypertrophy after portal vein embolization in patients with and without underlying liver disease

Author (year)	Baseline liver	PVE (n)	FLR (%) Pre	Post	DH (%)
Abdalla, 2002 [5]	Normal	18	18	25	8
Aoki, 2004 [72]	ICGR 15 <10%	8	40	51	11
	ICGR 15 >10%	9			
Azoulay, 2000 [75]	Mild or moderate	3	36	52	16
	fibrosis Cirrhosis	7			
Cotroneo, 2009 [104]	Normal	24	23	33	10
	Cirrhosis	7	31	40	9
Farges, 2003 [71]	Normal	13	31	47	16
	Cirrhosis	14	35	44	9
Ogata, 2006 [93]	Cirrhosis (PVE)	18	29	37	8
	Cirrhosis (TACE/PVE)	18	30	42	12
Ribero, 2007 [67]	Normal, fibrosis, Cirrhosis	112	–	–	9–11
Sugawara, 2002 [105]	Cirrhosis	40	35	48	13
Vauthey, 2000 [3]	Normal	12	26	36	10
Wakabayashi, 2002 [106]	Normal	17	27	36	9
	Hepatitis	26	33	40	7

PVE = portal vein embolization, (n) = number of patients, DH = degree of hypertrophy, TACE = transcatheter arterial chemoembolization, and ICGR 15 = indocyanine green retention at 15 min

HCC in patients with cirrhosis. PVE was performed when the FLR volume was predicted to be less than 40% and led to significant increases in the FLR volumes in all embolized patients. Importantly, none of 10 patients who underwent PVE had liver failure or death following resection whereas three of 19 patients in the non-PVE group suffered liver failure and one patient died. Overall survival (44% PVE vs. 53% no PVE), disease-free survival (21% PVE vs. 17% no PVE), and complication rates (56% PVE vs. 57% no PVE) were similar with or without PVE. Importantly, Wakabayashi and colleagues found that overall and disease-free survival rates remain similar between the groups even after adjustment for HCC stage (overall survival: 40% PVE vs. 46% no PVE; disease-free survival: 28% PVE vs. 13% no PVE; both $P =$ NS). Tanaka and colleagues [108] reported several benefits of PVE in a larger study of patients with HCC and cirrhosis. Disease-free survival rates were similar, but cumulative survival rates were significantly higher in the PVE group than in the non-PVE group. In addition, patients with recurrence following PVE plus resection were more often candidates for further treatments such as chemoembolization, an additional benefit of PVE in the long term (Table 11.2) [109–111].

Another study validated residual volume as the key to prediction of postoperative liver function and posthepatectomy course and the utility of PVE in patients with HCC. Palavecino and colleagues [112] evaluated 54 patients that underwent major hepatic resection for HCC between 1998 and 2007 and PVE was performed when the FLR volume was predicted to be insufficient [PVE group ($n = 21$), non-PVE group ($n = 33$)]. Both groups had similar rates of fibrosis or cirrhosis, HCV, HBV, American Joint Committee on Cancer stage, preoperative chemoembolization, overall postoperative complications and positive margin (P all non-significant). There were no perioperative deaths in the PVE group and six (18%) in the non-PVE group ($P = 0.038$). Excluding these perioperative deaths, the overall survival rates at 1, 3, and 5 years were 94, 82, and 72% in the PVE group and 93, 63, and 54% in the non-PVE group, respectively ($P = 0.35$). Similarly, disease-free survival was not significantly different between the groups, with 1-, 3- and 5-year disease-free survival of 84, 56, and 56% in the PVE group and 66%, 49% and 49% in the non-PVE group, respectively ($P = 0.38$). The authors concluded that PVE before major hepatectomy for HCC is associated with improved perioperative outcome. Further, excluding perioperative mortality, overall survival and disease-free survival rates were similar between patients with and without preoperative PVE.

Some data suggest that not only PVE provides an outcome benefit in patients with cirrhosis but the greatest outcome benefit may occur within the patient subset with worse liver function. In one study, multivariate analysis revealed that preoperative PVE was an independent predictor of survival following resection in patients with preoperative indocyanine green retention $\leq$ 13 (5-year overall survival rate, 52% PVE vs. 20% no PVE; $P = 0.002$) [108].

The combination of chemoembolization of the tumor followed by PVE before hepatectomy may further improve long-term outcomes after major resection for HCC. Aoki and colleagues reported on their experience with this strategy in 17 patients and found 5-year overall and disease-free survival rates of 56 and 47%,

Table 11.2 Patient mortality and postoperative complications after portal vein embolization (PVE) followed by major hepatectomy

Author (year)	Etiology	Baseline liver	PVE (n)	Major hepatectomy (%)	Postoperative complications/hepatic insufficiency	Mortality
Abdalla, 2002 [5]	Mixed	Normal	18	100	38%	0% (90 days)
Azoulay, 2000 [75]	HCC	Mild to moderate fibrosis	3	90	45%/0%	0% (ND)
		Cirrhosis	7			
Farges, 2003 [71]	Mixed	Combined	27	100	37%/4%	4% (in-hosp)
Hemming, 2003 [109]	Mixed	Combined	39	100	–	0% (30 days)
Imamura, 1999 [55]	Mixed	Combined	57	100	1.8%/1.8%	1.8% (30 days)
Ladurner, 2003 [110]	Mixed	Combined	19	68	–	0% (90 days)
Ribero, 2007 [67]	Mixed	Combined	78	100	21%/5.3%	3% (90 days)
Sugawara, 2002 [105]	HCC	Chronic hepatitis	50	64	19.7%/0%	0% (ND)
		Cirrhosis	16			
Takayama [2004]	Mixed	Combined	161	81	19%	1.2% (ND)
Tanaka, 2000 [108]	HCC	Cirrhosis	33	100	–	3% (30 days)
Vauthey, 2000 [3]	Mixed	Normal	12	100	–	0% (30 days)
Vauthey, 2004 [6]	Mixed	Normal	31	100	–	0% (30 days)
Wakabayashi, 2001 [111]	HCC	Cirrhosis	26	100	–/15.4%	12% (30 days)

PVE = portal vein embolization, n = number, HCC = hepatocellular carcinoma, ND = not defined

respectively. In a similar retrospective study, Ogata and colleagues [93] found that chemoembolization followed by PVE led to complete necrosis of the tumor in more than 80% of patients, compared to 5% with PVE alone. They also found that chemoembolization followed by PVE was associated with better 5-year disease-free survival rates than PVE alone (37% vs. 19%; $P = 0.04$), primarily due to lower rates of early recurrence in the liver.

The outcome from PVE and subsequent resection may be even more closely linked to the PVE technique in patients with otherwise normal livers than in patients with chronically diseased livers. In patients with cirrhosis, RPVE (without segment 4) is the most common technique used since extended hepatectomy is rarely indicated or possible. In patients without cirrhosis who have HCC [113], extended right or less commonly left hepatectomy is often indicated. In the case of extended right hepatectomy, owing to the consistently small volume of the left lateral liver (segments 2/3), preoperative PVE is frequently needed [69].

A recent report from M.D. Anderson Cancer Center considered 127 consecutive extended hepatectomies using standardized liver volume calculations to select patients for PVE [6]. In this series that was not limited to patients with HCC, 31 (24.4%) of the patients underwent PVE prior to extended hepatectomy. Only six patients (5%) experienced significant postoperative liver insufficiency (total bilirubin level >10 mg/dL or international normalized ratio >2). The postoperative complication rate was 30.7% (39/127), and only one patient (0.8%) died after hepatectomy. The median survival was 41.9 months, and the overall 5-year survival rate was 26% for the entire group. The low mortality rate following extended hepatectomy in this series reflects many factors, among which was the systematic attention to FLR volume and the use of PVE based on the indications reviewed above.

Conclusions

PVE is now a validated technique to increase the volume and function of the remnant liver prior to resection of hepatobiliary cancer. PVE increases the safety of major resection in patients with liver disease and extends the option of resection to patients with multiple hepatic metastases and limited parenchymal sparing from metastatic disease. Careful attention to key factors, such as the presence or absence of underlying liver disease, adjustment of liver size to patient size using proper techniques to measure the liver remnant, and recognition of the physiologic effect of the type of hepatic and extrahepatic procedure planned, permits the appropriate selection of patients for PVE. The FLR should be measured and standardized to the patient using the calculated FLR/TELV ratio, because this method produces a reproducible, accurate index of posthepatectomy liver function. Currently recommended thresholds prompting consideration of preoperative PVE are FLR/TELV ratios of ≤20% for patients with an otherwise normal liver, ≤30% for patients who have received high-dose chemotherapy, and <40% for patients with chronic liver disease. Continued critical analysis of the factors affecting liver hypertrophy in parallel with improvements in oncologic treatments will further improve the selection and outcomes of patients with liver cancer considered for PVE.

References

1. Tsao JI, Loftus JP, Nagorney DM, Adson MA, Ilstrup DM (1994) Trends in morbidity and mortality of hepatic resection for malignancy: matched comparative analysis. Ann Surg 220: 99–205

2. Shirabe K, Shimada M, Gion T et al (1999) Postoperative liver failure after major hepatic resection for hepatocellular carcinoma in the modern era with special reference to remnant liver volume. J Am Coll Surg 188:304–309

3. Vauthey JN, Chaoui A, Do KA et al (2000) Standardized measurement of the future liver remnant prior to extended liver resection: methodology and clinical associations. Surgery 127:512–519

4. Shoup M, Gonen M, D'Angelica M et al (2003) Volumetric analysis predicts hepatic dysfunction in patients undergoing major liver resection. J Gastrointest Surg 7:325–330

5. Abdalla EK, Barnett CC, Doherty D, Curley SA, Vauthey JN (2002) Extended hepatectomy in patients with hepatobiliary malignancies with and without preoperative portal vein embolization. Arch Surg 137:675–680

6. Vauthey JN, Pawlik TM, Abdalla EK et al (2004) Is extended hepatectomy for hepatobiliary malignancy justified? Ann Surg 239:722–730

7. Kubota K, Makuuchi M, Kusaka K et al (1997) Measurement of liver volume and hepatic functional reserve as a guide to decision-making in resectional surgery for hepatic tumors. Hepatology 26:1176–1181

8. Azoulay D, Castaing D, Smail A et al (2000) Resection of nonresectable liver metastases from colorectal cancer after percutaneous portal vein embolization. Ann Surg 231:480–486

9. Abdalla EK, Hicks ME, Vauthey JN. (2001) Portal vein embolization: rationale, technique and future prospects. Br J Surg 88:165–175

10. Makuuchi M, Thai BL, Takayasu K et al (1990) Preoperative portal vein embolization to increase safety of major hepatectomy for hilar bile duct carcinoma: a preliminary report. Surgery 107:521–527

11. de Baere T, Roche A, Vavasseur D et al (1993) Portal vein embolization: utility for inducing left hepatic lobe hypertrophy before surgery. Radiology 188:73–77

12. Nagino M, Nimura Y, Kamiya J et al (1995) Right or left trisegment portal vein embolization before hepatic trisegmentectomy for hilar bile duct carcinoma. Surgery 117:677–681

13. Nagino M, Kamiya J, Kanai M et al (2000) Right trisegment portal vein embolization for biliary tract carcinoma: technique and clinical utility. Surgery 127:155–160

14. Vauthey JN, Abdalla EK, Doherty DA et al (2002) Body surface area and body weight predict total liver volume in Western adults. Liver Transpl 8:233–240

15. Madoff DC, Abdalla EK, Vauthey JN (2005) Portal vein embolization in preparation for major hepatic resection: evolution of a new standard of care. J Vasc Interv Radiol 16: 779–790

16. Abulkhir A, Limongelli P, Healey AJ, Damrah O, Tait P, Jackson J, Habib N, Jiao LR (2008) Preoperative portal vein embolization for major liver resection: a meta-analysis. Ann Surg 247:49–57

17. Rous P, Larimore LD (1920) Relation of the portal blood flow to liver maintenance. A demonstration of liver atrophy conditional on compensation. J Exp Med 31:609–632

18. Schalm L, Bax HR, Mansens BJ (1956) Atrophy of the liver after occlusion of the bile ducts or portal vein and compensatory hypertrophy of the unoccluded portion and its clinical importance. Gastroenterology 31:131–155

19. Honjo I, Suzuki T, Ozawa K, Takasan H, Kitamura O, Ishikawa T (1975) Ligation of a branch of the portal vein for carcinoma of the liver. Am J Surg 130:296–302
20. Takayasu K, Matsumura Y, Shima Y, Moriyama N, Yamada T, Makuuchi M (1986) Hepatic lobar hypertrophy following obstruction of the ipsilateral portal vein from cholangiocarcinoma. Radiology 160:389–393
21. Kinoshita H, Sakai K, Hirohashi K, Igawa S, Yamasaki O, Kubo S (1986) Preoperative portal vein embolization for hepatocellular carcinoma. World J Surg 10:803–808
22. Koniaris LG, McKillop IH, Schwartz SI, Zimmers TA (2003) Liver regeneration. J Am Coll Surg 197:634–659
23. Ponfick VA (1890) Ueber Leberresection und Leberreaction. Verhandl Deutsch Gesellsch Chir 19:28 [German]
24. Michalopoulos GK, DeFrances MC (1997) Liver Regeneration. Science 276:60–66
25. Black DM, Behrns KE (2002) A scientist revisits the atrophy-hypertrophy complex: hepatic apoptosis and regeneration. Surg Oncol Clin N Am 11:849–864
26. Lee KC, Kinoshita H, Hirohashi K, Kubo S, Iwasa R (1993) Extension of surgical indication for hepatocellular carcinoma by portal vein embolization. World J Surg 17:109–115
27. Mizuno S, Nimura Y, Suzuki H, Yoshida S (1996) Portal vein branch occlusion induces cell proliferation of cholestatic rat liver. J Surg Res 60:249–257
28. Takeuchi E, Nimura Y, Mizuno S et al (1996) Ligation of portal vein branch induces DNA polymerases alpha, delta, and epsilon in nonligated lobes. J Surg Res 65:15–24
29. Kim RD, Stein GS, Chari RS (2001) Impact of cell swelling on proliferative signal transduction in the liver. J Cell Biochem 83:56–69
30. Nagy P, Teramoto T, Factor VM et al (2001) Reconstitution of liver mass via cellular hypertrophy in the rat. Hepatology 33:339–345
31. Komori K, Nagino M, Nimura Y (2006) Hepatocyte morphology and kinetics after portal vein embolization. Br J Surg 93:745–751
32. Kim RD, Kim JS, Watanabe G, Mohuczy D, Behrns KE (2008) Liver regeneration and the atrophy-hypertrophy complex. Seminars in Interventional Radiology 25:92–103
33. Starzl TE, Francavilla A, Porter KA, Benichou J, Jones AF (1978) The effect of splanchnic viscera removal upon canine liver regeneration. Surg Gynecol Obstet 147:193–207
34. Nagino M, Nimura Y, Kamiya J et al (1995) Changes in hepatic lobe volume in biliary tract cancer patients after right portal vein embolization. Hepatology 21:434–439
35. Kock NG, Hahnloser P, Roding B, Schenk WG Jr (1972) Interaction between portal venous and hepatic arterial blood flow: an experimental study in the dog. Surgery 72:414–419
36. Michalopoulos GK, Zarnegar R (1992) Hepatocyte growth factor. Hepatology 15:149–155
37. Bucher NLR, Swaffield MN (1975) Regulation of hepatic regeneration in rats by synergistic action of insulin and glucagon. Proc Natl Acad Sci USA 72:1157–1160
38. Fabrikant JI (1968) The kinetics of cellular proliferation in regenerating liver. J Cell Biol 36:551–565
39. Francavilla A, Porter KA, Benichou J et al (1978) Liver regeneration in dogs: morphologic and chemical changes. J Surg Res 25:409–419
40. Gaglio PJ, Baskin G, Bohm R Jr et al (2000) Partial hepatectomy and laparoscopic-guided liver biopsy in rhesus macaques (*Macaca mulatta*): novel approach for study of liver regeneration. Comp Med 50:363–368
41. Bucher NLR, Swaffield MN (1964) The rate of incorporation of labeled thymidine into the deoxyribonucleic acid of regenerating rat liver in relation to the amount of liver excised. Cancer Res 24:1611–1625
42. Duncan JR, Hicks ME, Cai SR, Brunt EM, Ponder KP (1999) Embolization of portal vein branches induces hepatocyte hypertrophy in swine: a potential step in hepatic gene therapy. Radiology 210:467–477
43. Goto Y, Nagino M, Nimura Y (1998) Doppler estimation of portal blood flow after percutaneous transhepatic portal vein embolization. Ann Surg 228:209–213

44. Yamanaka N, Okamoto E, Kawamura E et al (1993) Dynamics of normal and injured liver regeneration after hepatectomy as assessed on the basis of computed tomography and liver function. Hepatology 18:79–85
45. Shimamura T, Nakajima Y, Une Y et al (1997) Efficacy and safety of preoperative percutaneous transhepatic portal embolization with absolute ethanol: a clinical study. Surgery 121:135–141
46. Kawarada Y, Sanda M, Kawamura K, Suzaki M, Nakase I, Mizumoto R (1991) Simultaneous extensive resection of the liver and pancreas in dogs. Gastroenterol Jpn 6:747–756
47. Anderson CD, Meranze S, Bream P Jr et al (2004) Contralateral portal vein embolization for hepatectomy in the setting of hepatic steatosis. Am Surg 70:609–612
48. Veteläinen R, van Vliet AK, van Gulik TM (2007) Severe steatosis increases hepatocellular injury and impairs liver regeneration in a rat model of partial hepatectomy. Ann Surg 245: 44–50
49. Veteläinen R, Bennink RJ, van Vliet AK, van Gulik TM (2007) Mild steatosis impairs functional recovery after liver resection in an experimental model. Br J Surg 94:1002–1008
50. DeAngelis RA, Markiewski MM, Taub R, Lambris JD (2005) A high-fat diet impairs liver regeneration in C57BL/6 mice through overexpression of the NF-κB inhibitor, IκBα. Hepatology 42:1148–1157
51. Ijichi M, Makuuchi M, Imamura H, Takayama T (2001) Portal embolization relieves persistent jaundice after complete biliary drainage. Surgery 130:116–118
52. Uesaka K, Nimura Y, Nagino M (1996) Changes in hepatic lobar function after right portal vein embolization. An appraisal by biliary indocyanine green excretion. Ann Surg 223:77–83
53. Hirai I, Kimura W, Fuse A, Suto K, Urayama M (2003) Evaluation of preoperative portal embolization for safe hepatectomy, with special reference to assessment of nonembolized lobe function with 99mTc-GSA SPECT scintigraphy. Surgery 133:495–506
54. De Baere T, Roche A, Elias D, Lasser P, Lagrange C, Bousson V (1996) Preoperative portal vein embolization for extension of hepatectomy indications. Hepatology 24:1386–1391
55. Imamura H, Shimada R, Kubota M et al (1999) Preoperative portal vein embolization: an audit of 84 patients. Hepatology 29:1099–1105
56. Wakabayashi H, Okada S, Maeba T, Maeta H (1997) Effect of preoperative portal vein embolization on major hepatectomy for advanced-stage hepatocellular carcinomas in injured livers: a preliminary report. Surg Today 27:403–410
57. Shibayama Y, Hashimoto K, Nakata K (1991) Recovery from hepatic necrosis following acute portal vein embolism with special reference to reconstruction of occluded vessels. J Pathol 165:255–261
58. Ikeda K, Kinoshita H, Hirohashi K, Kubo S, Kaneda K (1995) The ultrastructure, kinetics and intralobular distribution of apoptotic hepatocytes after portal branch ligation with special reference to their relationship to necrotic hepatocytes. Arch Histol Cytol 58:171–184
59. Madoff DC, Hicks ME, Vauthey JN et al (2002) Transhepatic portal vein embolization: anatomy, indications, and technical considerations. Radiographics 22:1063–1076
60. Denys A, Madoff DC, Doenz F et al (2002) Indications for and limitations of portal vein embolization prior to major hepatic resection for hepatobiliary malignancy. Surg Oncol Clin N Am 11:955–968
61. Heymsfield SB, Fulenwider T, Nordlinger B et al (1979) Accurate measurement of liver, kidney, and spleen volume and mass by computerized axial tomography. Ann Intern Med 90:185–187
62. Soyer P, Roche A, Elias D, Levesque M (1992) Hepatic metastases from colorectal cancer: influence of hepatic volumetric analysis on surgical decision making. Radiology 184: 695–697
63. Ogasawara K, Une Y, Nakajima Y, Uchino J. (1995) The significance of measuring liver volume using computed tomographic images before and after hepatectomy. Surg Today 25:43–48
64. Makuuchi M, Kosuge T, Takayama T et al (1993) Surgery for small liver cancers. Semin Surg Oncol 9:298–304

65. Chun YS, Ribero D, Abdalla EK, Madoff DC, Mortenson MM, Wei SH, Vauthey JN (2008) Comparison of two methods of future liver remnant volume measurement. J Gastrointest Surg 12:123–128
66. Johnson TN, Tucker GT, Tanner MS, Rostami-Hodjegan A (2005) Changes in liver volume from birth to adulthood: a meta-analysis. Liver Transpl 11:1481–1493
67. Ribero D, Abdalla EK, Madoff DC, Donadon M, Loyer EM, Vauthey JN (2007) Portal vein embolization before major hepatectomy and its effects on regeneration, resectability and outcome. Br J Surg 94:1386–1394
68. Mitsumori A, Nagaya I, Kimoto S et al (1998) Preoperative evaluation of hepatic functional reserve following hepatectomy by technetium-99m galactosyl human serum albumin liver scintigraphy and computed tomography. Eur J Nucl Med 25:1377–1382
69. Abdalla EK, Denys A, Chevalier P, Nemr RA, Vauthey JN (2004) Total and segmental liver volume variations: implications for liver surgery. Surgery 135:404–410
70. Leelaudomlipi S, Sugawara Y, Kaneko J, Matsui Y, Ohkubo T, Makuuchi M (2002) Volumetric analysis of liver segments in 155 living donors. Liver Transpl 8:612–614
71. Farges O, Belghiti J, Kianmanesh R et al (2003) Portal vein embolization before right hepatectomy: prospective clinical trial. Ann Surg 237:208–217
72. Aoki T, Imamura H, Hasegawa K et al (2004) Sequential preoperative arterial and portal venous embolizations in patients with hepatocellular carcinoma. Arch Surg 139:766–774
73. Bedossa P, Dargere D, Paradis V (2003) Sampling variability of liver fibrosis in chronic hepatitis C. Hepatology 38:449–1457
74. Elias D, Lasser P, Spielmann M et al (1991) Surgical and chemotherapeutic treatment of hepatic metastases from carcinoma of the breast. Surg Gynecol Obstet 172:461–464
75. Azoulay D, Castaing D, Krissat J et al (2000) Percutaneous portal vein embolization increases the feasibility and safety of major liver resection for hepatocellular carcinoma in injured liver. Ann Surg 232:665–672
76. Kooby DA, Fong Y, Suriawinata A et al (2003) Impact of steatosis on perioperative outcome following hepatic resection. J Gastrointest Surg 7:1034–1044
77. Vauthey JN, Pawlik TM, Ribero D et al (2006) Chemotherapy regimen predicts steatohepatitis and an increase in 90-day mortality after surgery for hepatic colorectal metastases. J Clin Oncol 24:2065–2072
78. Adam R, Delvart V, Pascal G et al (2004) Rescue surgery for unresectable colorectal liver metastases downstaged by chemotherapy: a model to predict long-term survival. Ann Surg 240:644–657
79. Goere D, Farges O, Leporrier J, Sauvanet A, Vilgrain V, Belghiti J (2006) Chemotherapy does not impair hypertrophy of the left liver after right portal vein obstruction. J Gastrointest Surg 10:365–370
80. Beal IK, Anthony S, Papadopoulou A et al (2006) Portal vein embolisation prior to hepatic resection for colorectal liver metastases and the effects of periprocedure chemotherapy. Br J Radiol 79:473–478
81. Covey AM, Brown KT, Jarnagin WR et al (2008) Combined portal vein embolization and neoadjuvant chemotherapy as a treatment strategy for resectable hepatic colorectal metastases. Ann Surg 247:451–455
82. Zorzi D, Chun YS, Madoff DC, Abdalla EK, Vauthey JN (2008) Chemotherapy with bevacizumab does not affect liver regeneration after portal vein embolization in the treatment of colorectal liver metastases. Ann Surg Oncol 15:2765–2772
83. Denys AL, Abehsera M, Sauvanet A, Sibert A, Belghiti J, Menu Y (1999) Failure of right portal vein ligation to induce left lobe hypertrophy due to intrahepatic portoportal collaterals: successful treatment with portal vein embolization. AJR Am J Roentgenol 173:633–635
84. Azoulay D, Raccuia JS, Castaing D, Bismuth H. (1995) Right portal vein embolization in preparation for major hepatic resection. J Am Coll Surg 181:266–269
85. Di Stefano DR, de Baere T, Denys A et al (2005) Preoperative percutaneous portal vein embolization: evaluation of adverse events in 188 patients. Radiology 234:625–630

86. Nagıno M, Nimura Y, Kamiya J, Kondo S, Kanai M. (1996) Selective percutaneous transhepatic embolization of the portal vein in preparation for extensive liver resection: the ipsilateral approach. Radiology 200:559–563

87. Madoff DC, Hicks ME, Abdalla EK, Morris JS, Vauthey JN (2003) Portal vein embolization with polyvinyl alcohol particles and coils in preparation for major liver resection for hepatobiliary malignancy: safety and effectiveness – study in 26 patients. Radiology 227:251–260

88. Madoff DC, Abdalla EK, Gupta S et al (2005) Transhepatic ipsilateral right portal vein embolization extended to segment IV: improving hypertrophy and resection outcomes with spherical particles and coils. J Vasc Interv Radiol 16:215–225

89. Gibo M, Unten S, Yogi A et al (2007) Percutaneous ipsilateral portal vein embolization using a modified four-lumen balloon catheter with fibrin glue: initial clinical experience. Radiat Med 25:164–172

90. Tsuda M, Kurihara N, Saito H, et al (2006) Ipsilateral percutaneous transhepatic portal vein embolization with gelatin sponge particles and coils in preparation for extended right hepatectomy for hilar cholangiocarcinoma. J Vasc Interv Radiol 17:989–994

91. Nagino M, Kanai M, Morioka A et al (2000) Portal and arterial embolization before extensive liver resection in patients with markedly poor functional reserve. J Vasc Interv Radiol 11:1063–1068

92. Gruttadauria S, Luca A, Mandala' L, Miraglia R, Gridelli B (2006) Sequential preoperative ipsilateral portal and arterial embolization in patients with colorectal liver metastases. World J Surg 30:576–578

93. Ogata S, Belghiti J, Farges O, Varma D, Sibert A, Vilgrain V (2006) Sequential arterial and portal vein embolizations before right hepatectomy in patients with cirrhosis and hepatocellular carcinoma. Br J Surg 93:1091–1098

94. Perarnau JM, Daradkeh S, Johann M, Deneuville M, Weinling P, Coniel C (2003) Transjugular preoperative portal embolization (TJPE): a pilot study. Hepatogastroenterology 50:610–613

95. Capussotti L, Muratore A, Ferrero A, Anselmetti GC, Corgnier A, Regge D (2005) Extension of right portal vein embolization to segment IV portal branches. Arch Surg 140:1100–1103

96. Kishi Y, Madoff DC, Abdalla EK, Palavecino M, Ribero D, Chun YS, Vauthey JN (2008) Is embolization of segment 4 portal veins before extended right hepatectomy justified? Surgery 144:744–751

97. Elias D, De Baere T, Roche A, Ducreux M, Leclere J, Lasser P (1999) During liver regeneration following right portal embolization the growth rate of liver metastases is more rapid than that of the liver parenchyma. Br J Surg 86:784–788

98. Kokudo N, Tada K, Seki M et al (2001) Proliferative activity of intrahepatic colorectal metastases after preoperative hemihepatic portal vein embolization. Hepatology 34:267–272

99. Denys A, Lacombe C, Schneider F et al (2005) Portal vein embolization with N-butyl cyanoacrylate before partial hepatectomy in patients with hepatocellular carcinoma and underlying cirrhosis or advanced fibrosis. J Vasc Interv Radiol 16:1667–1674

100. Ogasawara K, Uchino J, Une Y, Fujioka Y (1996) Selective portal vein embolization with absolute ethanol induces hepatic hypertrophy and makes more extensive hepatectomy possible. Hepatology 23:338–345

101. Brown K, Brody L, Decorato D, Getrajdman G (2001) Portal vein embolization with use of polyvinyl alcohol. J Vasc Interv Radiol 12:882–886

102. Kodama Y, Shimizu T, Endo H, Miyamoto N, Miyasaka K (2002) Complications of percutaneous transhepatic portal vein embolization. J Vasc Interv Radiol 13:1233–1237

103. Knodell R, Ishak K, Black W et al (1981) Formulation and application of a numerical scoring system for assessing histological activity in asymptomatic chronic active hepatitis. Hepatology 1:431–435

104. Cotroneo AR, Innocenti P, Marano G, Legnini M, Iezzi R (2009) Pre-hepatectomy portal vein embolization: single center experience. Eur J Surg Oncol 35:71–78
105. Sugawara Y, Yamamoto J, Higashi H et al (2002) Preoperative portal embolization in patients with hepatocellular carcinoma. World J Surg 26:105–110
106. Wakabayashi H, Ishimura K, Okano K, Karasawa Y, Goda F, Maeba T, Maeta H (2002) Application of preoperative portal vein embolization before major hepatic resection in patients with normal or abnormal liver parenchyma. Surgery 131:26–33
107. Wakabayashi H, Yachida S, Maeba T, Maeta H (2000) Indications for portal vein embolization combined with major hepatic resection for advanced-stage hepatocellular carcinomas. A preliminary clinical study. Dig Surg 17:587–594
108. Tanaka H, Hirohashi K, Kubo S, Shuto T, Higaki I, Kinoshita H (2000) Preoperative portal vein embolization improves prognosis after right hepatectomy for hepatocellular carcinoma in patients with impaired hepatic function. Br J Surg 87:879–882
109. Hemming AW, Reed AI, Howard RJ et al (2003) Preoperative portal vein embolization for extended hepatectomy. Ann Surg 237:686–691
110. Ladurner R, Brandacher G, Riedl-Huter C et al (2003) Percutaneous portal vein embolisation in preparation for extended hepatic resection of primary nonresectable liver tumours. Dig Liver Dis 35:716–721
111. Wakabayashi H, Ishimura K, Okano K et al (2001) Is preoperative portal vein embolization effective in improving prognosis after major hepatic resection in patients with advanced-stage hepatocellular carcinoma? Cancer 92:2384–2390
112. Palavecino M, Chun YS, Madoff DC et al (2009) Major hepatic resection for hepatocellular carcinoma with or without portal vein embolization: perioperative outcome and survival. Surgery 145:399–405
113. Nzeako UC, Goodman ZD, Ishak KG (1996) Hepatocellular carcinoma in cirrhotic and non-cirrhotic livers. A clinico-histopathologic study of 804 North American patients. Am J Clin Pathol 105:65–75

Chapter 12
Laparoscopic Liver Resection for HCC: A European Perspective

Luca Viganò and Daniel Cherqui

Keywords Laparoscopic liver resection · HCC · Hepatic resection

Hepatocellular carcinoma (HCC), the most common primary liver cancer, occurs in >90% of the cases on an underlying hepatic disease [1]. Screening programs allow diagnosis at an early stage where curative treatments can be proposed. These include liver resection, percutaneous radiofrequency ablation, and liver transplantation [1, 2]. Even if liver transplantation is the best treatment for early HCC by removing both the tumor and the underlying liver disease, shortage of donor organs and dropout from the waiting list limit its efficacy [3]. In recent years liver resection in cirrhotic patients became safer [4, 5] and achieved a key role in HCC treatment: in advanced tumors it is the only therapeutic option, while in early tumor it can be proposed as an alternative or a bridge to liver transplantation [6–9].

The vast majority of hepatic resections for HCC are stand-alone procedures, without any need for reconstruction, which should make them good candidates for a laparoscopic approach. However, diffusion of laparoscopic liver resection is still limited and few centers worldwide regularly perform it [10]. The reasons for the limited development of such an approach to date are threefold. First, technical problems are anticipated and, indeed, the elementary maneuvers of open hepatic surgery (including manual palpation, organ mobilization, vascular control, and parenchymal transection) are thought to be difficult to reproduce laparoscopically. Second, there are anticipated hazards: hemorrhage may be more difficult to control laparoscopically, especially in cirrhotic livers, and the risk of gas embolism may be increased by the use of pneumoperitoneum. The third problem is a fear of oncological inadequacy and tumor spread. Although still limited in number of cases, publications about laparoscopic liver resection have increased in recent years and HCC has been one of the most common indications. In this chapter, we will review the various

D. Cherqui (✉)
Department of Surgery, New York-Presbyterian/Weill Cornell, New York, NY, USA

K.M. McMasters, J.-N. Vauthey (eds.), *Hepatocellular Carcinoma*,
DOI 10.1007/978-1-60327-522-4_12, © Springer Science+Business Media, LLC 2011

aspects of laparoscopic liver resection for HCC, including technical features, short- and long-term results. We will also briefly discuss the impact of laparoscopic liver resection on the treatment strategy of HCC.

Feasibility: Technique and Indications

In comparison with open hepatectomy series, the number of published papers about laparoscopic liver surgery is very low [10]. At present only 14 studies (including 1 multicentric) reported 50 or more cases [11–24] (Table 12.1). Interestingly the majority of them have been published in the last 2 years [11, 13, 18–24]. An increasing proportion of malignant diseases have been treated and HCC was the most common indication.

The feasibility of laparoscopic liver resection has been the main criterion studied to date. Despite the increasing number of reported series, in expert centers laparoscopic approach ranges from 5 to 30% [11, 13, 15, 16, 22] and only some recent series reported higher rates, reaching 50–80% [18, 20, 21]. On our part, over the past 12 years (1996–2008), we performed 174 laparoscopic liver resections out of 782 hepatectomies (22.3%) [25]. Considering HCC, the proportion of laparoscopic resection was higher, about 30% (69 of 229) and reached 39.4% in the last 4 years of our experience [25].

Table 12.1 Series of laparoscopic liver resections including more than 50 cases

Author	Year	#	Proportion of LLR on total LR	Malignant lesions	HCC
Descottes [14][a]	2003	87	NR	0%	0%
Mala [15]	2005	53	44%	89% (47)	2% (1)
Kaneko [16]	2005	52	17%	NR	77% (40)
Vibert [12]	2006	89	NR	73% (65)	18% (16)
Cai [17]	2006	62	NR	32% (20)	29% (18)
Dagher [11]	2007	70	15%	54% (38)	34% (24)
Koffron [18][b]	2007	273	NR	37% (103)	NR
Chen [19]	2008	116	NR	100% (116)	100% (116)
Topal [13]	2008	109	28%	71% (77)	NR
Buell [20]	2008	253	NR	42% (106)	14% (36)
Cho [21]	2008	128	NR	61% (78)	45% (57)
Sasaki [23]	2008	82	29%	93% (78)	45% (37)
Inagaki [24]	2009	68	NR	76% (52)	43% (36)
Cherqui [25]	2009	174	22%	63% (110)	40% (69)

[a]multicentric study
[b]only pure laparoscopic and hand-assisted laparoscopic hepatectomies included
NR: data not reported; LLR: laparoscopic liver resection; LR: liver resection

Surgical Technique

State-of-the-art equipment is required. The use of two monitors is recommended. Although some groups use 0° laparoscopes [11, 12], 30° laparoscopes are preferred by most authors.

Patient Positioning

We suggest two different positions according to lesion site. For lesions located in segments 2 through 5 (the majority of cases), the patient is placed in the supine position, with lower limbs apart (Fig. 12.1). The surgeon stands between the legs with one assistant on each side. For patients with lesions of segment 6 scheduled for atypical resection or segmentectomy, the left lateral decubitus position may be used in order to expose the lateral and posterior aspect of the right liver (Fig. 12.2). In this case the surgeon is on the ventral side of the patient. In case of laparoscopic right hepatectomy, supine position with lower limbs apart is preferred. Some authors prefer supine position with the surgeon stand on patient side and the assistant on the opposite one [18].

Pneumoperitoneum

A problem concerning laparoscopic liver surgery is the pneumoperitoneum itself. The risk of gas embolism due to hepatic vein lesions during parenchymal

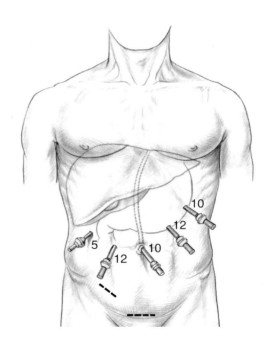

Fig. 12.1 Port placement for resection of lesions located in segments 2–5 and for right hepatectomy. The patient is in supine position with lower limbs apart and the surgeon between the legs. Numbers shown represent trocar sizes in millimeters

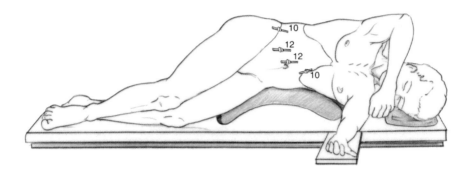

Fig. 12.2 Port placement for resection of lesions located in segment 6. The patient is in left lateral decubitus for right lobe mobilization and posterior exposure. The table can be turned to the right to reapply the right lobe and gain anterior access. Numbers shown represent trocar sizes in millimeters

transection has been suggested. Transesophageal echocardiography study in animal model demonstrated gas embolism in almost all animals undergoing laparoscopic liver resection with cardiac arrhythmia in two-thirds of cases [26]. In order to avoid it, gasless laparoscopy has been proposed [27]. However, gas embolism occurrence in clinical practice is extremely low [28]. In 2002, Biertho et al. reviewed published laparoscopic liver resections and reported only 2 cases of possible gas embolism over about 200 procedures [29]. In recent series [11, 18, 20, 30] and in our experience [22], few cases of transient mild cardiovascular alteration due to embolism occurred without clinical consequences. Carbon dioxide pneumoperitoneum minimizes risk of gas embolism as compared to air and low pneumoperitoneum pressure further reduces its incidence [31]. Electronic monitoring of intra-abdominal pressure is required and should be maintained at less than 14 mm Hg. Gas embolism occurrence has been also related to argon beam coagulation which increases endoabdominal pressure leading to increased risk of gas embolism [32]. To date CO_2 pneumoperitoneum is considered safe and gasless laparoscopy is no longer in use.

Port Sites Positioning and Hand Assistance

Positioning of port sites is different according to tumor site and it is shown in Figs. 12.1 and 12.2. Many variants have been described. The position of trocar for the laparoscope can be higher on the midline or more lateral on the right side in case of right liver resection [11, 12].

Hand-assisted laparoscopy is used by several authors [18, 33–35]. It consists in the placement through an 8-cm incision of a gas-tight port permitting the introduction of a hand in the abdomen. The assisting hand allows tactile feedback while palpating the liver and it may help in abdominal exploration, mobilizing the liver, provides gentle retraction, and helps during parenchymal transection. In addition, in case of bleeding hand compression allows easier hemostasis. For its proponents, this technique may render laparoscopic liver resection safer and more accessible. Koffron et al. recently proposed a wide use of hand assistance in order to increase the proportion of patients that can benefit from laparoscopic-assisted approach [18]. In our experience, hand assistance has been used in selected cases (about 10%) of right hepatectomies or limited resections of posterior right segments to facilitate when liver mobilization or parenchymal transection can be difficult.

Pedicle Clamping

Intermittent clamping (15-min clamping and 5-min release periods) can be performed whenever necessary. Our group demonstrated that in patients with normal cardiac function laparoscopic pedicle clamping is safe and well tolerated [36, 37]. However, it is used less often and the majority of recent resections have been performed without any clamping even in cirrhotic patients [25].

Liver Mobilization and Inflow/Outflow Control

Several techniques have been described which cannot be detailed here. Our usual technique is briefly depicted.

In left lateral sectionectomy, the round, falciform, and left triangular ligaments and the lesser omentum are divided. Dissection of the falciform ligament is continued to the level of the inferior vena cava and the insertions of the hepatic veins. Parenchymal transection is carried out until the portal pedicles of segments 2 and 3 are exposed. The pedicles are then divided using linear staplers. Left hepatic vein is divided at the end of parenchymal transection by linear stapler [38].

In limited resections, parenchymal transection is carried out along decided transection lines. Portal pedicles and hepatic veins are controlled as they are encountered during transection. In limited right-sided resections, the right triangular ligament is divided, taking advantage of the lateral position of the patient. Parenchymal transection is then carried out.

Laparoscopic right hepatectomy includes dorsal decubitus position, initial division of the right portal pedicle, right liver mobilization, taping of right hepatic vein if feasible and transection. Hand assistance can be used. Hand port is introduced through a right iliac or flank transverse incision. Surgeon's left hand or assistant's right hand helps mobilizing the liver and compresses in case of bleeding.

Parenchymal Transection

The main technical challenge of laparoscopic liver resection remains hemorrhage during parenchymal transection, especially in cirrhotic patients. Several devices have been developed with the aim to perform more bloodless and accurate parenchymal transection. These devices have not proved to be indispensable during open resections. However, in laparoscopic surgery, the simple principles of transection are more difficult to apply and some of the newly designed technologies are required.

The Ultrasonic Aspirator – The ultrasonic dissector selectively destroys liver parenchyma and spares vessels and bile ducts that can be selectively controlled. It does not have hemostatic properties. In our experience ultrasonic dissector is particularly useful in deep parenchymal transection, especially in right hepatectomy, to selectively identify and control vessels and bile ducts.

The Ultrasonic Scalpel – Also called harmonic scalpel, it has the major advantage to cut and coagulate at the same time. In the laparoscopic procedures, easy handling and rapid action are major advantages of this device. It can be particularly recommended for the superficial parts of transection (2 cm in depth). However, it is a blind instrument which should be used with caution when deeper liver parts are reached because of the risk of vascular injuries to larger vessels, especially to hepatic veins.

The Vessel Sealing System – The vessel sealing system uses low-frequency bipolar current and seals vessels up to 7 mm in diameter. Its use is rather similar to that of the ultrasonic scalpel, and it includes a knife that cuts after sealing.

Radiofrequency-Assisted Hepatic Resection (Habib Laparoscopic Sealer 4XL®) – The radiofrequency probe inserted along transection line generates pre-coagulation. Subsequent cut along coagulated line can be performed. Many advantages have been suggested: easy and bloodless transection, mainly in atypical resections; it can be helpful in wedge resections, in which visualization of transection planes and bleeding control may be more difficult; induced necrosis may improve safe surgical margins. Further studies are needed to evaluate its role in laparoscopic liver surgery.

Stapler Hepatectomy – Linear stapler devices are widely applied in laparoscopic liver surgery for portal pedicles and hepatic veins division. Recently, some authors proposed their use for parenchymal transection [39]. After the transection line is marked and the liver capsule is incised with diathermy, liver parenchyma can be divided with repeated applications of linear vascular staplers. According to its proponents, this technique allows fast and safe resection. However, vascular and biliary injuries can occur during blind transection and this technique does not allow fine control of margins and requires that tumors are located remotely from the transection line. In addition, the cost of this method is high and increases with the number of applications required. We have not favored this approach and further studies are necessary to clarify safety of stapler hepatectomy.

Other Devices – Many other devices have been proposed, such as water jet dissection, microwave-based devices, curettage and aspiration device, and monopolar irrigated coagulation devices, but available data do not allow any conclusive evaluation.

Specimen Extraction

In all cases, the specimen is placed in a plastic bag and extracted through a separate incision, either along a previous appendectomy incision or a new supra-pubic horizontal incision. Enlarged port site can also be utilized. Fragmentation must of course be avoided to allow proper pathological evaluation.

Indications

Indications to laparoscopic hepatectomy do not differ from those of open surgery. Technical feasibility has been reported as the only limiting factor [11, 12, 18, 20, 21, 40]. In order to select the best candidates for laparoscopic liver resection, two criteria have been considered by all authors.

Tumor Location

HCC located in antero-lateral segments of the liver (segments 2–6, so-called laparo-scopic segments, Fig. 12.3) and scheduled for wedges, segmentectomies, and left lateral sectionectomies are the best indications for laparoscopic approach [11, 12, 41]. Laparoscopic right hepatectomy can be planned for HCC located anywhere in the right lobe with the exception of those close to the hilum or the hepato-caval junc-tion, because of the risk of major vascular or biliary injury. The role of laparoscopy for lesions requiring resections of segments 7, 8, and 1 is not yet codified. Even if they have been traditionally considered non-laparoscopic segments because of diffi-cult visualization of surgical field, hand-assisted laparoscopy and thoracoscopy have been proposed in such location [18, 19, 23, 34, 42]. Cho et al. recently reported a series of 36 patients with lesions located in postero-superior segments (Sg7-8-4a-1) treated by pure laparoscopic approach [21, 43]. Even if 30% of cases underwent a right hepatectomy, anatomic segmentectomies, atypical resections, and right poste-rior sectionectomies have also been performed. Similarly, laparoscopic resections of segment 1 have been recently reported [13, 18, 20]. Further studies are necessary to confirm feasibility and reproducibility of these procedures.

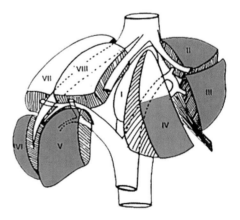

Fig. 12.3 The "laparoscopic segments." *Shaded areas* are considered consistent with laparoscopic resection

Tumor Size

Except for exophytic lesions which are easy to resect by laparoscopy, even if large in size, laparoscopy is usually not recommended for HCC exceeding 5 cm of diameter [11, 19, 21–23, 44, 45]. Even if some authors did not adopt this criterion [12, 18, 20], laparoscopic liver resection cannot be recommended for large intrahepatic lesions because of difficult tumor mobilization and risks of rupture or inadequate margin.

Liver Function

Liver function is an essential component of selection of patients considered for liver resection for HCC. Results of liver surgery in cirrhotic patients significantly improved thanks to a strict patient selection based on their liver function and future remnant liver volume [4, 5, 46]. In open surgery only Child–Pugh A patients with a future remnant liver over 40% are considered for liver resection. Presence of portal hypertension is not an absolute contraindication to liver surgery but indications have to be cautiously discussed on a case-by-case basis, and we would only consider a limited resection for such patients [3, 47, 48]. The same criteria should be adopted for laparoscopic liver resection. In case of peripheral nodules requiring atypical resections, some authors proposed laparoscopic liver resection in patients with poor liver function (Child–Pugh B) [24, 34, 49, 50]. Laparoscopic approach allows easy

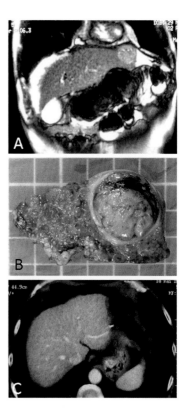

Fig. 12.4 Laparoscopic atypical resection of segment 2 as a "bridge" to liver transplantation for HCC in Child–Pugh B patient. (**a**) Preoperative MRI. (**b**) The specimen. (**c**) Postoperative CT scan, 1 month after the laparoscopic resection

resection of peripheral nodules preserving the abdominal wall and its collateral veins and reducing fluid dispersion. Good outcomes have been reported, but further data are required to codify these indications. In our center few Child–Pugh B patients have been treated (Fig. 12.4); indications are discussed on a case-by-case basis and retained in a limited number of cases.

Evaluation of Laparoscopic Liver Resection

No randomized study on the efficacy of laparoscopic liver resection has so far been published. Studies on laparoscopy in other areas of abdominal surgery may provide a worthwhile analogy. There are few randomized trials even for common operations that compare open and laparoscopic approaches and even fewer that have demonstrated any superiority of laparoscopy; conversely, none has demonstrated any superiority of laparotomy.

For example, randomized studies comparing laparoscopy and mini-laparotomy for cholecystectomy have failed to demonstrate the superiority of one approach over the other [51, 52]. However, few would dispute that laparoscopy is now the standard approach for elective cholecystectomy. This suggests that in the absence of a clear difference between laparotomy and laparoscopy and provided that the same result can be achieved, surgeons favor laparoscopy. Another analogy can be drawn from the COST randomized trial of open vs laparoscopic colectomy for colon cancer [53]. This study was designed as a non-inferiority trial and enrolled 872 patients. It demonstrated similarity for recurrence and survival and a slight advantage to laparoscopy for hospital stay and analgesic requirements (1 day reduction for each item). The conclusion was that the laparoscopic approach is an acceptable alternative to open surgery for colon cancer.

A randomized study of open vs laparoscopic liver resection is of course desirable, but it will be difficult to conduct because of the variability of the indications, types of resections, and types of techniques used. It will also require a large number of patients which will be difficult to accrue. At the present time only retrospective and case–control comparisons are available.

An increasing number of papers reported outcomes of laparoscopic liver resections. The majority of them are focused on short-term outcomes, such as hospital stay and analgesic requirements. These are important but vary according to local practice. Other outcome measures, such as re-operations, incisional hernias, and bowel obstructions, are potential advantages which remain to be demonstrated. Finally, there are very few oncological results available.

Short-Term Outcomes

Few papers have been specifically addressed on HCC. We will consider our own experience and the literature on laparoscopic liver resection presently available focusing on HCC or including HCC cases.

Table 12.2 Short-term results of laparoscopic liver resection in patients affected by HCC (series including more than 10 patients)

Author	Year	#	Major hep	Mortality	Morbidity	Conversion
Shimada [45]	2001	17	0%	0%	6% (1)	0%
Teramoto [42][a]	2003	11	0%	0%	18% (2)	1 converted case excluded
Kaneko [57]	2005	30	0%	0%	10% (3)	3% (1)
Tang [30]	2006	17	0%	0%	NR	NR
Vibert [12]	2006	16	NR	6% (1)	NR	NR
Belli [61]	2007	23	0%	4% (1)	22% (5)	4% (1)
Cai [62]	2008	24	NR	0%	0%	NR
Dagher [58]	2008	32	13% (4)	3% (1)	25% (8)	9% (3)
Cho [21]	2008	57	18% (10)	0%	16% (9)	5% (3)
Chen [19]	2008	116	3% (4)	0%	6% (7)	5% (6)
Buell [20]	2008	36	9.7% (3/31)[b]	9.7% (3/31)[b]	29% (9/31)[b]	NR
Sasaki [23]	2008	37	0%	0%	3% (1)	0%
Santambrogio [59]	2009	19	0%	0%	11% (2)	1 converted case excluded
Huang [35]	2009	27	NR	0%	19% (5)	NR
Lai [60]	2009	25	4% (1)	0%	16% (4)	4% (1)
Inagaki [24]	2009	36	0%	0%	NR	NR
Cherqui [25]	2009	69	7% (5)	0%	22% (15)	13% (9)

[a]Laparoscopic and thoracoscopic resections;
[b]Data detailed only for cirrhotic patients (31/36 HCC)
NR: data not reported

In cirrhotic patients, liver resections, even minor ones, carry a high risk of complications, including ascites, jaundice, and encephalopathy [54, 55]. Specific benefits from laparoscopic approach have been suggested: it might offer the advantage of preserving the abdominal wall and its collateral veins resulting in less portal hypertension, less need for fluids, and improved re-absorption of ascites [40]. Short-term results of series including more than 10 consecutive laparoscopic liver resections for HCC are detailed in Table 12.2.

Across more than 2000 published laparoscopic liver resections, 10 postoperative deaths have been reported (less than 0.5%) [11–13, 20, 21, 44, 56]. Six out of ten deaths occurred in cirrhotic patients [11, 12, 20, 44]. Buell et al. [20] recently reported more than 250 laparoscopic liver resections and observed a significantly increased mortality in cirrhotic patients in comparison with non-cirrhotic ones (9.7% vs 0.3%). These data underline that liver surgery in cirrhotic patients has to be considered at increased risk, even if laparoscopically performed.

In the literature, morbidity rates after laparoscopic liver surgery ranged from 5 to 20% [11, 13, 14–23]. Considering cirrhotic patients they tended to be higher, about 10–30% [19, 21, 25, 35, 42, 45, 57–62]. In the above-mentioned series of Buell et al., morbidity was 29% in cirrhotics vs 14% in non-cirrhotics ($p = 0.02$) [20]. Morino et al. observed increased hospital stay and blood loss in case of cirrhosis [63]. In our series of 174 laparoscopic resections, mortality was nil and morbidity occurred in 14.4% of cases [25]. Considering the 69 patients affected by HCC morbidity rate was 21.7%, but it significantly decreased in the second half of our series (lower than 10%) [25].

Two complications are commonly feared in laparoscopic liver surgery: gas embolism and bleeding. As previously discussed, gas embolism is rarely reported and is usually without any clinical consequences, except for transient cardiovascular alterations. On the other side, hemorrhagic complications can occur during parenchymal transection and may lead to urgent conversion. In the literature some severe hemorrhagic complications have been reported, mainly related to hepatic veins injuries [11, 12, 22, 64]. These have been usually managed either laparoscopically or by conversion to laparotomy without reported consequences except for two cases: one brain death [12] and one hypovolemic shock with postoperative renal failure requiring hemodialysis for 4 months [64]. No intraoperative death has been reported. In the published series, hemorrhagic risk was not increased in cirrhotic patients.

In the literature, reported conversion rate is about 5–15% [11–13, 15, 22, 65]. Similar data have been reported in HCC cases [19, 21, 23, 25, 45, 57–61]. The reasons for conversion are essentially two. The first reason is, of course, bleeding. The second is a technical one, a composite association of difficult exposure, insufficient or poor quality view, fragile tumor with risk of rupture or uncertainty about the distance between the tumor and the transection plane. In our series, the conversion rate was 9.8% in the whole series and 13% in HCC cases, with two-thirds for technical reasons and one-third for bleeding [25]. In our experience, massive bleeding requiring rapid conversion never occurred; they were rather situations that were difficult to control by laparoscopy and that, by their persistence, hampered the progress of the operation and were leading to a significant blood loss.

Comparison with Open Liver Resections

Three case–control studies (one from our group) [44, 60, 66] compared outcomes of laparoscopic and open liver resections in cirrhotic patients. Two comparative studies without any matching criteria compared laparoscopic and open resections for HCC [45, 57]. The outcomes of these studies are summarized in Table 12.3.

Reduced morbidity, especially rare occurrences of postoperative ascites, was observed in patients operated through a laparoscopic approach [44, 66]. Operative time of laparoscopic resections was longer in two studies [45, 66], while a trend toward reduced blood loss has been reported [44, 45, 66]. Hospital stay was shorter in laparoscopic group [40, 45, 60].

Learning Curve

In surgical procedures the so-called learning curve effect has been described, demonstrating improvement in results along with experience [67, 68]. In laparoscopic liver surgery series, some authors reported reduced operative times, blood

Table 12.3 Studies comparing laparoscopic vs open liver resection for HCC

Author	Year	# L	# O	Operative time (min) L	Operative time (min) O	Blood loss (mL) L	Blood loss (mL) O	Blood tr. L	Blood tr. O	Morbidity L	Morbidity O	Hospital stay (days) L	Hospital stay (days) O
Case–control studies													
Laurent [66]	2003	13	14	**267 ± 79**	**182 ± 57**	620 ± 130	720 ± 240	8%	29%	36%	50%	15.3 ± 8.6	17.3 ± 18.9
Belli [44]	2007	23	23	**148 ± 30**	**125 ± 17**	260 ± 127	377 ± 114	**0%**	**17%**	**13%**	**48%**	**8.2 ± 2.6**	**12.0 ± 4.0**
Lai [60]	2009	25	33	150 (75–210)	135 (50–120)	NR		NR		16%	15%	**7 (4–11)**	**9 (5–37)**
Comparative studies													
Shimada [45]	2001	17	38	325	280	400	800	6%	11%	6%	11%	**12 ± 5**	**22 ± 8**
Kaneko [57]	2005	30	28	182 ± 38	210 ± 40	350 ± 210	505 ± 185	NR		10%	18%	**14.9 ± 7.1**	**21.6 ± 8.8**

L.: laparoscopic resections; O: open resections; Blood tr.: blood transfusion; Bold typed data $p < 0.05$;
NR: data not reported

loss, and conversion rate when comparing early and late cases of their series [11, 16, 38, 69]. Our group recently studied the learning curve effect along our experience of laparoscopic liver resections [25]. We split our series of 69 laparoscopic liver resections for HCC into three groups of 23 consecutive cases. Conversion rate progressively decreased (26.1, 8.7, and 4.3%). A significant decrease of pedicle clamping rate (from 100 to 17.4%), clamping duration when used (60 to 20 min), operative time (240 to 150 minutes), and blood loss (400 to 100 cc) was observed. Morbidity decreased from 43.5 to 13.0 and 8.7% and hospital stay passed from 9 to 7 and 6 days, respectively.

Left Lateral Sectionectomy

Left lateral sectionectomy has a privileged place in laparoscopic resections (Fig. 12.5). Our group demonstrated by a case–control study that, despite longer operative times, laparoscopy is associated with reduced blood loss and morbidity, especially in cirrhotic patients [70]. A further analysis on 36 laparoscopic left lateral sectionectomies reported no mortality and no liver-specific morbidity, low blood loss, and no transfusion [38]. Conversion occurred only in one patient during our experience. In addition a clear learning curve effect was demonstrated: operative time, use of Pringle maneuver, and hospital stay were significantly reduced in the last 18 patients. All these data have been confirmed by further recent studies [71–73]. Laparoscopy can be recommended as the routine approach to left lateral sectionectomy.

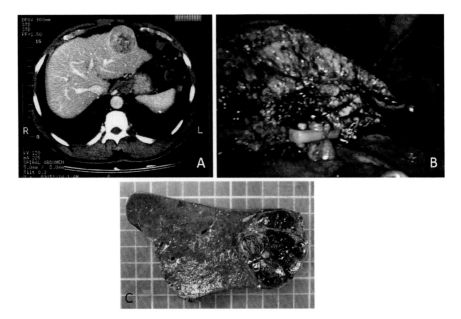

Fig. 12.5 Laparoscopic left lateral sectionectomy for HCC. (**a**) Preoperative CT scan. (**b**) The surgical field at the end of parenchymal transection. (**c**) The specimen

Other Minor Resections

Antero-lateral liver segments (segments 2–6) are the so-called laparoscopic liver segments. Their non-anatomical resections are commonly reported in the literature and are associated with excellent outcomes [11–20, 22, 23] (Fig. 12.6). Even if no studies specifically compared their results with those of open counterparts, equivalence between the two procedures can be postulated and advantages of laparoscopic approach can be hypothesized. In fact, together with left lateral sectionectomies, they represent the majority of cases included in case–control studies comparing open and laparoscopic liver surgery.

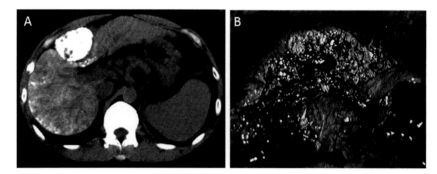

Fig. 12.6 Laparoscopic segmentectomy 4b for HCC. (**a**) Preoperative CT scan. (**b**) The surgical field at the end of parenchymal transection

As mentioned above, non-anatomical resections of segments 7, 8, and 1 have been usually excluded from laparoscopic approach because of difficult visualization of surgical field. Similarly right liver segmental anatomic resections present many problems, mainly related to adequate exposure, the need for two transection planes, and the difficulties to check margin adequacy [40]. Increased risk of intraoperative bleeding and positive surgical margin can be feared. Recently feasibility of these procedures has been reconsidered and successful laparoscopic cases have been reported, especially applying hand assistance [19, 21, 34, 74] (Fig. 12.7). Laparoscopic right posterior sectionectomies and caudate lobectomies have been performed with good outcomes [18, 20, 21, 43, 74]. Cho et al. compared outcomes of laparoscopic approach for lesion in antero-lateral segments vs. postero-superior ones and they did not report any differences, except for longer operative time and higher transfusion rate in the second group [21, 43]. Despite these positive results, little data are presently available and further studies are necessary to validate outcome of these procedures.

Major Hepatectomy

An increasing number of laparoscopic major hepatectomies have been reported in the literature [11–13, 18, 20–22, 56, 69, 75–77], including large series in the past

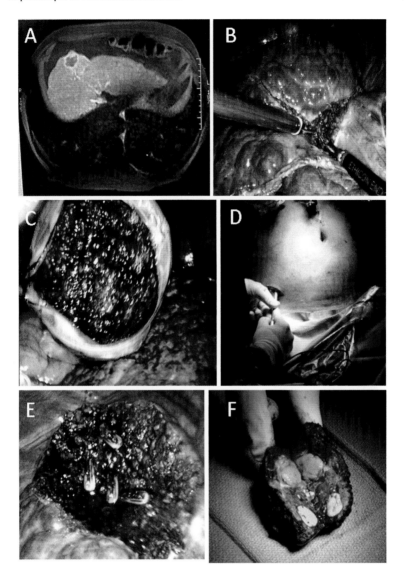

Fig. 12.7 Laparoscopic atypical resection of segment 8 for HCC. (**a**) Preoperative MRI. (**b**) Liver transection performed with harmonic scalpel. (**c**) Specimen is placed in a plastic bag. (**d**) Specimen extraction through a separate incision. (**e**) The surgical field at the end of parenchymal transection. (**f**) The specimen

2 years [11, 13, 18, 20–22, 75]. The majority of procedures were right or left hepatectomies. However, few specific data about these procedures are available and only a limited number of cases have been performed in patients with HCC [19–21, 25, 58, 60] (Table 12.2). Even if some authors suggest feasibility of right hepatectomy by

pure laparoscopic approach [75–77], the hand assistance can be useful in selected cases. It may help to mobilize the liver, to perform parenchymal transection and to control bleeding.

At present, laparoscopic major hepatectomies are still limited to few expert centers and cannot be considered standard procedures. Further evaluation and technical refinements are required before laparoscopic major liver resections can be recommended.

Oncological Results

Controversy about laparoscopy in cancer patients arose from unacceptable peritoneal and port site seeding in early patients with incidental gallbladder cancer or with colon cancer [78, 79]. Proper use of oncological surgical principles has reduced this problem to the point that there are no more differences as compared to open surgery. It is highly important that oncological principles are strictly followed: "no touch", no direct manipulation of the tumor, immediate conversion in case of locally advanced cancer, and protection for extraction.

Up to December 2008, 12 papers (two from our group) specifically focused on laparoscopic resection of HCC [19, 42, 45, 57–61, 66, 80, 81]. Further data on HCC are included among other laparoscopic series [12, 20, 21, 23, 24, 30, 35, 62]. Published series including more than 10 patients are detailed in Table 12.4.

Surgical margin width was adequate in the majority of cases: its median was over 1 cm in almost all series and few positive surgical margins have been reported [19–23, 30, 42, 45, 58, 59, 61]. Three-year overall and disease-free survival rates were about 65–75% and 50–70%, respectively [12, 19, 22, 23, 42, 57–59, 62]. In our series, 64 patients with HCC underwent laparoscopic liver resection: the mean surgical margin width was 13 mm and 5-year overall and disease-free survival rates were 65% and 34%, respectively [22]. These outcomes are similar or even better than those reported in open series, although high recurrence rates are observed at 5 years as expected with underlying chronic liver hepatitis or cirrhosis [23, 82–84].

No port site recurrences imputable to laparoscopy were noted. Direct comparison in case–control studies between laparoscopic and open resection for HCC reported no differences in terms of surgical margin width and midterm results [44, 60, 66].

Most recurrences observed in our experience occurred in a remote segment suggesting multicentric carcinogenesis due to underlying liver disease. Most were amenable to treatment including reresection, ablation, TACE, or transplantation. These results warrant close postoperative follow-up to allow early detection of recurrences. Indeed, 34% of patients with recurrences underwent salvage liver transplantation [22].

Laparoscopic approach may have a role even in recurrent HCC. A recent paper by Belli et al. demonstrated feasibility of redo laparoscopic treatment (12 resections and 3 radiofrequency ablations), even in patients with previous open resection

Table 12.4 Laparoscopic liver resections for HCC (series including more than 10 patients). Overall and disease-free survival rates are reported only if detailed data were available in the paper (i.e., percentages or events with follow-up duration)

Author	Year	#	Diameter (cm)	Surgical margin (mm)	Overall survival	Disease-free survival
Shimada [45]	2001	17	2.6 ± 0.9	8 ± 7	NS vs open control group	
Teramoto [42][a]	2003	11	NR	82% negative	5 yr 75%	5 yr 38.2%
Kaneko [57]	2005	40	NR	NR	5 yr 61%	5 yr 31%
Tang [30]	2006	17	NR	70.6% > 10 mm	2 yr 59%	NR
Vibert [12]	2006	16	6.5	NR	3 yr 66%	3 yr 68%
Belli [61]	2007	23	3.1 ± 0.7	91.4% > 10 mm	NS vs open control group	
Cai [62]	2008	24	NR	NR	5 y 56.2%	NR
Dagher [58]	2008	32	3.8 ± 2	10.4 ± 9	3 yr 72%	3 yr 55%
Cho [21]	2008	57	3.5 ± 2.0[b] 2.9 ± 1.3[c]	16.4 ± 15.0[b] 15.8 ± 18.8[c]	NR	
Chen [19]	2008	116	2.1 ± 0.8[d] 3.2 ± 1.9[e]	100% >10 mm	5 yr 59%[d] 5 yr 62%[e]	NR
Buell [20]	2008	36	4.6	7 mm (100% R0)	NR[g]	
Sasaki [23]	2008	37	3.5 ± 3.7	8.7 ± 7.1	5 yr 52.7%	NR
Santambrogio [59]	2009	19	2.8 ± 1.0	100% > 5 mm	4 yr 50%	4 yr 24%
Huang [35]	2009	27	2.5 (2–4)	NR	NR[g]	NR[g]
Lai [60]	2009	25	2.5 (1–7)	88% R0	3 yr 60%	3 yr 52%
Inagaki [24]	2009	36	NR	NR	5 yr 79.3%	NR
Bryant[f] [22]	2009	64	4.4 ± 2.6	13 ± 12	5 yr 65%	5 yr 34%

[a]Laparoscopic and thoracoscopic resections
[b]HCC in antero-lateral liver segments
[c]HCC in postero-superior liver segments
[d]patients with resection of ≤ 2 segments
[e] patients with resection of > 2 segments
[f]Author's series
[g]Insufficient follow-up data in the paper
NR: data not reported; NS: not significant

[81]. Previous laparoscopic resection enabled easier procedures thanks to fewer adhesions.

Resection and Liver Transplantation: Does Laparoscopy Modify the Picture?

The treatment of patients with HCC within Milan criteria is debated, because both liver transplantation and liver resection can be proposed. Liver transplantation is the ideal treatment by removing both the tumor and the underlying liver disease, but shortage of donors and its consequent dropout on the waiting list due to progression limit the number of patients who can receive it [3]. By contrast, liver resection is readily available, but is associated to high recurrence rates [8, 82–84]. In a modern view, liver resection and transplantation should not be considered competitive but complementary and treatment should be tailored to each patient case. Resection can be used before liver transplantation in three different strategies: first, resection as primary therapy considering "salvage" liver transplantation in case of recurrence or liver failure [8]; second, resection as tool to select patients for the liver transplantation on the basis of pathological data of the tumor and the surrounding parenchyma [85–87]; finally, "bridge" resection, i.e., resection as treatment on the waiting list.

The advantages and the disadvantages of these options are not the topic of this chapter, but it should be emphasized that the laparoscopic approach could enhance the role of liver resection in case of peripheral nodules. It allows easy resections with early recovery and low morbidity. Oncological results are not inferior to open resections. Complete pathological data of both tumor and parenchyma can be safely obtained. Indications can be extended even to patients with mild compromised liver function (Child–Pugh B). Laparoscopic liver resection is also complementary to radiofrequency ablation which is associated with a higher risk of seeding in superficial lesions. Therefore, laparoscopic limited resection could be used in peripheral lesions and radiofrequency in deeply located nodules, which would otherwise require major liver resection.

The main criticism to liver resection are the difficulties encountered at the subsequent liver transplantation if required. Adam et al. reported poor outcomes of salvage liver transplant after previous hepatectomy because of adhesions related to primary treatment and increased blood loss [88]. In our center, 12 patients underwent bridge or salvage transplantation after primary laparoscopic resection with no mortality. When transplantation was performed, they benefitted from the absence of adhesions and, in comparison with 12 transplantations after open hepatectomies, we observed lower operative time, blood loss, and transfusion rate [89]. Reduced adherences after laparoscopic liver surgery have been confirmed by Belli et al. in the analysis of the redo surgery [81].

Conclusions

For laparoscopic liver resection to be effective, specific training and access to adequate technology are required. Patient selection must be accurate, and the availability of laparoscopy should not change the indications for resection. The rules of oncological surgery must be followed for minimally invasive operations, just as in their open counterparts. At present, good candidates for laparoscopic liver resection are patients with peripheral HCC requiring limited hepatectomy or left lateral sectionectomy. In these cases surgery can be performed with early recovery and low morbidity. Oncological results appear to be similar to open surgery but further studies are necessary. The laparoscopic approach strengthens the role of liver resection in the treatment strategy of peripheral HCC within Milan criteria. In the perspective of liver transplantation, laparoscopic liver resection enables easier transplantation in comparison with open resection.

References

1. Bruix J, Sherman M, Llovet JM, et al (2001) Clinical management of hepatocellular carcinoma. Conclusions of the Barcelona-2000 EASL conference. European Association for the Study of the Liver. J Hepatol 35:421–30
2. Bruix J, Sherman M (2005) Management of hepatocellular carcinoma. AASLD practice guideline. Hepatology 42:1208–1235
3. Llovet JM, Fuster J, Bruix J (1999) Intention-to-treat analysis of surgical treatment for early hepatocellular carcinoma: resection versus transplantation. Hepatology 30:1434–1440
4. Torzilli G, Makuuchi M, Inoue K et al (1999) No-mortality liver resection for hepatocellular carcinoma in cirrhotic and noncirrhotic patients: is there a way? A prospective analysis of our approach. Arch Surg 134:984–992
5. Fan ST, Lo CM, Liu CL, Lam CM, Yuen WK, Yeung C, Wong J (1999) Hepatectomy for hepatocellular carcinoma: toward zero hospital deaths. Ann Surg 229:322–330
6. Abdalla EK, Denys A, Hasegawa K et al (2008) Treatment of large and advanced hepatocellular carcinoma. Ann Surg Oncol 15:979–985
7. Capussotti L, Ferrero A, Viganò L, Polastri R, Tabone M (2009) Liver resection for HCC with cirrhosis: surgical perspectives out of EASL/AASLD guidelines. Eur J Surg Oncol 35:11–5
8. Cherqui D, Laurent A, Mocellin N et al (2009) Liver resection for transplantable hepatocellular carcinoma: long-term survival and role of secondary liver transplantation. Ann Surg 250:738–746
9. Cha CH, Ruo L, Fong Y et al (2003) Resection of hepatocellular carcinoma in patients otherwise eligible for transplantation. Ann Surg 238:315–323
10. Viganò L, Tayar C, Laurent A, Cherqui D (2009) Laparoscopic liver resection: a systematic review. J Hepatobiliary Pancreat Surg 16:410–421
11. Dagher, I, Proske, JM, Carloni, A, Richa, H, Tranchart, H, Franco, D (2007) Laparoscopic liver resection: results for 70 patients. Surg Endosc 21:619–624
12. Vibert E, Perniceni T, Levard H, Denet C, Shahri NK, Gayet B (2006) Laparoscopic liver resection. Br J Surg 93:67–72
13. Topal B, Fieuws S, Aerts R, Vandeweyer H, Penninckx F (2008) Laparoscopic versus open liver resection of hepatic neoplasms: comparative analysis of short-term results. Surg Endosc 22:2208–2213
14. Descottes B, Glineur D, Lachachi F et al (2003) Laparoscopic liver resection of benign liver tumors. Surg Endosc 17:23–30
15. Mala T, Edwin B, Rosseland AR, Gladhaug I, Fosse E, Mathisen O (2005) Laparoscopic liver resection: experience of 53 procedures at a single center. J Hepatobiliary Pancreat Surg 12:298–303
16. Kaneko H (2005) Laparoscopic hepatectomy: indications and outcomes. J Hepatobiliary Pancreat Surg 12:438–443
17. Cai XJ, Yu H, Liang X et al (2006) Laparoscopic hepatectomy by curettage and aspiration. Experiences of 62 cases. Surg Endosc 20:1531–1535
18. Koffron AJ, Auffenberg G, Kung R, Abecassis M (2007) Evaluation of 300 minimally invasive liver resections at a single institution: less is more. Ann Surg 246:385–392
19. Chen HY, Juan CC, Ker CG (2008) Laparoscopic liver surgery for patients with hepatocellular carcinoma. Ann Surg Oncol 15:800–806
20. Buell JF, Thomas MT, Rudich S et al (2008) Experience with more than 500 minimally invasive hepatic procedures. Ann Surg 248:475–486
21. Cho JY, Han HS, Yoon YS, Shin SH (2008) Experiences of laparoscopic liver resection including lesions in the posterosuperior segments of the liver. Surg Endosc 22:2344–2349
22. Bryant R, Laurent A, Tayar C, Cherqui D (2009) Laparoscopic liver resection-understanding its role in current practice: the Henri Mondor Hospital experience. Ann Surg 250:103–111
23. Sasaki A, Nitta H, Otsuka K, Takahara T, Nishizuka S, Wakabayashi G (2009) Ten-year experience of totally laparoscopic liver resection in a single institution. Br J Surg 96:274–279

24. Inagaki H, Kurokawa T, Yokoyama T, Ito N, Yokoyama Y, Nonami T (2009) Results of laparoscopic liver resection: retrospective study of 68 patients. J Hepatobiliary Pancreat Surg 16:64–68

25. Viganò L, Laurent A, Tayar C, Tomatis M, Ponti A, Cherqui D (2009) The learning curve in laparoscopic liver resection: improved feasibility and reproducibility. Ann Surg 250:772–778

26. Schmandra TC, Mierdl S, Bauer H, Gutt C, Hanisch E (2002) Transoesophageal echocardiography shows high risk of gas embolism during laparoscopic hepatic resection under carbon dioxide pneumoperitoneum. Br J Surg 89:870–876

27. Watanabe Y, Sato M, Ueda S et al (1997) Laparoscopic hepatic resection: A new and safe procedure by abdominal wall lifting method. Hepatogastroenterology 44:143–47

28. Farges O, Jagot P, Kirstetter P, Marty J, Belghiti J (2002) Prospective assessment of the safety and benefit of laparoscopic liver resections. J Hepatobiliary Pancreat Surg 9:242–248

29. Biertho L, Waage A, Gagner M (2002) Laparoscopic hepatectomy Ann Chir 127:164–170

30. Tang CN, Tsui KK, Ha JP, Yang GP, Li MK (2006) A single-centre experience of 40 laparoscopic liver resections. Hong Kong Med J 12:419–425

31. Bazin JE, Gillart T, Rasson P, Conio N, Aigouy L, Schoeffler P (1997) Haemodynamic conditions enhancing gas embolism after venous injury during laparoscopy: a study in pigs. Br J Anaesth 78:570–575

32. Palmer M, Miller CW, van Way CW 3rd, Orton EC (1993) Venous gas embolism associated with argon-enhanced coagulation of the liver. J Invest Surg 6:391–399

33. Fong Y, Jarnagin W, Conlon KC, DeMatteo R, Dougherty E, Blumgart LH (2000) Hand-assisted laparoscopic liver resection: lessons from an initial experience. Arch Surg 135:854–859

34. Huang MT, Lee WJ, Wang W, Wei PL, Chen RJ (2003) Hand-assisted laparoscopic hepatectomy for solid tumor in the posterior portion of the right lobe: initial experience. Ann Surg 238:674–679

35. Huang MT, Wei PL, Wang W, Li CJ, Lee YC, Wu CH (2009) A series of laparoscopic liver resections with or without HALS in patients with hepatic tumors. J Gastrointest Surg 13:896–906

36. Decailliot F, Cherqui D, Leroux B et al (2001) Effects of portal triad clamping on haemodynamic conditions during laparoscopic liver resection. Br J Anaesth 87:493–496

37. Decailliot F, Streich B, Heurtematte Y, Duvaldestin P, Cherqui D, Stéphan, F (2005) Hemodynamic effects of portal triad clamping with and without pneumoperitoneum: an echocardiographic study. Anesth Analg 100:617–622

38. Chang S, Laurent A, Tayar C, Karoui M, Cherqui D (2007) Laparoscopy as a routine approach for left lateral sectionectomy. Br J Surg 94:58–63

39. Schemmer P, Friess H, Hinz U et al (2006) Stapler hepatectomy is a safe dissection technique: analysis of 300 patients. World J Surg 30:419–430

40. Cherqui D, Husson E, Hammoud R et al (2000) Laparoscopic liver resections: a feasibility study in 30 patients. Ann Surg 232:753–762

41. Cherqui D (2003) Laparoscopic liver resection. Br J Surg 90:644–646

42. Teramoto K, Kawamura T, Takamatsu S et al (2005) Laparoscopic and thoracoscopic approaches for the treatment of hepatocellular carcinoma. Am J Surg 189:474–478

43. Cho JY, Han HS, Yoon YS, Shin SH (2008) Feasibility of laparoscopic liver resection for tumors located in the posterosuperior segments of the liver, with a special reference to overcoming current limitations on tumor location. Surgery 144:32–38

44. Belli G, Fantini C, D'Agostino A et al (2007) Laparoscopic versus open liver resection for hepatocellular carcinoma in patients with histologically proven cirrhosis: short- and middle-term results. Surg Endosc 21:2004–2011

45. Shimada M, Hashizume M, Maehara S et al (2001) Laparoscopic hepatectomy for hepatocellular carcinoma. Surg Endosc 15:541–544

46. Abdalla EK, Hicks ME, Vauthey JN (2001) Portal vein embolization: rationale, technique and future prospects. Br J Surg 88:165–175

47. Torzilli G, Donadon M, Marconi M et al (2008) Hepatectomy for stage B and stage C hepato-cellular carcinoma in the Barcelona Clinic Liver Cancer classification: results of a prospective analysis. Arch Surg 143:1082–1090

48. Capussotti L, Ferrero A, Viganò L, Muratore A, Polastri R, Bouzari H (2006) Portal hypertension: contraindication to liver surgery? World J Surg 30:992–999

49. Abdel-Atty MY, Farges O, Jagot P, Belghiti J (1999) Laparoscopy extends the indications for liver resection in patients with cirrhosis. Br J Surg 86:1397–400

50. Jiao LR, Ayav A, Navarra G et al (2008) Laparoscopic liver resection assisted by the laparoscopic Habib Sealer. Surgery 144:770–774

51. Ros A, Gustafsson L, Krook H et al (2001) Laparoscopic cholecystectomy versus mini-laparotomy cholecystectomy: a prospective, randomized, single-blind study. Ann Surg 234:741–749

52. McMahon AJ, Russell IT, Baxter JN et al (1994) Laparoscopic versus minilaparotomy cholecystectomy: a randomised trial. Lancet 343:135–138

53. Fleshman J, Sargent DJ, Green E et al (2007) Laparoscopic colectomy for cancer is not infe-rior to open surgery based on 5-year data from the COST Study Group trial. Ann Surg 246: 655–662

54. Belghiti J, Hiramatsu K, Benoist S, Massault P, Sauvanet A, Farges O (2000) Seven hundred forty-seven hepatectomies in the 1990s: an update to evaluate the actual risk of liver resection, J Am Coll Surg 191:38

55. Lai EC, Fan ST, Lo CM, Chu KM, Liu CL, Wong J (1995) Hepatic resection for hepatocellular carcinoma. An audit of 343 patients. Ann Surg 221:291–298

56. Huscher CG, Lirici MM, Chiodini S (1998) Laparoscopic liver resections. Semin Laparosc Surg 5:204–210

57. Kaneko H, Takagi S, Otsuka Y, et al (2005) Laparoscopic liver resection of hepatocellular carcinoma. Am J Surg 189:190–194

58. Dagher I, Lainas P, Carloni A et al (2008) Laparoscopic liver resection for hepatocellular carcinoma. Surg Endosc 22:372–378

59. Santambrogio R, Aldrighetti L, Barabino M et al (2009) Laparoscopic liver resections for hepatocellular carcinoma. Is it a feasible option for patients with liver cirrhosis? Langenbecks Arch Surg 394:255–264

60. Lai EC, Tang CN, Ha JP, Li MK (2009) Laparoscopic liver resection for hepatocellular carcinoma: ten-year experience in a single center. Arch Surg 144:143–147

61. Cai XJ, Yang J, Yu H et al (2008) Clinical study of laparoscopic versus open hepatectomy for malignant liver tumors. Surg Endosc 22:2350–2356

62. Belli G, Fantini C, D'Agostino A, Belli A, Russolillo N (2004) Laparoscopic liver resections for hepatocellular carcinoma (HCC) in cirrhotic patients. HPB 6:236–46

63. Morino M, Morra I, Rosso E, Miglietta C, Garrone C (2003) Laparoscopic vs open hepatic resection: a comparative study. Surg Endosc 17:1914–1918

64. Troisi R, Montalti R, Smeets P et al (2008) The value of laparoscopic liver surgery for solid benign hepatic tumors. Surg Endosc 22:38–44

65. Simillis C, Constantinides VA, Tekkis PP et al (2007) Laparoscopic versus open hepatic resections for benign and malignant neoplasms – a meta-analysis. Surgery 141:203–211

66. Laurent A, Cherqui D, Lesurtel M, Brunetti F, Tayar C, Fagniez PL (2003) Laparoscopic liver resection for subcapsular hepatocellular carcinoma complicating chronic liver disease. Arch Surg 138:763–769

67. Tekkis PP, Senagore AJ, Delaney CP, Fazio VW (2005) Evaluation of the learning curve in laparoscopic colorectal surgery: comparison of right-sided and left-sided resections. Ann Surg 242:83–91

68. Schlachta CM, Mamazza J, Seshadri PA, Cadeddu M, Gregoire R, Poulin EC (2001) Defining a learning curve for laparoscopic colorectal resections. Dis Colon Rectum 44:217–222

69. Dulucq JL, Wintringer P, Stabilini C, Berticelli J, Mahajna A. (2005) Laparoscopic liver resections: a single center experience. Surg Endosc 19:886–891

70. Lesurtel M, Cherqui D, Laurent A, Tayar C, Fagniez PL (2003) Laparoscopic versus open left lateral hepatic lobectomy: a case-control study. J Am Coll Surg 196:236–242

71. Abu Hilal M, McPhail MJ, Zeidan B et al (2008) Laparoscopic versus open left lateral hepatic sectionectomy: A comparative study. Eur J Surg Oncol 34:1285–1288

72. Aldrighetti L, Pulitanò C, Catena M et al (2008) A prospective evaluation of laparoscopic versus open left lateral hepatic sectionectomy. J Gastrointest Surg 12:457–462

73. Belli G, Fantini C, D'Agostino A, Belli A, Cioffi L, Russolillo N (2006) Laparoscopic left lateral hepatic lobectomy: a safer and faster technique. J Hepatobiliary Pancreat Surg 13: 149–154

74. Robles R, Marín C, Abellán B, López A, Pastor P, Parrilla P (2008) A new approach to hand-assisted laparoscopic liver surgery. Surg Endosc 22:2357–2364

75. Gayet B, Cavaliere D, Vibert E et al (2007) Totally laparoscopic right hepatectomy. Am J Surg 194:685–689

76. O'Rourke N, Fielding G (2004) Laparoscopic right hepatectomy: surgical technique. J Gastrointest Surg 8:213–216

77. Dagher I, Caillard C, Proske JM, Carloni A, Lainas P, Franco D (2008) Laparoscopic right hepatectomy: original technique and results. J Am Coll Surg 206:756–760

78. Fong Y, Brennan MF, Turnbull A et al (1993) Gallbladder cancer discovered during laparoscopic surgery–potential for iatrogenic dissemination. Arch Surg 128:1054–1056

79. Johnstone PA, Rohde DC, Swartz SE, Fetter JE, Wexner SD (1996) Port site recurrences after laparoscopic and thoracoscopic procedures in malignancy. J Clin Oncol 14:1950–1956

80. Cherqui D, Laurent A, Tayar C et al (2006) Laparoscopic liver resection for peripheral hepatocellular carcinoma in patients with chronic liver disease: midterm results and perspectives. Ann Surg 243:499–506

81. Belli G, Cioffi L, Fantini C et al (2009) Laparoscopic redo surgery for recurrent hepatocellular carcinoma in cirrhotic patients: feasibility, safety, and results. Surg Endosc 23:1807–1811

82. Jaeck D, Bachellier P, Oussoultzoglou E, Weber JC, Wolf P (2004) Surgical resection of hepatocellular carcinoma. Post-operative outcome and long-term results in Europe: an overview. Liver Transpl 10(2 Suppl 1):S58–S63

83. Fong Y, Sun RL, Jarnagin W, Blumgart LH (1999) An analysis of 412 cases of hepatocellular carcinoma at a Western center. Ann Surg 229:790–799

84. Poon RT, Fan ST, Lo CM et al (2001) Improving survival results after resection of hepatocellular carcinoma: a prospective study of 377 patients over 10 years. Ann Surg 234:63–70

85. Sala M, Fuster J, Llovet JM et al (2004) High pathological risk of recurrence after surgical resection for hepatocellular carcinoma: an indication for salvage liver transplantation. Liver Transpl 10:1294–1300

86. Scatton O, Zalinski S, Terris B et al (2008) Hepatocellular carcinoma developed on compensated cirrhosis: resection as a selection tool for liver transplantation. Liver Transpl 14:779–88

87. Hoshida Y, Villanueva A, Kobayashi M et al (2008) Gene expression in fixed tissues and outcome in hepatocellular carcinoma. N Engl J Med 359:1995–2004

88. Adam R, Azoulay D, Castaing D et al (2003) Liver resection as a bridge to transplantation for hepatocellular carcinoma on cirrhosis: a reasonable strategy? Ann Surg 238:508–518

89. Laurent A, Tayar C, Andréoletti M, Lauzet JY, Merle JC, Cherqui D (2009) Laparoscopic liver resection facilitates salvage liver transplantation for hepatocellular carcinoma. J Hepatobiliary Pancreat Surg 16:310–314

Chapter 13
Laparoscopic Liver Surgery for the Management of Hepatocellular Carcinoma: The American Perspective

Kadiyala V. Ravindra and Joseph F. Buell

Keywords Laparoscopic liver surgery · Laparoscopic liver resection · HCC · Hepatic resection · Patient selection

Despite better understanding and advances in oncology, the best available therapeutic option for the management of hepatocellular carcinoma (HCC) is surgical – either liver transplantation or resection. Liver transplantation appears most attractive since it treats the primary tumor and the field defect associated with the underlying liver disease. However, this option is feasible only when there are an adequate number of organs available and when the disease and patient meet certain stringent criteria. Most centers abide by the Milan criteria [1] to determine candidacy for liver transplantation. These are a single tumor ≤5 cm, two or three tumors all <3 cm, absence of major vascular invasion, and no extrahepatic disease. Unfortunately, only a minority of hepatoma patients fit these morphological parameters. Many other cirrhotic patients do not fulfill the requirements for transplantation due to comorbidity or psychosocial reasons. A few centers have attempted to expand transplantation to patients with greater tumor burden. These criteria were developed by the UCSF group and consist of solitary tumor ≤6.5 cm, or three or fewer nodules with the largest lesion ≤4.5 cm, and total tumor diameter ≤8 cm, without gross vascular invasion [2].

Hepatic resection should be considered for patients deemed unsuitable for transplantation. However, proper selection of patients is required to avoid postoperative liver failure. On rare occasions, laparoscopic resection has been utilized to select patients for liver transplantation – particularly when there is a question of major vascular invasion arising in the presence of small tumors. When patients are unable to undergo resection, they are then considered for ablative strategies including radiofrequency ablation [3], cryoablation [4], percutaneous alcohol injection [5], microwave ablation [6], laser ablation [7], chemoembolization [8], chemotherapeutic beads, and infusion of yttrium microspheres [9].

K.V. Ravindra (✉)
Department of Surgery, Duke University Medical Center, Durham, NC, USA

K.M. McMasters, J.-N. Vauthey (eds.), *Hepatocellular Carcinoma*,
DOI 10.1007/978-1-60327-522-4_13, © Springer Science+Business Media, LLC 2011

Hepatic resection poses several important challenges. In the setting of normal parenchyma, resection maybe limited only by the presence of extrahepatic spread, bi-lobar disease, or major vascular extension. These criteria serve only as relative contraindications and should be considered on a case-by-case basis. Major liver resection in a patient with normal parenchyma is tolerated down to a functional liver remnant of only two or three segments. However, in the setting of a diseased liver, resection is an entirely different proposition. A fibrotic or cirrhotic liver has poor and unpredictable ability to regenerate with resultant liver failure. This is a deterrent to major liver resection in hepatoma occurring against the background of cirrhosis.

Various methods have been used to guide the extent of possible resection in this situation. These include the Child's status, ICG excretion test [10], and evidence of portal hypertension (platelet count, wedged hepatic venous pressure gradient) [11] (Table 13.1). Despite these tools, planning and executing liver resection in cirrhosis continues to be a serious undertaking. Recent advances in the care of cirrhotic patients have enabled mortality rates as low as 3% [12].

Table 13.1 Selection criteria for liver resection for hepatocellular carcinoma in chronic liver disease

For a major resection (≥ three segments)
Child-Pugh class A
Indocyanine green retention at 15 min <15%
No esophageal varices
Platelets >100,000/mm^3
Transaminases ≤ two times normal
Hypertrophy of liver after portal vein embolization
Functional residual liver volume > 50%

For a limited resection (<three segments)
Child-Pugh class A
Child-Pugh class B for a peripheral tumorectomy
Esophageal varices grade 2 maximum

With permission from Bryant et al. [11]

Liver surgery has evolved significantly over the last two decades. It is well standardized and has excellent results largely due to advances in the techniques of liver surgery aided by knowledge of the segmental anatomy of liver, improved imaging techniques, better intra- and postoperative management of these patients, particularly cirrhotics. Almost concurrent with the advance in liver surgery, the field of minimally invasive surgery exploded and caused a major surgical revolution. It was inevitable that liver surgeons would apply these techniques. Large series of laparoscopic hepatic resections [13–15] have been reported and have encouraged wider application of the technique even in patients with malignant neoplasms.

Selection of Patients for Surgery

The decision to operate on a patient with hepatoma is largely determined by the morphological evaluation of the tumor on imaging and an evaluation of the functional reserve of the liver. The indications for surgery are as follows:

1) Diagnostic: while evaluating a hypervascular lesion in a cirrhotic – to differenti-
    ate neoplasia from a regenerative nodule
2) Resection of the lesion with intent to cure
3) Assessment of histological features for transplant indications
4) Ablation of the lesion at surgery by use of RF or microwave energy

Imaging

Evaluation of lesions developing in a background of cirrhosis remains a challenge
when the lesions are small. A variety of techniques such as ultrasound, triple phase
CT scan, and MR imaging are essential in guiding therapy. The latter two are
comparable and must be chosen based on local expertise and equipment. CT imaging characteristics that are diagnostic include intense enhancement on late arterial
phase, washout on portal/delayed phase, and a late capsule/pseudo capsule enhancement. MR may be preferred in differentiating regenerative nodules from tumors
when the lesions are small. However, the presence of renal impairment (not uncommon in cirrhotics) precludes the use of gadolinium. Lesions less than 1 cm are
difficult to characterize on imaging studies and may be followed by serial imaging in 3–6 months to detect an increase in size. This information helps stage the
disease based on the number of lesions, size of individual lesions, presence of major
vascular invasion, and extrahepatic disease. Imaging of the lungs and bone scans are
routinely performed at most centers prior to planning surgical resection to rule out
metastatic disease.

Additionally, CT volumetry permits calculation of the residual liver volume
(the volume of liver remaining after resection). Preoperative volumetric analysis
is essential to ensure sufficient functional liver parenchyma remains. The functional
residual liver volume is calculated by the formula: volume of residual liver/volume
of total liver – volume of the tumor. Vauthey [16] demonstrated that a future liver
remnant of <25% was associated with increased complications following extended
liver resections in patients without underlying disease. However, in the presence of
parenchymal liver disease this figure may need to be higher than 50% [11].

Functional Reserve of Liver

This is an extremely important component of liver resection in cirrhotics. Many
methods have been utilized to estimate the functional reserve and guide the extent
of liver resection. Typically liver resections are contemplated only in Child's
A or early B cirrhosis. But the assessment of the liver reserve based on synthetic function of the liver (serum albumin, prothrombin time) has not been very
reliable. Dynamic assessment of complex liver functions such as clearance of sub-
stances (ICG – indocyanine green) or the formation of metabolites (lidocaine to

monoethylglycinexylidide [MEGX] or 14C-aminopyrine) has been used to more accurately delineate the functional reserve in patients with liver disease.

In the Far East, the indocyanine green (ICG) retention test has been used with success in selecting candidates for liver resection [17]. ICG is an infrared absorbing fluorescent agent which is almost exclusively eliminated by the liver into the bile. Following the intravenous injection of 0.5 mg/kg of ICG the rate of disappearance from the plasma is calculated. A retention of >15% of the injected dye at 15 min indicates poor liver reserve and predicts poor outcome with liver resections involving three or more segments.

The ICG retention test proved to be the best discriminating preoperative test in patients with hepatoma prior to hepatectomy [10]. However, this test has not been widely used in the West to guide liver surgery. The guidelines listed in a recent review summarize the criteria used by major centers to select patients for liver resection in the presence of chronic liver disease [11]. A gross rule of thumb for what would be considered possibly safe is lobar resection for Child-Pugh class A patients, a 15% resection for class B, and a 5% resection for class C.

Laparoscopic Liver Resection for Hepatoma

The debate about the feasibility and safety of laparoscopic liver surgery is slowly but surely being put to rest. Large series of liver resections performed laparoscopically have been published and have matched the results of open surgery. Laparoscopic methods have the potential to lower the stress posed by liver surgery. Whether a significant reduction in morbidity actually is achieved has yet to be conclusively determined.

History

A multicenter European study published in 2002 was the first to present the results of laparoscopic liver resection for malignant liver tumors [18]. However, the retrospective study involving 11 centers contained only 10 patients with hepatoma, 9 of whom were cirrhotic. The next significant data came from the Henri Mondor Hospital in Paris in 2006 [19]. This single center prospective study included 27 patients who were followed for a mean period of 2 years. The paper conclusively demonstrated the feasibility and the midterm safety of laparoscopic resection. Subsequent papers from Italy [20] and Taiwan [21] have corroborated this concept.

Technique

There are three different terminologies that have been used with regard to laparoscopic liver resections:

1. Pure laparoscopic
2. Hand-assisted laparoscopic resection
3. Laparoscopic-assisted (hybrid) open resection

There is no clear advantage of one approach over the others. All aim to reduce the surgical trauma by minimizing the length of surgical incision. An incision is often required to extract the tumor specimen and one may as well make this incision at the beginning if it will aid the dissection. Poon [22] has reported the following advantages with the insertion of a hand port:

1. Palpation with the hand and the use of intraoperative ultrasonography through the hand port improve the staging of tumor and permit better delineation of resection margin
2. The hand is the best retractor
3. Manual compression in the event of major bleeding
4. Hand assistance in intracorporeal suturing
5. Specimen retrieval through the hand port

The position of the patient is supine when performing resections on the left lobe segments. The French surgeons utilize the lithotomy position with the surgeon standing between the legs during the surgery. The left lateral decubitus with a steep reverse Trendelenburg position is ideal for lesions in the right lobe – particularly those requiring mobilization of the right lobe to gain access to the posterior surface. When a hand port is inserted, the location has varied in different series. It may be placed in the midline close to the xiphoid with a lateral extension or in the midclavicular line at or above the plane of the umbilicus [23] (Fig. 13.1). The exact position varies with the individual anatomy, the size of the liver, and location of the tumor(s).

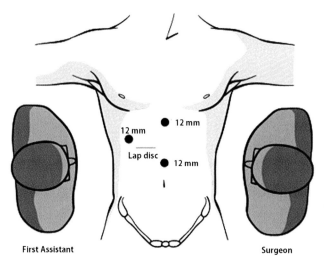

Fig. 13.1 Port placement and surgeon positioning during laparoscopic liver resection (right-sided resection). With permission from Buell et al. [23]

Typically the procedure is initiated with the placement of a trocar inferior to the umbilicus. Incisions through or above the umbilicus are not recommended in order to avoid collaterals in the falciform ligament. After a preliminary examination, an ultrasound of the liver is performed. Laparoscopic ultrasound has been used extensively in most series. This helps in confirming the site and size of the lesion, detecting additional lesions, identifying the vascular structures in proximity to the lesion, and guiding the placement of biopsy needle or radiofrequency probe.

The majority of liver resections performed for hepatoma in cirrhotics have involved one or two segments or non-anatomical resections [24] (Table 13.2). In

Table 13.2 Findings and results from literature [24]

Variable	Results	Index number of analyzable patients (% out of 300 patients)
Sex ratio M/F	132/58	190 (68%)
Mean age	61.8 (34–76)	175 (62%)
Liver cirrhosis	156 (78%)	201 (72%)
Child-Pugh classification: A/B/C	130/28/4	169 (60%)
Mean tumor size (mm)	33.6 (9–75)	188 (70%)
Location (Couinaud segments)		
2/3 s	81 (38%)	
4 s	38 (18%)	
5/6 s	85 (39%)	
7 s	8 (4%)	
8 s	3 (1%)	
LUS used	200 (83%)	240 (85%)
Type of resection		211 (75%)
Atypical	121 (57%)	
Segmentectomy	35 (17%)	
Left Lobectomy	40 (19%)	
Left Hepatectomy	7 (3%)	
Right Hepatectomy	4 (2%)	
Mesohepatectomy	3 (1%)	
Bisegementectomy (5/6 s)	1	
Pringle maneuver	62 (38%)	162 (58%)
Pringle maneuver (mean duration)	50.6 (15–17)	
Perioperative complications	17 (10%)	169 (60%)
Conversion to laparoscopy	24 (9%)	262 (93%)
Mean operative time (min)	216.8 (50–680)	175 (62%)
Mean blood losses (ml)	401 (0–1,700)	155 (55%)
Transfusion rate	17 (11%)	161 (57%)
Surgical margins (>1 cm)	77 (65%)	118 (42%)
Operative mortality	5 (1.7%)	281 (100%)
Postoperative complications	42 (20%)	211 (70%)
Reoperation	2 (0.9%)	214 (76%)
Mean postoperative hospital stay (days)	12.3 (2–76)	161 (57%)
Mean follow-up time (months)	19.6	102 (36%)
Alive without recurrence	86 (57%)	151 (54%)

With permission from Santambrogio et al. [24]

a review of 300 undergoing laparoscopic hepatectomy for hepatoma in cirrhotics, only 11 involved resection of an entire lobe. This illustrates the difficulty of major liver resections in cirrhotics. The location of the hepatoma determines the feasibility and ease of laparoscopic resection. When the lesion is located peripherally in the anterior and inferior aspects (segments 2, 3, 4b, 5, or 6) surgical resection is easier. Lesions located on the superior and posterior parts (segments 1, 4a, 7, or 8) pose a challenge.

Depending on the location of the liver, the mobilization of the liver is performed – the falciform and the appropriate triangular ligaments are divided. For lesions in the posterior right lobe, the bare area of the liver will often have to be freed with exposure of the retrohepatic inferior vena cava. The option of a Pringle maneuver has been utilized by some centers to reduce bleeding during the resection. However, this is not mandatory.

Transecting the liver parenchyma with minimal blood loss is a challenge, especially in the cirrhotic liver. This has led to development of a variety of devices which utilize different types of energy to dissect the liver and seal the blood vessels. These include the ultrasonic dissector (Harmonic Scalpel^{TM}), bipolar diathermy, water jet dissector (Helix Hydro-jet^{TM}), dissecting sealer (Tissuelink^{TM} and Aquamantys^{TM}), Habib 4X^{TM}, radiofrequency device. The caliber of the vessels traversing the most superficial 2–3 cm of the parenchyma is small and hence any of the above devices can be successfully employed. As the depth increases, larger vessels (those associated with the Glissonian pedicle and the hepatic veins) are encountered. We believe that these are most safely and expeditiously dealt with by the use of a vascular stapler. As experience with vascular staplers has grown, it is being widely used even to divide the parenchyma without isolation of major blood vessels. As no single device has been shown superior to the others, it is best to develop expertise depending on the devices available at each center. However, it should be noted that the cirrhotic parenchyma poses specific challenges for laparoscopic resection related to the stiffness of the liver, which impairs mobility, and fibrosis, which can limit the use of vascular staplers.

Preferred Technique at Our Center

The positioning of the patient is crucial for performing laparoscopic liver resections. For lesions in the right lobe, particularly in the posterior or superior segments, the patient is positioned in the left lateral decubitus with the table in steep reverse Trendelenburg position. We find that this greatly facilitates the mobilization of the right lobe of liver and exposure of the retrohepatic vena cava. For lesions in the left lobe we prefer the supine position. We do not utilize the hand port as a routine. Typically peripheral lesions involving segments 2, 3, 4b, 5, or 6 can be resected by the pure laparoscopic technique. We utilize the hand port for lesions involving the caudate lobe, the posterior surface, or the superior segments 4a, 7, and 8. The hand port is inserted through a transverse incision in the right upper abdomen – the exact site depends on the size and location of the liver lesion.

Our preference is to delineate the margins of the lesion with the help of intra-operative ultrasound. When a lobectomy is performed, our preference is to avoid extensive hilar dissection. We prefer to staple the major vessels in the parenchyma. If easily accessible, the right hepatic vein may be stapled outside the liver. We use the harmonic scalpel to mark a 1 cm margin around the lesion. The hepatotomy is then initiated with the harmonic device. After a depth of 2 cm is reached we prefer to complete the parenchymal transection with the help of vascular staplers. The specimen is delivered out of the hand port if one has been placed. Otherwise it is placed in an endopouch and retrieved. After the specimen is removed, hemostasis of the raw surface is achieved using diathermy, argon beam coagulation, and intra-corporeal suturing to control more significant bleeding. We utilize a "quick stitch" to control active bleeders or sites of bile leak. This involves the use of a 15 cm long 2-0 silk swaged suture with clips on one end which serve to anchor the suture at the liver surface. After the site of bleeding is controlled with the suturing, clips are placed at the exit site to lock the stitch in place. After satisfactory hemo- and bile stasis has been attained, we apply topical sealants to the raw surface. These include BioGlu (Cryolife), Tisseel (Baxter), and Co-seal (Baxter).

The CVP is maintained less than 5 throughout the procedure. This reduces the bleeding during transection and from the resulting raw surface. There has been con-troversy regarding the use of Argon beam at laparoscopy. We have not encountered gas embolism and believe the practice is safe – particularly when the intraabdominal pressure does not exceed 15 mmHg.

Despite the best of precautions, the liver surgeon will often be faced with seri-ous challenges. The most common is bleeding. Pressure either with an instrument or with the hand will achieve temporary hemostasis. After stabilizing the patient and ensuring the availability of a good suction device, an attempt must be made to identify the cause of the bleeding. The most troublesome bleeding comes from the veins which often retract into the liver. We employ different techniques as outlined above including the quick stitch. If the bleeding continues, a hand port may have to be inserted if not already present. We have found that reapplication of the vascular stapler to excise an additional margin of liver tissue is often successful in achieving hemostasis.

Laparoscopic resection for hepatocellular cancer as with open resection for this disease is complicated. Cirrhosis has historically portended higher operative mor-bidity and mortality. When our group approaches a cirrhotic we recognize and adhere to our principles of low CVP, in conjunction with a pure laparoscopic approach, when feasible. We also recognize and continue to debate over the pri-mary thermal technology utilized to transect hepatic parenchyma. Mobilization and division of the major inflow and outflow vessels are performed only when necessary for margins. Intrahepatic division is often preferred for these vessels. When inade-quate control of major vascular structures is encountered, use of the "Koffron quick stitch" is employed. This is a pre-cut length of silk or prolene with two 10 mm clips on the end. This allows primary closure of vessels. When this is not easily achieved, conversion to a hand-assist approach is employed. This allows direct digital control of bleeding without the need for complete conversion to laparotomy. This maneuver in itself often obviates major hemorrhage. Lastly, use of endovascular staplers are used when the remaining vascular pedicle of the tumor is identified when greater than 90% of the tumor is resected. Liberal application of staplers in a cirrhotic liver often results in deformed staplers and incomplete staple formation, hence should be averted till essential.

A margin of 1 cm is considered satisfactory. However, depending on the location of the lesion (e.g., when tumor abuts major vessels), a smaller margin may be acceptable as long as the tumor does not extend to the resection margins. If the lesion is not deemed resectable or additional lesions are found, radiofrequency ablation of the lesion is commonly performed. The RFA probe is placed in the center of the tumor and treated as per the device protocol.

Results

The skepticism surrounding the advent of laparoscopic liver surgery for hepatoma had to do mainly with the fear of complications and oncological integrity. The safety on both these counts has now been demonstrated in large series.

In the preliminary data from a multicenter study from Europe [18], of the 9 cirrhotic patients (Child's A = 5; B = 4) undergoing laparoscopic liver resection for hepatoma, 5 developed transient liver failure and ascites. Perioperative complications, such as bleeding, need for blood transfusion, need for portal triad clamping, and conversion to open resection, were higher in the hepatoma group as compared to patients with liver metastasis undergoing laparoscopic resection. A tumor-free margin of at least 1 cm was obtained in 70% of patients. No port site metastasis was detected and the disease-free survival was 44% at a mean follow-up of 14 months. Although this study demonstrated the feasibility of laparoscopic liver resection, it did not convince most physicians about a future role in HCC therapy.

The first prospective study [19] with a reasonable follow-up included 27 Child's A cirrhotic patients with solitary peripheral lesions up to 5 cm. The resections included 17 anatomic and 10 non-anatomic resections; the rate of conversion to open resection was 26%. Most of the conversions were required for lesions in segment 6 of the liver. Postoperative complications were noted in 33%, and 15 patients had a surgical margin less than 1 cm. During a mean follow-up of 2 years 8 patients (30%) developed recurrence (includes 3 with local recurrence) and the overall and disease-free 3-year survival rates were 93 and 64%, respectively.

A recent study from Italy [20] retrospectively compared laparoscopic and open liver resection for hepatoma in cirrhotic patients. Although the mean operating time was longer in the laparoscopic group, this group required significantly less blood transfusion and use of a Pringle maneuver and had reduced hospital stay and postoperative complications compared to the open resection group. The resection margin was greater than 1 cm in 92% of the laparoscopic group. The mortality rate and 2-year survival were similar in both groups.

The largest single center report of laparoscopic liver resections for HCC is a retrospective study from Taiwan [21]. This included 116 cirrhotic patients of whom 18 were Child's status B/C. Major resections (>2 segments) were performed in 19 patients. A hand port device was used for lesions in segments 7 and 8. Conversion to open resection was necessary in 5.2% of patients and the need for blood transfusion was low (6.9%). An extremely low complication rate of 6% was reported. A 5-year survival rate of 60% was reported with a complete absence of port site recurrences.

An updated European multicenter study (Dagher, personal communication) included 163 resections (cirrhotic: 120; fibrosis: 11, and normal: 32). A pure laparoscopic approach was used in 95% of cases but required a lower abdominal incision for specimen retrieval. Major resections were done in 10%. The rate of conversion to open resection and the need for blood transfusion were 9.2 and 9.8%, respectively. There were 2 postoperative deaths and the morbidity was detailed as liver specific in 11.6% and nonspecific in 10.4%. The mean surgical margin was 14.2 ± 10.6 mm and exceeded 5 mm in 83.4%. At a mean follow-up of 30.4 months, tumor recurrence in the liver was noted in 39.2% (local in 17% and distant 83%).

A summary of the majority of reports in the literature is contained in Table 13.2.

The above results strongly support the feasibility and safety of the laparoscopic technique in the surgical treatment of hepatoma of the liver in cirrhotics.

Summary

Laparoscopic resection of liver for hepatoma is a safe option. In centers with the necessary expertise results are equivalent to open surgery. The advantages of small incisions minimizing the incidence of ascites and adhesions are likely to increase the use of this option in the cirrhotic population (Child's A/B). This is crucially important in those likely to need liver transplantation in the future.

References

1. Mazzaferro V, Regalia E, Doci R, et al (1996) Liver transplantation for the treatment of small hepatocellular carcinomas in patients with cirrhosis. N Engl J Med 334:693–699
2. Yao FY, Ferrell L, Bass NM, et al (2001) Liver transplantation for hepatocellular carcinoma: expansion of the tumor size limits does not adversely impact survival. Hepatology 33:1394–1403
3. Livraghi T, Goldberg SN, Lazzaroni S, Meloni F, Solbiati L, Gazelle GS, et al (1999) Small hepatocellular carcinoma: treatment with radio-frequency ablation versus ethanol injection. Radiology 210:655–661
4. Zhou XD, Tang ZY (1998) Cryotherapy for primary liver cancer. Semin Surg Oncol 14:171–174
5. Shiina S, Tagawa K, Niwa Y, et al (1993) Percutaneous ethanol injection therapy for hepatocellular carcinoma: results in 146 patients. AJR Am J Roentgenol 160(5):1023–1028
6. Matsukawa T, Yamashita Y, Arakawa A, et al (1997) Percutaneous microwave coagulation therapy in liver tumors. A 3-year experience. Acta Radiol 38:410–415

7. Pacella CM, Bizzarri G, Guglielmi R, et al (2001) Laser thermal ablation in the treatment of small hepatocellular carcinoma: results in 74 patients. Radiology 221:712–720

8. Llovet JM, Bruix J (2003) Systematic review of randomized trials for unresectable hepatocellular carcinoma: Chemoembolization improves survival. Hepatology 37:429–442

9. Salem R, Lewandowski RJ, Atassi B, et al (2005) Treatment of unresectable hepatocellular carcinoma with use of 90Y microspheres (TheraSphere): safety, tumor response, and survival. J Vasc Interv Radiol 16:1627–1639

10. Lau H, Man K, Fan ST, Yu WC, Lo CM, Wong J (1997) Evaluation of preoperative hepatic function in patients with hepatocellular carcinoma undergoing hepatectomy. Br J Surg 84:1255–1259

11. Bryant R, Laurent A, Tayar C, et al (2008) Liver resection for hepatocellular carcinoma. Surg Oncol Clin N Am 17:607–633, ix

12. Lau WY (1997) The history of liver surgery. J R Coll Surg Edinb 42:303–309

13. Buell JF, Thomas MT, Rudich S, et al (2008) Experience with more than 500 minimally invasive hepatic procedures. Ann Surg 248:475–486

14. Koffron AJ, Auffenberg G, Kung R, Abecassis M (2007) Evaluation of 300 minimally invasive liver resections at a single institution: less is more. Ann Surg 246:385–392

15. Nguyen KT, Gamblin TC, Geller DA (2008) Laparoscopic liver resection for cancer. Future Oncol 4:661–670

16. Vauthey JN, Chaoui A, Do KA, et al (2000) Standardized measurement of the future liver remnant prior to extended liver resection: methodology and clinical associations. Surgery 127:512–519

17. Makuuchi M, Sano K (2004) The surgical approach to HCC: our progress and results in Japan. Liver Transpl 10(2 Suppl 1):S46–S52

18. Gigot JF, Glineur D, Santiago Azagra J, et al (2002) Laparoscopic liver resection for malignant liver tumors: preliminary results of a multicenter European study. Ann Surg 236:90–97

19. Cherqui D, Laurent A, Tayar C, et al (2006) Laparoscopic liver resection for peripheral hepatocellular carcinoma in patients with chronic liver disease: midterm results and perspectives. Ann Surg 243:499–506

20. Belli G, Fantini C, D'Agostino A, et al (2007) Laparoscopic versus open liver resection for hepatocellular carcinoma in patients with histologically proven cirrhosis: short- and middle-term results. Surg Endosc 21:2004–2011

21. Chen HY, Juan CC, Ker CG (2008) Laparoscopic liver surgery for patients with hepatocellular carcinoma. Ann Surg Oncol 15:800–806

22. Poon RT (2007) Current role of laparoscopic surgery for liver malignancies. Surg Technol Int 16:73–81

23. Buell JF, Koffron AJ, Thomas MJ, et al (2005) Laparoscopic liver resection. J Am Coll Surg 200:472–480

24. Santambrogio R, Aldrighetti L, Barabino M, et al (2009) Laparoscopic liver resections for hepatocellular carcinoma. Is it a feasible option for patients with liver cirrhosis? Langenbecks Arch Surg 394:255–264

Chapter 14
Liver Transplant for Hepatocellular Carcinoma

Thomas A. Aloia, A. Osama Gaber, and R. Mark Ghobrial

Keywords Liver cancer · Liver transplantation · Immunosuppression · Outcomes · Prognostic factors

History of Liver Transplant for HCC

From the start of liver transplantation, treatment of hepatocellular carcinoma (HCC) has played a central role. Following the unsuccessful transplant of a child with biliary atresia in 1963, the second and third attempts at liver transplantation at the University of Colorado were in adults with advanced HCC. At autopsy, both recipients were found to have micrometastatic disease [1]. As liver transplantation proceeded in an experimental environment, the high mortality procedure was frequently reserved for patients with advanced malignancy. In 1967, a 19-month-old child with primary liver cancer became the first liver transplant recipient to achieve prolonged survival, but recurred within 4 months and died of disseminated cancer at 400 days [2]. As the procedure and immunosuppression were refined, patient and allograft survivals improved to the point that oncologic recurrence and survival rates could be determined [3, 4].

This initial experience clearly showed that, in the immunosuppressed state following liver transplantation, patients with advanced stage HCC had extraordinarily high recurrence rates [5]. As more experience was gained and allograft outcomes continued to improve, the non-oncologic indications for liver transplantation were expanded and, appropriately, oncologic indications were constricted [6]. In 1989, a moratorium on liver transplantation for HCC was put in place.

Following this, enthusiasm waned and few guidelines directed the listing and transplantation of patients with HCC until the publication of the "Milan criteria"

R.M. Ghobrial (✉)
Department of Surgery, Weill-Cornell Medical College, The Methodist Hospital, Houston, TX, USA

K.M. McMasters, J.-N. Vauthey (eds.), *Hepatocellular Carcinoma*,
DOI 10.1007/978-1-60327-522-4_14, © Springer Science+Business Media, LLC 2011

[7]. The Milan experience, which identified a subset of early HCC patients with strict tumor number (≤ 3) and tumor size (≤ 3 cm) criteria who had both excellent allograft and oncologic outcomes, rekindled interest in liver transplantation for malignant disease. Over the next decade the percentage of cadaveric liver transplants for patients with HCC steadily rose, and 5-year post-transplant patient survival rates of 60% and HCC recurrence rates of less than 15% were finally achieved [8–14].

The re-expansion of liver transplantation into the HCC recipient pool was temporally correlated with two other shifts in liver transplantation practice. First, in Western countries with significant rates of hepatitis C virus infection and obesity, the acute rise in the incidence of HCC cases has focused the hepatology and transplant community on the problem of effective treatments [15, 16]. Additionally, more standardized screening recommendations have allowed diagnosis of earlier stage patients with HCC who more likely benefit from liver transplantation [17]. Second, in 2002, the United Network for Organ Sharing (UNOS) instituted the model for end-stage liver disease (MELD) waitlist rank system and created MELD exception algorithms that advantage waitlisted patients with UNOS T2-3 criteria HCC [18]. Together, these two factors have contributed to a sharp rise in the percentage of US liver transplants performed for HCC [19].

Currently, liver transplantation stands as the best treatment modality for early-stage HCC in patients with decompensated cirrhosis, giving patients the opportunity to be free from the potentially lethal complications of both cancer and their underlying liver disease [11, 12, 20–22]. In settings where the number of patients with HCC and cirrhosis exceeds the availability of cadaveric liver allografts, alternative strategies are required. These include more liberal use of liver resection, interventional and systemic treatments, public health campaigns for organ donation awareness, and living-related liver transplantation.

The Role of HCC Staging Systems in Pre-transplant Decision-Making

Multiple staging systems have been proposed for the stratification of prognosis and treatment of patients with HCC. Although both the American Joint Committee on Cancer (AJCC) staging system (6th Edition) and the Pittsburg modified tumor-node-metastasis staging systems have a strong correlation with outcomes in patients with HCC, their reliance on pathological information (i.e., microvascular invasion) limits their utility in cirrhotic pre-transplant patients. With only radiologic staging information available for most patients, US transplant programs have relied on the American Liver Tumor Study Group/UNOS staging system to determine transplant candidacy and MELD point allocation (Table 14.1). This system relies on the accuracy of contrast-enhanced cross-sectional imaging modalities, including computed tomography (CT) and magnetic resonance imaging (MRI). Under UNOS criteria, liver masses in cirrhotic patients with vascular phase blush in the absence of gross

Table 14.1 Modified UNOS staging system for HCC

UNOS HCC tumor stage	Radiographic criteria (liver mass with vascular blush on CT, MR, or angiogram
T1	Solitary, <2 cm
T2	Solitary, 2–5 cm 2–3 tumors, all less than 3 cm
T3	Solitary, 5–6 cm 2–3 tumors, at least one >3 cm, none greater than 5 cm, aggregate not greater than 9 cm
T4a	Solitary, >6 cm 2–3 tumors, any greater than 5 cm and/or aggregate greater than 9 cm >3 tumors
T4b	T2, T3, T4a plus gross intrahepatic portal or hepatic vein involvement

American Liver Tumor Study Group [97] and Yao [10], with T3 modification to account for Regional T3 MELD exception criteria.

vascular invasion are eligible to be staged with this system. Many centers have added further imaging criteria, including washout of contrast on venous phase imaging and the presence of T2 signal on MRI, in order to proceed to transplant listing with an HCC indication without tissue biopsy. These noninvasive criteria have been validated, obviating the need for tissue biopsy and the risk of immediate complication or tumor seeding [23–25]. Using these criteria, in the absence of complete response to neoadjuvant therapies, remarkably few patients will have a negative pathology specimen at explant.

In Europe, the Barcelona Clinic Liver Cancer Staging and Treatment Approach has been popularized [26, 27]. This system uniquely integrates clinical tumor staging, degree of cirrhotic complications as measured by the Child-Turcotte-Pugh (CTP) score, portal pressure measurement, performance status, and comorbidities to assign various treatments to HCC patients. In this algorithm, liver transplantation is reserved for Conventional Milan Criteria (CMC) HCC patients with preserved performance status and cirrhosis with portal hypertension. HCC patients transplanted under this algorithm are reported to have 5-year post-transplant survivals of 60–70%.

Despite advances in radiologic staging there continues to be a considerable difference between preoperative clinical staging and postoperative tumor staging. Exclusive of histopathologic variables such as vascular invasion and tumor differentiation, the simple measurements of tumor number and maximal tumor dimension that make up the foundation of UNOS, Conventional Milan Criteria (CMC), and University of California at San Francisco (UCSF) criteria can lead to pathological upstaging in as many as 30% of recipients [14, 22, 28–32]. Predictably, patient and oncologic outcomes post-transplant correlate more closely with the pathological stage of disease. For example, one European study identified 39 patients with HCC pathologically staged between CMC and within UCSF criteria. These patients demonstrated similar and favorable survival compared to pathologically staged CMC patients; however, survival for the 44 patients who were clinically staged prior to transplant between CMC and UCSF criteria experienced a 5-year survival rate of only 48%. This example highlights the importance of precise preoperative liver imaging and clinical staging prior to liver transplantation.

The Clinical Significance of Serum Alpha-Fetoprotein

Serum alpha-fetoprotein (AFP) measurement is commonly used as a screening tool for HCC in patients with cirrhosis and a staging tool in patients with suspected or proven HCC. In general, the test has little accuracy. Most patients with early-stage HCC do not have elevated AFP levels. Rarely, patients with negative radiographic metastatic survey will have AFP levels above 200 ng/mL, raising the suspicion of occult metastases. Although some studies report a correlation between elevated pre-transplant AFP, poor tumor differentiation, and post-transplant recurrence [33, 34], in the absence of radiographic evidence for vascular invasion or metastatic disease, AFP elevation should not be a contraindication to transplantation.

In practical terms for liver transplantation, the AFP level is useful in only two settings. First, under UNOS guidelines patients with macronodular cirrhosis (that makes radiographic differentiation between dysplastic nodules and early HCC difficult) who also have an AFP level >500 in the absence of radiographic evidence for liver malignancy may receive additional MELD exception points. Second, in patients with early T-stage HCC and an elevated or rising AFP level, complete metastatic survey including bone scan is advisable and should be repeated every 3 months while on the transplant waitlist.

Pre- and Post-transplant Metastasis Screening

As HCC is most likely to metastasize to lung and bone, traditional metastasis screening consists of chest CT and bone scan with either nuclear isotope or magnetic resonance. A shared experience that bone metastases are rare in UNOS T1 and T2 patients has lead to UNOS no longer requiring metastatic survey of the skeleton as a criteria for liver transplant listing with HCC MELD exception. For patients with either elevated AFP and/or UNOS T3 stage disease, bone survey remains a prudent staging study. While on the waitlist, restaging with chest and liver imaging is typically repeated every 3 months.

Of HCC patients who recur following liver transplant, 90% will do so within 2 years of the transplant procedure [35–39]. Therefore, radiological and biochemical staging during this critical period is performed every 3 months. Thereafter, restaging intervals can reasonably be lengthened to 6–12 month intervals.

Neoadjuvant Therapies

As liver transplant waitlist times have increased and interventional radiology techniques have improved, many liver transplant teams have employed neoadjuvant therapies in an effort to decrease waitlist dropout and to potentially reduce the rate of post-transplant recurrence [40, 41]. These include transarterial chemoembolization (TACE), percutaneous ethanol injection, radiofrequency ablation (RFA), cryoablation, and more recently, radioembolization with yttrium-90, microwave ablation, and systemic chemotherapy.

TACE

Given its wide therapeutic window in cirrhotic patients and relatively simple delivery, the most frequently used neoadjuvant therapy in waitlisted HCC patients has been TACE. The chemotherapeutic agent is typically doxorubicin or cisplatin, and the embolic agent is variable, typically consisting of gelfoam, polyvinyl alcohol, embospheres, or glass beads. Lipiodol is also frequently added as a radiographic marker. Multiple publications report large experiences with TACE in the pre-transplant setting [37, 40–48]. Although TACE has been shown to lengthen survival in patients with unresectable and nontransplantable bulky disease [49], it has been difficult to show a benefit in early-stage patients awaiting transplant, either in terms of reducing waitlist dropout rates or in post-transplant survival.

Based on a review of the published outcomes data, the opinion that TACE has no role in the neoadjuvant treatment of pre-transplant HCC patients was recently proposed [50]. This opinion contrasted with a shared experience among many centers that TACE, while rarely curative, is frequently able to maintain a stable disease pattern during prolonged wait times and is frequently associated with significant tumoral necrosis in explanted liver pathology analyses.

One explanation for the inability of many studies to prove a TACE benefit is that, like most other chemotherapies, there is a finite therapeutic window for TACE in patients with HCC. Also similar to systemic chemotherapy for most solid tumors, only a small percentage of patients achieve a complete response (i.e., cure), with most patients' responses distributed equally between progression, stable disease, and partial response. This pattern would predict a finite interval in which TACE would have maximal benefit. This hypothesis is supported by a recent analysis of the reported literature indicating that centers reporting outcomes in the setting of median waitlist times between 4 and 9 months showed a benefit to neoadjuvant TACE, while programs with shorter (<4 mo) and longer (>9 mo) median waitlist times found no benefit from TACE [51]. These data suggest that HCC patients

listed at programs with waitlist times between 4 and 9 months should be offered
neoadjuvant TACE therapy.

HCC Tumor Ablation

Following TACE, ablation treatments are the second most frequently used
neoadjuvant therapy in patients with transplantable HCC. The most experience is
with radiofrequency ablation and to a lesser extent cryoablation. Their application
can be limited by anatomic tumor characteristics (location, size over 3 cm, and
tumor number) and the condition of the cirrhotic liver. However, those patients who
are candidates for ablative treatments typically benefit from this approach. Liver
explant data suggest that individually treated tumors, particularly those less than
3 cm, frequently have extensive necrosis [52, 53]. Like TACE, radiofrequency ablation does appear to have a finite therapeutic window with patients recurring at the
ablation site or elsewhere in the liver within 6 months [54]. The complication rates
tend to be higher for ablation than for TACE, but in general, this modality is well
tolerated in CTP class A patients with low to mid MELD scores. More recently,
microwave ablation has been proposed as a novel ablative modality, but not enough
clinical experience has been gained to comment on the utility of this therapy for
HCC patients awaiting transplant.

Radioembolization with Y-90

Following the large experience with transarterial chemotherapy delivery to HCC
patients, the use of radioembolization as a neoadjuvant therapy for patients with
HCC has gained favor. Two products are available for this application. Unlike
TACE, which is most effectively given in a selective application to the artery directly
feeding the liver tumor, yttrium-90 (Y-90) particles are generally directed either to
one hemi-liver or to the whole liver. Given the broader dispersion, pretreatment
testing with nuclear colloid scan to rule out hepatopulmonary shunts and arteriogram to identify and embolize accessory hepatic arteries to extrahepatic structures
is mandatory.

Selected centers have report excellent short-term results in nontransplantable
HCC patients [55], as well as a smaller subset of patients awaiting transplant
[56, 57]. Typically, patients who have received this therapy prior to transplant yield
a liver explant specimen with significant tumor necrosis. Although it has not been
determined whether there is a post-transplant survival advantage for neoadjuvant
Y-90 over TACE, radiotherapy is appealing for patients with multifocal HCC where
a broader dispersion of therapeutic agent is likely to achieve a more durable tumor
effect. Caution is required in patients with advanced cirrhosis, in whom the radiation
hepatitis induced by the therapy can lead to early and/or delayed liver failure.

Systemic Chemotherapy

Traditionally, there have been few effective systemic chemotherapy options for patients with HCC, regardless of stage [58, 59]. More recently, the oral multi-kinase inhibitor of the vascular endothelial growth factor receptor, sorafenib, was shown to have a small but measurable survival benefit in patients with Stage IV HCC [60, 61]. The trial that established this effect focused mainly on CTP class A patients.

Subsequently, off-label use of this drug has entered the liver transplant arena. Some patients with unsuspected advanced pathologic stage HCC have been treated with sorafenib post-transplant. There is a limited but growing experience with the drug in the pre-transplant setting. Few objective reports on this experience are available, but multiple trials have been initiated to determine its impact on patients with HCC [62], either as a routine neoadjuvant therapy in early-stage patients or as a modality to downstage UNOS T3-4 patients to transplantable criteria, usually in combination with other interventional neoadjuvant approaches such as TACE. The impact that sorafenib delivered immediately prior to liver transplant has (as seen sometimes in the neoadjuvant setting) on wound healing, liver regeneration, and/or hepatic artery thrombosis is unknown.

Experience with Liver Transplantation in the Post "Milan Criteria" Era

As clinical staging and pathological staging are discordant in as many as 30% of HCC liver transplant recipients, it has been noted that selected patients with pathologic staging that unexpectedly exceeded the CMC have achieved favorable oncologic outcomes post-transplant. These data have encouraged several programs to implement and investigate expanded HCC criteria. The goal of these expanded criteria systems has been to identify a subset of patients outside of the CMC who would share equivalent survival rates, thereby increasing the pool of patients who may benefit from transplantation.

The most frequently used set of extended HCC criteria are the UCSF criteria [10]. These criteria modestly expand the tumor size criteria beyond CMC to include those patients with solitary HCC lesions up to 6.5 cm and patients with 2–3 tumors to have an individual upper size limit of 4.5 cm and an aggregate upper size limit of 8 cm. In large studies, these expanded criteria capture an additional 10–20% of patients beyond CMC alone [32, 63, 64].

In limited application, the UCSF group and others have found equivalent survival rates for patients in CMC and those between CMC and UCSF (Table 14.2) [22, 32, 63, 64]. Patients with final pathologic staging in excess of UCSF criteria do consistently have higher recurrence rates and poorer survival post-transplant (Fig. 14.1) Further pathological analysis indicates that tumor size and number that exceed

Table 14.2 Comparison of post-liver transplant survivals for patients with pathological staging within conventional Milan criteria, within UCSF criteria, and beyond UCSF criteria

	Milan		UCSF		Beyond UCSF	
UCLA [22]	$N = 126$	86%	$N = 208$	81%	$N = 133$	32%
French Multicenter [32]	$N = 184$	70%	$N = 39$	64%	$N = 238$	34%
UCSF [10]	–	–	$N = 60$	75%	$N = 10$	<30%
Spain [63]	$N = 33$	68%	$N = 26$	67%	$N = 6$	48%

Fig. 14.1 [Post-transplant] survival estimate by preoperative imaging assessment [22]

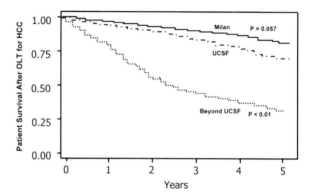

UCSF criteria serve as surrogates for microvascular invasion and poor tumor differentiation, which may biologically explain the relationship between the advanced staging and the poor outcomes [65].

These data are compelling and have supported the development of Regional "T3" MELD exception criteria. Typically, these criteria do not advantage waitlisted patients to the degree that UNOS T2 (CMC) patients are advantaged, but depending on median MELD scores in the region, these MELD exception points may facilitate transplantation for this subset of patients.

As with any staging system there are certain patients who, from a prognostic standpoint, are not appropriately accounted for. In the case of HCC both the CMC and the UCSF criteria are fairly rigid. In response to this rigidity, the Milan group has recently reported on a multicenter experience with liver transplantation for HCC tumors outside of CMC and has developed more flexible criteria that combine tumor number with maximal tumor diameter in centimeters. This analysis has found that post-transplant survivals for patients with a score of 7 or less (e.g., two tumors with maximal diameter of 5 cm or five tumors with maximal diameter of 2 cm) are similar and oncologically acceptable (Fig. 14.2) [66]. This rule of seven transplant eligibility criteria requires validation in other settings but is appealing in its flexibility, allowing a more clinically applicable system that would be fair to HCC patients.

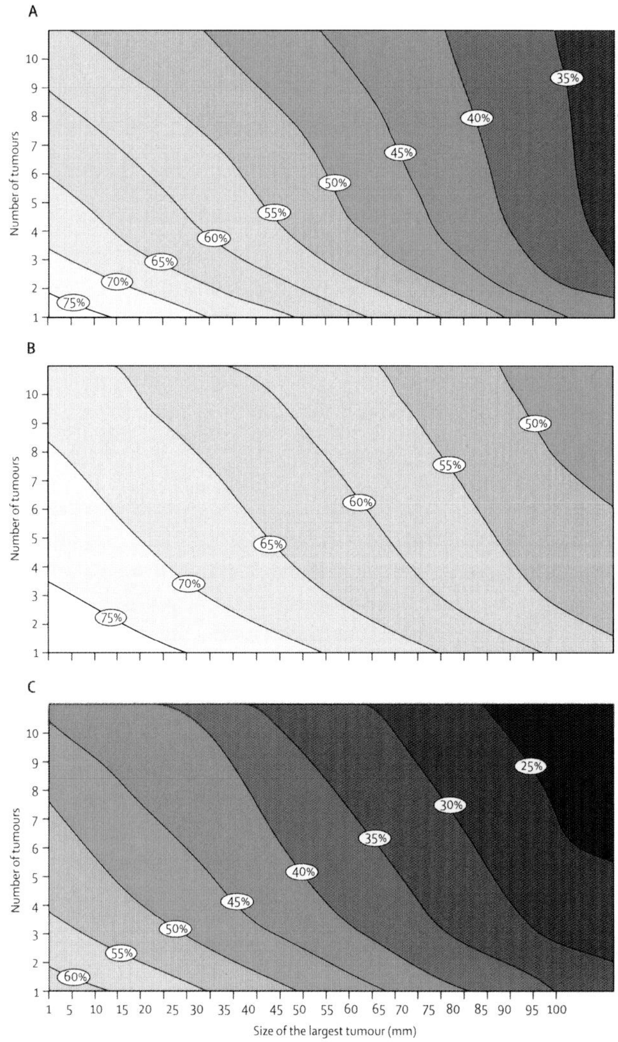

Fig. 14.2 Contour plot of the 5-year overall-survival probability according to size of the largest tumor, number of tumors, and presence or absence of microvascular invasion [66]

While UNOS, regional liver transplant committees, and individual liver transplant programs struggle with the equitable application of these various staging systems, what is apparent is that there is no currently used component to account for tumor biology. For example, patients with T3 lesions who remain stable over long waitlist times or achieve downstaging via dramatic responses to neoadjuvant treatments have no mechanism to advance on the liver transplant waitlist. Recent studies have shown that patients downstaged to T2 criteria may share similar post-transplant outcomes with those who started in T2 criteria [29, 38, 67, 68]. If confirmed in controlled trials, downstaging criteria may need to be accounted for in future clinical staging systems and MELD exception criteria proposals [69].

Current practice

Current regional practice regarding the management of HCC patients in the pre-transplant setting has been dictated by the median MELD score for transplantation and the regional MELD exception point criteria, which vary across regions. In general, patients with HCC within CMC (UNOS T2 stage) receive MELD exception to 22 points. Variable upgrades to 25 or more points are granted on an every 3-month basis provided that the disease remains stable on serial radiographic imaging. For a program with a median laboratory MELD score of 20, this point allocation schema yields short waitlist times. In contrast, urban programs in competitive markets that transplant at median MELD scores above 26 may have HCC patients routinely waiting over 6 months for allograft offer.

In the setting of long waitlist times, several programmatic strategies have been developed. First, programs with extended waitlist times typically develop a broad array of neoadjuvant treatment modalities to prevent disease progression and, therefore, limit waitlist dropout. These modalities include repetitive transarterial chemoembolization, intraarterial radiotherapy, and systemic chemotherapy. Second, several programs have shifted their practice to living-related liver transplants. This serves to shorten the wait times and to convert the procedure into an elective oper-ation. Of course, this requires additional resources and assumes the medical risk for a living donor. Third, programs have sought to use extended criteria cadaveric allografts. These organs so-called orphan livers have unique risk profiles and should be considered on a case-by-case basis. In the setting of advanced malignancy in the liver, they offer a viable option despite higher risks of early allograft dysfunction.

The role of liver resection in the pre-transplant setting remains controversial. Although liver resection has been proposed as a bridge therapy to transplantation [70], this strategy is associated with high recurrence rates [20, 71, 72] and has not been embraced within the USA. In general, the US experience suggests that CTP class A patients without portal hypertension rarely present with HCC at a resectable stage of disease. For patients with more advanced liver disease, the US medico-legal environment tends to dissuade surgeons from assuming the morbidity and mortality risk associated with liver resection. In addition, there remains concern that the pre-vious procedure may unacceptably increase the complication rate associated with repeat laparotomy for transplantation [73].

Living Donor Liver Transplantation for HCC

The role of living donor liver transplantation in HCC treatment developed in response to the wide gap between the number of patients with transplantable HCC and the lack of available cadaveric donor allografts. In Asia, multiple centers have published large series of HCC patients receiving living donor liver allografts. In the USA, early living donor liver transplant programmatic development was stunted in 2002 by a highly publicized donor death. In addition, several data sources suggested that HCC recipient outcomes may be inferior to those of deceased donor transplantation. This may be related to rapid transplantation of patients with aggressive tumor biology that would have been "declared" during an interval of time on the waitlist. In addition, US living donor liver transplantation has been characterized by the tendency to reserve the procedure for recipients with HCC beyond CMC [20, 74, 75].

In addition, initial OPTN/UNOS data suggested that living donor allografts had worse survival rates, although this may have been related to a learning curve effect [76]. In 2007, the nine member A2ALL consortium also reported a learning curve effect on mortality risk with living donor liver transplantation [75]. Although their comparison to deceased donor transplantation found an association between living liver donor transplantation and higher HCC recurrence rates independent of disease stage, overall 3-year mortality rates were similar.

In contrast to these data, the world experience would suggest that living donor liver transplantation performed in experienced centers with low donor complication rates offers an acceptable option for patients with both CMC and extended (T3) stage HCC [39, 77, 78]. It can serve to expand the donor pool and offers the advantages of an elective operation performed earlier in the course of disease, thereby limiting the possibility of disease progression during prolonged waitlist intervals [78, 79]. In the USA, clinical studies aimed at defining the HCC stage that most benefits from the technique are ongoing.

Outcomes and Determinants for Recurrence Following Liver Transplantation for HCC

Multiple patient, tumor, and transplant-related variables have been investigated for their ability to predict recurrence of HCC following liver transplantation. As is true for the prognosis of all patients under treatment for HCC, the presence of vascular invasion, typically into portal venous and/or hepatic venous structures, consistently ranks as the highest risk factor for tumor recurrence [12, 13, 22, 80–85]. Three decades of experience with liver transplantation have reinforced this concept to the point that pre-transplant radiographic evidence of gross vascular invasion is considered an absolute contraindication to liver transplantation. For patients with unsuspected microvascular invasion in the explanted liver, the recurrence rate may be as high as 60% at 1-year, mandating vigilant follow-up and consideration of adjuvant chemotherapy aimed at forestalling recurrence.

The dominant influence of microvascular invasion on post-transplant outcomes also emphasizes the need for improvements in pre-transplant staging modalities. For each clinical HCC staging system currently in use, there continues to be a consistent degree of prognostic inaccuracy based on the absence of information regarding vascular invasion. Even the Modified Milan Rule of 7 system shows a significant shift

of the isograms depending on the presence of vascular invasion in the explant specimens (Fig. 14.2) [66]. For the field to progress more precise imaging modalities,
perhaps with functional correlates to vascular invasion, are required.

Secondary, but still significant, risk factors for HCC recurrence following transplant include elevated pre-transplant AFP levels, multifocality/satellitosis, and poor
tumor differentiation. Although increased tumor number and particularly maximal
tumor size are associated with higher HCC recurrence rates, these factors have
not consistently been found to be prognostic independent of their relationship with
microvascular invasion and tumor differentiation [12, 22, 80–82, 86, 87]. Based on
these data, in the absence of radiologic or biopsy evidence for vascular invasion,
there are few objective criteria that reliably predict recurrence following transplant
for HCC. For patients with "high-risk" HCC (i.e., size >5 cm, >3 tumors, poor
differentiation) further development of measures that identify favorable individual
tumor biology are needed to optimize liver transplant candidacy.

The suspected relationship between hepatitis C virus infection on poor post-
transplant oncologic outcomes in HCC patients has also been investigated. Although
hepatitis C patients tend to have worse patient and allograft survival rates compared
to non-hepatitis C patients, analyses show that this effect is independent of HCC
and oncologic outcomes [83, 84].

In summary, patients with UNOS T2 HCC and no evidence for microvascular
invasion in the explanted tumor site are frequently cured of HCC and have recurrence rates less than 20% at 5 years. Although the all-stage patient survival curve

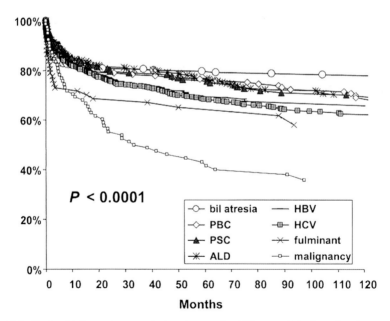

Fig. 14.3 Kaplan-Meier patient survival estimates for different etiologies of end-stage liver
disease [88]

for patients transplanted for HCC is poorer than for other indications (5 yr 60%), this rate is far superior to the historical survival rate of similar stage patients who do not undergo transplant (Fig. 14.3) [88]. In addition, this general survival curve represents a mixture of clinical and pathologic disease stages. As stated above, for patients with favorable pathologic staging in the absence of vascular invasion, liver transplant can achieve excellent patient, allograft, and oncologic outcomes. In the absence of reliable indicators for favorable vs. unfavorable tumor biology, the indications for transplant in patients with "high-risk" HCC remain controversial.

Immunosuppression Following Liver Transplantation for HCC

From the beginning of liver transplantation, transplant physicians have feared that immunosuppression given to induce tolerance of the foreign allograft in the recipient collaterally reduces the ability of the immune system to fight malignant cancer. Liver transplant recipients with a history of HCC are not only at high risk for HCC tumor recurrence but also have elevated rates of skin and colorectal cancer. With regard to specific immunosuppression medications, limited data suggest that cyclosporine may be associated with a more aggressive pattern of HCC recurrence in preclinical and patient studies [89–91].

   In this setting, novel immunosuppression protocols have been tested in patients transplanted with HCC indications [92]. The most commonly advocated regimen calls for a transition from calcineurin inhibitors (e.g., cyclosporine or tacrolimus) to the bacterial macrolide, sirolimus. Despite serving as an effective immuno-suppressant to prevent allograft rejection, there is preclinical data to support the simultaneous tumoricidal effect of this agent, which may help to prevent recurrence [93, 94]. The drug has been used in a compassionate setting post-liver transplant with a good safety profile [95]. The US Food and Drug Administration has warned that patients given sirolimus immediately after transplant may have an elevated risk of hepatic artery thrombosis and those taking the combination of sirolimus and cal-cineurin inhibitor may be at higher risk for post-transplant infections. With these caveats in mind, the use of sirolimus and other allograft immunosuppressive agents with tumoricidal properties remain under investigation in patients transplanted for HCC.

Future Perspectives

The history of liver transplantation for HCC has been characterized by constant clinical and scientific investigation. Transplant clinicians continue to try to appro-priately allocate the scarce resource of donor liver allografts to the most deserving patients, in many cases relying on imperfect staging information to make these difficult decisions. This environment naturally leads to controversy (Table 14.3).

Table 14.3 Major controversial areas in liver transplantation for HCC

Improving the accuracy of pre-transplant staging (i.e., tumor size, tumor number, microvascular invasion, prognostic molecular signature)

Integration of tumor biology in candidate selection (i.e., response to neoadjuvant therapy and downstaging)

Establishing criteria for organ allocation to patients exceeding Conventional Milan Criteria who may have similar survivals (i.e., UCSF criteria)

Optimal application of neoadjuvant therapies

Refining criteria for allocation of living donor liver transplants

Integration of new technologies (i.e., systemic sorafenib and radioembolization) pre- and post-transplant

Immunosuppression modulation in HCC recipients

Independent of liver transplantation, the HCC field is moving toward molecular staging. There is promising data that certain proteomic and molecular profiles correlate with survival in patients with HCC [96]. If validated, these data may support a renewed interest in pre-transplant tumor biopsy as a means to provide tissue for prognostic value. Ultimately, a novel staging system that accounts for an individual tumor's molecular profile may be used to determine liver transplant candidacy. In addition to molecular staging, certain stipulations may be added to allocation algorithms that account for tumor biology over time. Until such time, tumor number and tumor size, serving as surrogates for the likelihood of poor cellular differentiation and microvascular invasion, remain the cornerstones for the clinical staging of HCC patients being considered for liver transplantation.

References

1. Starzl TE, Marchioro TL, Vonkaulla KN, Hermann G, Brittain RS, Waddell WR (1963) Homotransplantation of the liver in humans. Surg Gynecol Obstet 117:659–676
2. Starzl TE (1992) The puzzle people: memoirs of a transplant surgeon. University of Pittsburg Press, Pittsburgh, PA
3. Starzl TE, Iwatsuki S, Van Thiel DH et al (1982) Evolution of liver transplantation. Hepatology 2:614–636
4. Iwatsuki S, Gordon RD, Shaw BW, Jr, Starzl TE (1985) Role of liver transplantation in cancer therapy. Ann Surg 202:401–407
5. Klintmalm GB, Stone MJ (1990) Liver transplantation for malignancy. Transpl Rev 4: 52–58
6. Ringe B, Pichlmayr R, Wittekind C, Tusch G (1991) Surgical treatment of hepatocellular carcinoma: experience with liver resection and transplantation in 198 patients. World J Surg 15:270–285
7. Mazzaferro V, Regalia E, Doci R et al (1996) Liver transplantation for the treatment of small hepatocellular carcinomas in patients with cirrhosis. N Engl J Med 334:693–699
8. Yoo HY, Patt CH, Geschwind JF, Thuluvath PJ (2003) The outcome of liver transplantation in patients with hepatocellular carcinoma in the United States between 1988 and 2001: 5-year survival has improved significantly with time. J Clin Oncol 21:4329–4335
9. Sala M, Varela M, Bruix J (2004) Selection of candidates with HCC for transplantation in the MELD era. Liver Transpl 10(10 Suppl 2):S4–S9

10. Yao FY, Ferrell L, Bass NM et al (2001) Liver transplantation for hepatocellular carcinoma: expansion of the tumor size limits does not adversely impact survival. Hepatology 33: 1394–1403

11. Shetty K, Timmins K, Brensinger C et al (2004) Liver transplantation for hepatocellular carcinoma validation of present selection criteria in predicting outcome. Liver Transpl 10:911–918

12. Hemming AW, Cattral MS, Reed AI, Van Der Werf WJ, Greig PD, Howard RJ (2001) Liver transplantation for hepatocellular carcinoma. Ann Surg 233:652–659

13. Jonas S, Bechstein WO, Steinmuller T et al (2001) Vascular invasion and histopathologic grading determine outcome after liver transplantation for hepatocellular carcinoma in cirrhosis. Hepatology 33:1080–1086

14. Bruix J, Fuster J, Llovet JM (2003) Liver transplantation for hepatocellular carcinoma: Foucault pendulum versus evidence-based decision. Liver Transpl 9:700–702

15. McGlynn KA, Tarone RE, El-Serag HB (2006) A comparison of trends in the incidence of hepatocellular carcinoma and intrahepatic cholangiocarcinoma in the United States. Cancer Epidemiol Biomarkers Prev 15:1198–1203

16. El-Serag HB (2002) Hepatocellular carcinoma and hepatitis C in the United States. Hepatology 36(5 Suppl 1):S74–S83

17. Bruix J, Sherman M (2005) Management of hepatocellular carcinoma. Hepatology 42: 1208–1236

18. Freeman RB, Jr, Wiesner RH, Harper A et al (2002) The new liver allocation system: moving toward evidence-based transplantation policy. Liver Transpl 8:851–858

19. Ioannou GN, Perkins JD, Carithers RL, Jr (2008) Liver transplantation for hepatocellular carcinoma: impact of the MELD allocation system and predictors of survival. Gastroenterology 134:1342–1351

20. Poon RT, Fan ST, Lo CM, Liu CL, Wong J (2007) Difference in tumor invasiveness in cirrhotic patients with hepatocellular carcinoma fulfilling the Milan criteria treated by resection and transplantation: impact on long-term survival. Ann Surg 245:51–58

21. Bigourdan JM, Jaeck D, Meyer N et al (2003) Small hepatocellular carcinoma in Child A cirrhotic patients: hepatic resection versus transplantation. Liver Transpl 9: 513–520

22. Duffy JP, Vardanian A, Benjamin E et al (2007) Liver transplantation criteria for hepatocellular carcinoma should be expanded: a 22-year experience with 467 patients at UCLA. Ann Surg 246:502–511

23. Forner A, Vilana R, Ayuso C et al (2008) Diagnosis of hepatic nodules 20 mm or smaller in cirrhosis: Prospective validation of the noninvasive diagnostic criteria for hepatocellular carcinoma. Hepatology 47:97–104

24. Louha M, Nicolet J, Zylberberg H et al (1999) Liver resection and needle liver biopsy cause hematogenous dissemination of liver cells. Hepatology 29:879–882

25. Stigliano R, Burroughs AK (2005) Should we biopsy each liver mass suspicious for HCC before liver transplantation?–no, please don't. J Hepatol 43:563–568

26. Llovet JM, Fuster J, Bruix J (2004) The Barcelona approach: diagnosis, staging, and treatment of hepatocellular carcinoma. Liver Transpl 10(2 Suppl 1):S115–S120

27. Llovet JM, Di Bisceglie AM, Bruix J et al (2008) Design and endpoints of clinical trials in hepatocellular carcinoma. JNCI 100:698–711

28. Kaihara S, Kiuchi T, Ueda M et al (2003) Living-donor liver transplantation for hepatocellular carcinoma. Transplantation 75(3 Suppl):S37–S40

29. Ravaioli M, Grazi GL, Piscaglia F et al (2008) Liver transplantation for hepatocellular carcinoma: results of down-staging in patients initially outside the Milan selection criteria. Am J Transplant 8:2547–2557

30. Herrero JI, Sangro B, Quiroga J et al (2001) Influence of tumor characteristics on the outcome of liver transplantation among patients with liver cirrhosis and hepatocellular carcinoma. Liver Transpl 7:631–636

31. Yao FY, Kerlan RK, Jr, Hirose R et al (2008) Excellent outcome following down-staging of hepatocellular carcinoma prior to liver transplantation: an intention-to-treat analysis. Hepatology 48:819–827

32. Decaens T, Roudot-Thoraval F, Hadni-Bresson S et al (2006) Impact of UCSF criteria according to pre- and post-OLT tumor features: analysis of 479 patients listed for HCC with a short waiting time. Liver Transpl 12:1761–1769

33. Ravaioli M, Ercolani G, Cescon M et al (2004) Liver transplantation for hepatocellular carcinoma: further considerations on selection criteria. Liver Transpl 10:1195–1202

34. Yang SH, Suh KS, Lee HW et al (2007) A revised scoring system utilizing serum alphafetoprotein levels to expand candidates for living donor transplantation in hepatocellular carcinoma. Surgery 141:598–609

35. Marsh JW, Dvorchik I, Subotin M et al (1997) The prediction of risk of recurrence and time to recurrence of hepatocellular carcinoma after orthotopic liver transplantation: a pilot study. Hepatology 26:444–450

36. Schwartz M (2004) Liver transplantation for hepatocellular carcinoma. Gastroenterology 127(5 Suppl 1):S268–S276

37. Fisher RA, Maluf D, Cotterell AH et al (2004) Non-resective ablation therapy for hepatocellular carcinoma: effectiveness measured by intention-to-treat and dropout from liver transplant waiting list. Clin Transplant 18:502–512

38. Cillo U, Vitale A, Bassanello M et al (2004) Liver transplantation for the treatment of moderately or well-differentiated hepatocellular carcinoma. Ann Surg 239:150–159

39. Todo S, Furukawa H (2004) Living donor liver transplantation for adult patients with hepatocellular carcinoma: experience in Japan. Ann Surg 240:451–461

40. Yao FY, Bass NM, Nikolai B et al (2003) A follow-up analysis of the pattern and predictors of dropout from the waiting list for liver transplantation in patients with hepatocellular carcinoma: implications for the current organ allocation policy. Liver Transpl 9:684–692

41. Maddala YK, Stadheim L, Andrews JC et al (2004) Drop-out rates of patients with hepatocellular cancer listed for liver transplantation: outcome with chemoembolization. Liver Transpl 10:449–455

42. Porrett PM, Peterman H, Rosen M et al (2006) Lack of benefit of pre-transplant locoregional hepatic therapy for hepatocellular cancer in the current MELD era. Liver Transpl 12:665–673

43. Oldhafer KJ, Chavan A, Fruhauf NR et al (1998) Arterial chemoembolization before liver transplantation in patients with hepatocellular carcinoma: marked tumor necrosis, but no survival benefit? J Hepatol 29:953–959

44. Decaens T, Roudot-Thoraval F, Bresson-Hadni S et al (2005) Impact of pretransplantation transarterial chemoembolization on survival and recurrence after liver transplantation for hepatocellular carcinoma. Liver Transpl 11:767–775

45. Roayaie S, Frischer JS, Emre SH et al (2002) Long-term results with multimodal adjuvant therapy and liver transplantation for the treatment of hepatocellular carcinomas larger than 5 centimeters. Ann Surg 235:533–539

46. Graziadei IW, Sandmueller H, Waldenberger P et al (2003) Chemoembolization followed by liver transplantation for hepatocellular carcinoma impedes tumor progression while on the waiting list and leads to excellent outcome. Liver Transpl 9:557–563

47. Hayashi PH, Ludkowski M, Forman LM et al (2004) Hepatic artery chemoembolization for hepatocellular carcinoma in patients listed for liver transplantation. Am J Transpl 4:782–787

48. Varela M, Real MI, Burrel M et al (2007) Chemoembolization of hepatocellular carcinoma with drug eluting beads: efficacy and doxorubicin pharmacokinetics. J Hepatol 46:474–481

49. Llovet JM, Bruix J (2003) Systematic review of randomized trials for unresectable hepatocellular carcinoma: Chemoembolization improves survival. Hepatology 37:429–442

50. Lesurtel M, Mullhaupt B, Pestalozzi BC, Pfammatter T, Clavien PA (2006) Transarterial chemoembolization as a bridge to liver transplantation for hepatocellular carcinoma: an evidence-based analysis. Am J Transplant 6:2644–2650

51. Aloia TA, Fahy BN (2008) A decision analysis model predicts the optimal treatment pathway for patients with colorectal cancer and resectable synchronous liver metastases. Clin Colorectal Cancer 7:197–201
52. Lu DS, Yu NC, Raman SS et al (2005) Percutaneous radiofrequency ablation of hepatocellular carcinoma as a bridge to liver transplantation. Hepatology 41:1130–1137
53. Lu DS, Yu NC, Raman SS et al (2005) Radiofrequency ablation of hepatocellular carcinoma: treatment success as defined by histologic examination of the explanted liver. Radiology 234:954–960
54. Mazzaferro V, Battiston C, Perrone S et al (2004) Radiofrequency ablation of small hepatocellular carcinoma in cirrhotic patients awaiting liver transplantation: a prospective study. Ann Surg 240:900–909
55. Salem R, Thurston KG (2006) Radioembolization with yttrium-90 microspheres: a state-of-the-art brachytherapy treatment for primary and secondary liver malignancies: part 3: comprehensive literature review and future direction. J Vasc Interv Radiol 17:1571–1593
56. Kulik LM, Atassi B, van Holsbeeck L et al (2006) Yttrium-90 microspheres (TheraSphere) treatment of unresectable hepatocellular carcinoma: downstaging to resection, RFA and bridge to transplantation. J Surg Oncol 94:572–586
57. Riaz A, Kulik L, Lewandowski RJ et al (2009) Radiologic-pathologic correlation of hepatocellular carcinoma treated with internal radiation using yttrium-90 microspheres. Hepatology 49:1185–1193
58. Lo CM, Liu CL, Chan SC et al (2007) A randomized, controlled trial of postoperative adjuvant interferon therapy after resection of hepatocellular carcinoma. Ann Surg 245:831–842
59. Simonetti RG, Liberati A, Angiolini C, Pagliaro L (1997) Treatment of hepatocellular carcinoma: a systematic review of randomized controlled trials. Ann Oncol 8:117–136
60. Abou-Alfa GK, Schwartz L, Ricci S et al (2006) Phase II study of sorafenib in patients with advanced hepatocellular carcinoma. J Clin Oncol 24:4293–4300
61. Llovet JM, Ricci S, Mazzaferro V et al (2008) Sorafenib in advanced hepatocellular carcinoma. N Engl J Med 359:378–390
62. Llovet JM, Bruix J (2008) Molecular targeted therapies in hepatocellular carcinoma. Hepatology 48:1312–1327
63. Fernandez JA, Robles R, Marin C et al (2003) Can we expand the indications for liver transplantation among hepatocellular carcinoma patients with increased tumor size? Transplant Proc 35:1818–1820
64. Leung JY, Zhu AX, Gordon FD et al (2004) Liver transplantation outcomes for early-stage hepatocellular carcinoma: results of a multicenter study. Liver Transpl 10:1343–1354
65. Yao FY, Ferrell L, Bass NM, Bacchetti P, Ascher NL, Roberts JP (2002) Liver transplantation for hepatocellular carcinoma: comparison of the proposed UCSF criteria with the Milan criteria and the Pittsburgh modified TNM criteria. Liver Transpl 8:765–774
66. Mazzaferro V, Llovet JM, Miceli R et al (2009) Predicting survival after liver transplantation in patients with hepatocellular carcinoma beyond the Milan criteria: a retrospective, exploratory analysis. Lancet Oncol 10:35–43
67. Majno PE, Adam R, Bismuth H et al (1997) Influence of preoperative transarterial lipiodol chemoembolization on resection and transplantation for hepatocellular carcinoma in patients with cirrhosis. Ann Surg 226:688–701
68. Yao FY, Hirose R, LaBerge JM et al (2005) A prospective study on downstaging of hepatocellular carcinoma prior to liver transplantation. Liver Transpl 11:1505–1514
69. Llovet JM, Schwartz M, Fuster J, Bruix J (2006) Expanded criteria for hepatocellular carcinoma through down-staging prior to liver transplantation: not yet there. Semin Liver Dis 26:248–253
70. Belghiti J, Cortes A, Abdalla EK et al (2003) Resection prior to liver transplantation for hepatocellular carcinoma. Ann Surg 238:885–893
71. Fong Y, Sun RL, Jarnagin W, Blumgart LH (1999) An analysis of 412 cases of hepatocellular carcinoma at a Western center. Ann Surg 229:790–800

72. Ercolani G, Grazi GL, Ravaioli M et al (2003) Liver resection for hepatocellular carcinoma on cirrhosis: univariate and multivariate analysis of risk factors for intrahepatic recurrence. Ann Surg 237:536–543
73. Adam R, Azoulay D, Castaing D et al (2003) Liver resection as a bridge to transplantation for hepatocellular carcinoma on cirrhosis: a reasonable strategy? Ann Surg 238:508–519
74. Kulik L, Abecassis M (2004) Living donor liver transplantation for hepatocellular carcinoma. Gastroenterology 127(5 Suppl 1):S277–S282
75. Fisher RA, Kulik LM, Freise CE et al (2007) Hepatocellular carcinoma recurrence and death following living and deceased donor liver transplantation. Am J Transplant 7: 1601–1608
76. Thuluvath PJ, Yoo HY (2004) Graft and patient survival after adult live donor liver transplantation compared to a matched cohort who received a deceased donor transplantation. Liver Transpl 10:1263–1238
77. Hwang S, Lee SG, Joh JW, Suh KS, Kim DG (2005) Liver transplantation for adult patients with hepatocellular carcinoma in Korea: comparison between cadaveric donor and living donor liver transplantations. Liver Transpl 11:1265–1272
78. Lo CM, Fan ST, Liu CL, Chan SC, Wong J (2004) The role and limitation of living donor liver transplantation for hepatocellular carcinoma. Liver Transpl 10:440–447
79. Sarasin FP, Majno PE, Llovet JM, Bruix J, Mentha G, Hadengue A (2001) Living donor liver transplantation for early hepatocellular carcinoma: A life-expectancy and cost-effectiveness perspective. Hepatology 33:1073–1079
80. Zavaglia C, De Carlis L, Alberti AB et al (2005) Predictors of long-term survival after liver transplantation for hepatocellular carcinoma. Am J Gastroenterol 100:2708–2716
81. Margarit C, Charco R, Hidalgo E, Allende H, Castells L, Bilbao I (2002) Liver transplantation for malignant diseases: selection and pattern of recurrence. World J Surg 26:257–263
82. Schlitt HJ, Neipp M, Weimann A et al (1999) Recurrence patterns of hepatocellular and fibrolamellar carcinoma after liver transplantation. J Clin Oncol 17:324–331
83. Shimoda M, Ghobrial RM, Carmody IC et al (2004) Predictors of survival after liver transplantation for hepatocellular carcinoma associated with Hepatitis C. Liver Transpl 10:1478–1486
84. Thuluvath PJ, Maheshwari A, Thuluvath NP, Nguyen GC, Segev DL (2009) Survival after liver transplantation for hepatocellular carcinoma in the model for end-stage liver disease and pre-model for end-stage liver disease eras and the independent impact of hepatitis C virus. Liver Transpl 15:754–762
85. Klintmalm GB (1998) Liver transplantation for hepatocellular carcinoma: a registry report of the impact of tumor characteristics on outcome. Ann Surg 228:479–490
86. Pawlik TM, Delman KA, Vauthey JN et al (2005) Tumor size predicts vascular invasion and histologic grade: Implications for selection of surgical treatment for hepatocellular carcinoma. Liver Transpl 11:1086–1092
87. Esnaola NF, Lauwers GY, Mirza NQ et al (2002) Predictors of microvascular invasion in patients with hepatocellular carcinoma who are candidates for orthotopic liver transplantation. J Gastrointest Surg 6:224–232
88. Busuttil RW, Farmer DG, Yersiz H et al (2005) Analysis of long-term outcomes of 3200 liver transplantations over two decades: a single-center experience. Ann Surg 241:905–918
89. Vivarelli M, Bellusci R, Cucchetti A et al (2002) Low recurrence rate of hepatocellular carcinoma after liver transplantation: better patient selection or lower immunosuppression? Transplantation 74:1746–1751
90. Vivarelli M, Cucchetti A, Piscaglia F et al (2005) Analysis of risk factors for tumor recurrence after liver transplantation for hepatocellular carcinoma: key role of immunosuppression. Liver Transpl 11:497–503
91. Guba M, von Breitenbuch P, Steinbauer M et al (2002) Rapamycin inhibits primary and metastatic tumor growth by antiangiogenesis: involvement of vascular endothelial growth factor. Nat Med 8:128–135

92. Aloia TA, Goss JA (2009) A report of outcomes after orthotopic liver transplant with allografts from heparin antibody-positive donors. Exp Clin Transplant 7:13–17
93. Guba M, Steinbauer M, Ruhland V et al (2002) Elevated MIA serum levels are predictors of poor prognosis after surgical resection of metastatic malignant melanoma. Oncol Reports 9:981–984
94. Schumacher G, Oidtmann M, Rosewicz S et al (2002) Sirolimus inhibits growth of human hepatoma cells in contrast to tacrolimus which promotes cell growth. Transplant Proc 34:1392–1393
95. Kneteman NM, Oberholzer J, Al Saghier M et al (2004) Sirolimus-based immunosuppression for liver transplantation in the presence of extended criteria for hepatocellular carcinoma. Liver Transpl 10:1301–1311
96. Marsh JW, Finkelstein SD, Demetris AJ et al (2003) Genotyping of hepatocellular carcinoma in liver transplant recipients adds predictive power for determining recurrence-free survival. Liver Transpl 9:664–671
97. UNOS/OPTN policy 3.6.4.4. http://www.optn.org. Accessed November 2009

Chapter 15
Vascular Resection for Hepatocellular Carcinoma

Robin D. Kim and Alan W. Hemming

Keywords Vascular resection · Vascular reconstruction · HCC · Intraoperative strategies for hepatic/vascular resections · *Ante situm* procedure

Introduction

Liver surgery has progressed over the last two decades to become a distinct area of specialization. Strategies such as portal vein embolization (Chapter 11) to induce growth of the planned liver remnant permit more aggressive resections, and improved imaging allows the surgeon to assess tumor position in relation to the intrahepatic vasculature. Liver transplantation has also progressed, but has been limited by the shortage of cadaveric donors. The development of live donor liver transplantation in response to this organ shortage has, in turn, led to techniques that can also be applied in non-transplant liver surgery. Resection and reconstruction of portal vein, hepatic artery, bile duct, and hepatic veins, all standard components of live donor liver transplantation, can be used in resecting complex HCC lesions by surgeons experienced in techniques developed for both liver resection and transplantation. Vascular resection and reconstruction is utilized to both achieve adequate oncologic tumor clearance and also preserve uninvolved hepatic parenchyma when vascular inflow or outflow is involved. In this chapter, we examine the role and techniques of vascular resection and reconstruction for HCC.

A.W. Hemming (✉)
Division of Transplantation and Hepatobiliary Surgery, Department of Surgery, University of California, San Diego, CA, USA

K.M. McMasters, J.-N. Vauthey (eds.), *Hepatocellular Carcinoma*,
DOI 10.1007/978-1-60327-522-4_15, © Springer Science+Business Media, LLC 2011

The Pathophysiology of Vascular Invasion in HCC

Vascular invasion is an important characteristic of HCC as not only may it require vascular resection/reconstruction, but it is also a significant predictor of recurrence following resection [1, 2]. In one series of 322 patients who underwent curative resection for HCC, macroscopic vascular invasion (that which is visible on gross section) and microscopic vascular invasion (that which is detected at histology) were detected in 15.5% and 59.0%, respectively [2]. The pathophysiology of vascular invasion has been elucidated by histologic studies of early cases. Immunohistochemistry studies of tumors using CD31, a marker for endothelial cells, show that in most cases invasion begins when tumor nests surrounded by sinusoidal vessels extend into the portal and hepatic veins. These endothelial-coated tumor emboli enter the circulation, adhere to local tributaries and proliferate, and can embolize to distant sites once entering the systemic circulation [3]. This mechanism is invasion independent as it does not depend on the invasive activity of tumor cells but rather a relationship with endothelial progenitors [4]. This intravasation of tumor nests by tumor vessels explains the shunting seen in the arterial phase of CT scans, as the contrast that is delivered arterially is shunted to neighboring hepatic or portal veins through a well-vascularized tumor (Fig. 15.1).

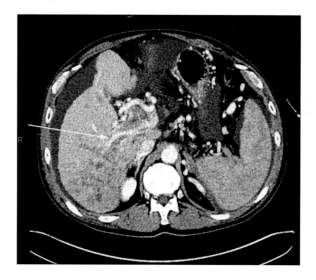

Fig. 15.1 Arterial phase CT demonstrating arterial flow within the portal vein, indicating vascularized tumor within the portal vein

Hepatocellular cancer invades either portal or hepatic veins by local extension through the above mechanism, ultimately occluding and expanding the vascular space. In portal vein invasion, tumor cells may disseminate into distal branches resulting in intrahepatic metastases. This event is responsible for the tumor satellitosis that accompanies a dominant tumor within the same segment. Others have used radiopaque injection of tumors to confirm that the portal vein may act as an efferent vessel in the setting of portal hypertension, thus explaining the tumor emboli found in the rectal veins and esophageal varices in autopsy studies [3, 5]. One large series of 1023 patients who underwent resections for HCC found macroscopic portal vein tumor thrombus in 54 patients (5.4%) [6]. In hepatic vein invasion, the tumor may grow and extend into the inferior vena cava and the right atrium, and when large may create an arterio-venous shunt bypassing the sinusoidal filter. Tumor dissemination from hepatic vein invasion is significant when cells are released as multicellular tumor nests with preserved cell–cell and cell–matrix interactions [7]. Unlike single cells, these clusters can survive anoikis, mechanical disruption, and host defenses to metastasize distant sites such as the lungs [8].

Some of the risk factors of vascular invasion in HCC include tumor size [2, 9, 10], tumor number, [9, 11], histologic grade [9, 10, 12], and elevated alpha-fetoprotein level [2, 11]. It is essential to understand the pathophysiology that accompanies the need for vascular resection in HCC and weigh the risk of recurrence against the increased technical demands and risks of any proposed procedure.

Evaluation and Work-Up of the Patient with HCC for Resection

Underlying Liver Disease in the Patient with HCC

A careful assessment of the patients underlying liver function is needed to determine the operative risk liver failure and death following resection for HCC (Chapter 9). In general, Child–Pugh class C is a contraindication to resection, and early class B patients without portal hypertension may undergo minor resections from wedge resection to a single segmentectomy. Child–Pugh class A patients that are considered for major hepatectomy (resection of four or more segments) should undergo assessment of both liver and physiologic status [13, 14]. In addition, strategies such as pre-operative portal vein embolization (PVE) to increase the future liver remnant (FLR) have been associated with decreased complications and extended surgical options for HCC patients (Chapter 11) [15–18].

Other risk factors are associated with liver failure and death following resection of HCC. Portal hypertension (PH) is a contraindication to liver resection as it has been associated with increased morbidity and mortality following major resection [19]. PH is defined as a hepatic vein pressure gradient (HVPG) greater than 10 mm Hg, and some associated signs include esophageal varices, anatomic portosystemic shunts, and ascites [20]. Thrombocytopenia with platelet counts <100,000 cells/mm^2 has been associated with portal hypertension and an increased in-hospital mortality following liver resection [13]. There are occasional cases in which portal hypertension exists in the setting of a non-cirrhotic liver secondary to either partial portal vein or hepatic vein occlusion by tumor. In rare instances resection can be considered in these situations if the surgeon is convinced that the underlying liver is non-cirrhotic with the assumption that portal pressures and liver function will improve after resection and the mechanical problem caused by tumor obstruction is relieved. Active viral hepatitis is another risk factor for liver failure and death following HCC resection and is suggested by serum alanine aminotransferase levels (fourfold in one series) [21, 22].

For major hepatectomies that involve vascular resection, particularly of the hepatic veins and inferior vena cava (IVC), it will be the rare patient that has any significant degree of cirrhosis that would be considered for resection. Cirrhotic patients with portal vein involvement requiring tumor thrombectomy or portal vein resection that otherwise meet standard resection criteria can be considered for resection.

Pre-operative Imaging

Pre-operative imaging is required to stage the tumor, to assess its position in relation to hepatic vasculature, and to plan the liver resection to achieve an R0 resection while preserving adequate liver remnant. Accurate imaging of the intrahepatic architecture enhanced with three-dimensional reconstruction is important to assess the possible need for vascular reconstruction. For example, imaging may clarify the venous anatomy in the setting where a tumor in segment 7 or 8 requires sacrifice of the main right hepatic vein and yet segment 6 requires preservation. Accurate imaging may indicate the need for or obviate vascular reconstruction such as a large inferior hepatic vein draining segment 6 that makes reconstruction of the main right hepatic vein unnecessary. Alternatively, anatomy may be discovered that requires vascular reconstruction such as a large segment 6 tributary to the middle hepatic vein that would require reconstruction in an extended left hepatectomy [23].

Triphasic spiral computed tomography (CT) of the liver with concurrent assessment of the chest is the most widely used modality for planning surgery and staging for HCC. The classic appearance of a lesion hyper-enhancing on the arterial phase with subsequent hypo-enhancement ("washout") in the portal venous phase in the setting of underlying liver disease is diagnostic, with some variability depending on size, location, and level of fat or fibrosis of the surrounding liver. In addition, gross vascular invasion can be visualized by local extension and expansion of tumor thrombus in a hepatic or portal vein from the tumor and by the shunting of contrast through the thrombus during the arterial phase (Fig. 15.1). Despite its popularity, CT is limited in detecting macroscopic vascular invasion as the findings may be subtle. One group has reported that CT scan detected 68% of portal vein thrombi associated with HCC and correctly characterized 68% as malignant following pathologic examination [24].

Magnetic resonance imaging (MRI) with gadolinium for MR angiography and venography may further demonstrate the hepatic veins, particularly when all three are involved resulting in outflow obstruction that prevents adequate flow of contrast into the hepatic veins during CT. In addition, MRI with agents such as supermagnetic iron oxide has been shown to detect even microvascular invasion with sensitivity, specificity, and accuracy rates of 82, 84, and 86%, respectively [25].

Three-dimensional reconstruction of axial images and volumetric assessment of the total and planned liver remnant have been found to be more accurate than axial imaging before liver resection [26, 27]. These imaging techniques coupled with computer-aided functional remnant predictions, based on not only spared liver parenchyma but also simulated inflow/outflow changes, have been shown to not only alter surgery extent but also the need for vascular reconstruction [28]. Although a remnant liver volume of 25% after resection is generally adequate in the uninjured liver, extended liver resections for HCC generally occur in the setting of compromised liver due to fibrosis. If the FLR is projected to be less that 40%, pre-operative PVE can be used to increase the size of the liver remnant. In addition, with vascular reconstruction and the possible use of cold perfusion the liver receives an additional ischemic injury beyond that of standard liver resection. We have arbitrarily chosen to use PVE in any patient requiring major hepatectomy with vascular reconstruction who has an FLR <40% even in the setting of normal hepatic parenchyma. The lack of adequate growth following PVE is a sign of severe liver injury and inadequate regenerative capacity which precludes extended resection [17].

Intraoperative Strategies for Hepatic/Vascular Resections

Both low central venous pressure (CVP) and inflow occlusion (Pringle maneuver) are strategies used in standard liver resections to minimize blood loss [29]. Low central venous pressure (CVP <6 mm Hg) can be achieved by positioning the patient in reverse Trendelenburg position [30], fluid restriction, diuresis and vasodilators. Low CVP during parenchymal transection decreases back-bleeding from the hepatic veins and their tributaries and is useful when extensive dissection of the hepatic veins is needed in preparation for vascular resection.

Inflow occlusion (Pringle maneuver) decreases blood loss during liver transection and is achieved by occluding the hepatic artery and portal vein using a large atraumatic vascular clamp or tourniquet. Although normal livers can tolerate up to 60 min of continuous inflow occlusion/warm ischemia [31], injured livers (from cirrhosis, biliary obstruction, or chemotherapy) tolerate significantly less ischemia before irreversible injury ensues [32]. Intermittent inflow occlusion for 15 min with 5 min breaks has been suggested to reduce liver injury [33] and may be used in complex resections in which the parenchymal transection may be prolonged or when hepatic venous reconstruction are required at the completion of the liver transection. Despite these efforts, these complex cases are particularly at risk for ischemic injury as they are associated with underlying liver injury, greater blood loss at surgery, and longer periods of ischemia during vascular resection/reconstructions.

Ischemic preconditioning (IP) has been suggested by some to protect the liver from subsequent ischemic injury [34]. Ischemic preconditioning is performed by applying the Pringle maneuver for 10 min and then reperfusing the liver for at least 10 min prior to reapplying inflow occlusion for the liver transection. The mechanisms by which ischemic preconditioning protects the liver include the upregulation of the protective signals such as IL-6 and STAT3, alterations in energy metabolism, and abrogation of injurious events such as neutrophil accumulation, microcirculatory disturbance, and reactive oxygen species, and proinflammatory mediators [35]. The benefits of IP for liver resections have not been found consistently. A recent meta-analysis has shown that in non-cirrhotic patients, IP before liver resection was associated with a decrease in blood transfusions but did not change mortality, liver failure, morbidity, or length of stay [36]. Although we use both the Pringle maneuver (15 min on, 5 min off) and ischemic preconditioning when necessary, our standard practice is to use no inflow occlusion at all during the hepatic parenchymal transection phase of the procedure if vascular reconstruction is planned. Ideally the hepatic transection is done preserving perfusion to the remnant liver until the time that blood flow must be interrupted to resect and reconstruct the involved vessel. This minimizes the ischemic time and reduces liver injury.

Technical Considerations for Hepatic Resection with Vascular Reconstruction and Published Experience

Lesions Involving the Hilar Vessels

Tumors of all types may involve the hilar vessels by extrinsic compression, and in the case of adenocarcinomas may invade from the outside. Hepatocellular cancer behaves in a different fashion. Although HCC may cause extrinsic compression due to size, this process rarely leads to invasion of the vessel wall. Instead, HCC has a propensity to invade nearby portal veins by extending tumor thrombi into sinusoids, then into the portal vein branch lumen itself, and this thrombus may extend to the ipsilateral, then main and contralateral portal veins.

Generally, the hilar vessels are addressed after liver mobilization and ultrasonography and before parenchymal transection to minimize blood loss. When pre-operative and intraoperative imaging rule out tumor thrombus in the case of extrinsic compression, the portal vein can be separated from the compressed hepatic parenchyma surrounding the tumor and still obtain adequate though small margins. However, when a tumor thrombus involves the main trunk of the right or left portal vein or extends down into the main portal vein or across to the contralateral portal vein, then proximal and distal control must be achieved without amputating the thrombus and creating a tumor embolus. The main and contralateral portal veins are dissected out well beyond tumor to prevent amputation and embolization of tumor at the time of clamp placement. The ipsilateral portal vein can be transected and the tumor thrombus extracted in most cases. The proximal and distal remnant portal veins are then flushed, and the ipsilateral stump closed. In cases where the tumor is adherent to the vein wall, the section of portal vein can be resected and in general a primary end-to-end anastomosis performed between the main portal vein to right or left branch (Fig. 15.2a–c). Up to 2 cm of vein can be resected without the use of a graft. Blood flow to the liver is maintained through the hepatic artery, and the portal vein clamp time is short. Although portal vein resections and reconstructions

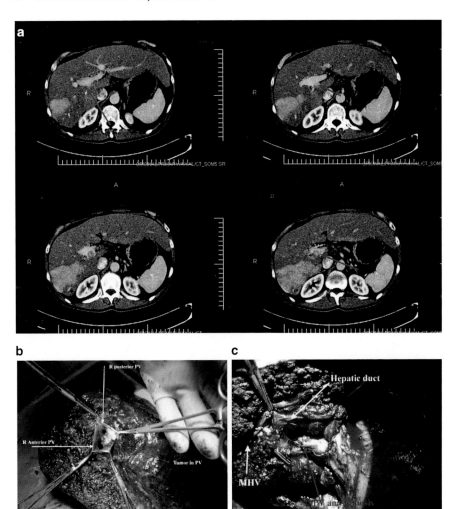

Fig. 15.2 (a) Hepatocellular carcinoma (HCC) extending from the posterior branch of the right portal vein into the main right portal vein and into the main portal vein. (b) Resection specimen demonstrating tumor extending down from the posterior branch of the portal vein (PV) to the main right portal vein with tumor adherence to the vein wall. (c) Patient side of Fig. 15.2b with the left portal vein anastomosed to the main portal vein. The left hepatic duct and bile duct have been elevated and rotated to the left to provide access to the portal vein but do not require division. MHV = middle hepatic vein

have been described for HCC tumor thrombi, they are rarely necessary and offer no survival advantage to thrombectomy as described above as long as the whole thrombus is extracted [6]. If thrombectomy alone can be achieved with no residual tumor on the vein wall then resection can be avoided. In the rare case that both hepatic artery and portal vein require reconstruction they can be performed alternately, maintaining flow through one vessel while reconstructing the other.

Hepatic Vein and IVC Involvement

Similar to their effects on hilar vessels, large HCC lesions involving the hepatic veins or retrohepatic vena cava by external compression rarely invade the vessels walls. However, hepatic veins are more likely to require resection and reconstruction since they are thin walled and lack the protective Glissonian extensions that envelop hilar vessels. In addition, tumors centrally involving hepatic veins that also drain peripheral uninvolved segments may need reconstruction in order to maintain outflow in parenchyma preserving resections. One example is the reconstruction of a right hepatic vein in order to resect a tumor in segments 7 and 8 while preserving the outflow to segment 6 (Fig. 15.3a, b).

a   **b**

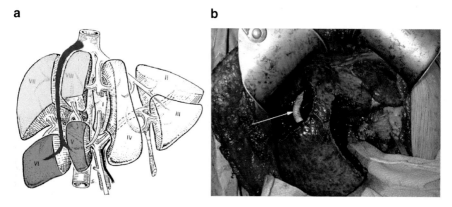

Fig. 15.3 (**a**) Resection of tumor in segment 7 or 8 may require sacrifice of the right hepatic vein and preservation of venous outflow to segment 6 by reconstructing the right hepatic vein may be required if significant alternative venous outflow does not exist. (**b**) Resection of segment 7, part of 8 and 5 for HCC in a cirrhotic liver. The right hepatic vein has been reconstructed using 8 mm ringed Gortex since no inferior hepatic vein was present. Notice the significant volume of liver that segment 6 represents in this case

Hepatocellular cancer may also cause tumor thrombi in the hepatic veins in 11–23% (Fig. 15.4a–c) [37, 38], the IVC in 9–26% [37–39], and further extend into the right atrium in 2.4% to 6.3% of cases [37, 38, 40]. Although rare, there have been 87 case reports of HCC with intracavitary cardiac involvement [39]. In these extreme cases, complications may include heart failure, tricuspid stenosis or insufficiency, ventricular outflow tract obstruction, ball valve thrombus syndrome, sudden cardiac death, secondary Budd–Chiari syndrome, pulmonary embolism, and pulmonary metastasis [39]. We have in rare cases resected HCC with extension of tumor into the right atrium under cardiopulmonary bypass with hypothermic arrest. This is obviously an extreme measure that really cannot be considered curative although it is life prolonging in some cases.

There are a number of options for reconstructing the resected vasculature. Hepatic veins can be reconstructed using autologous vein graft from such sites as the

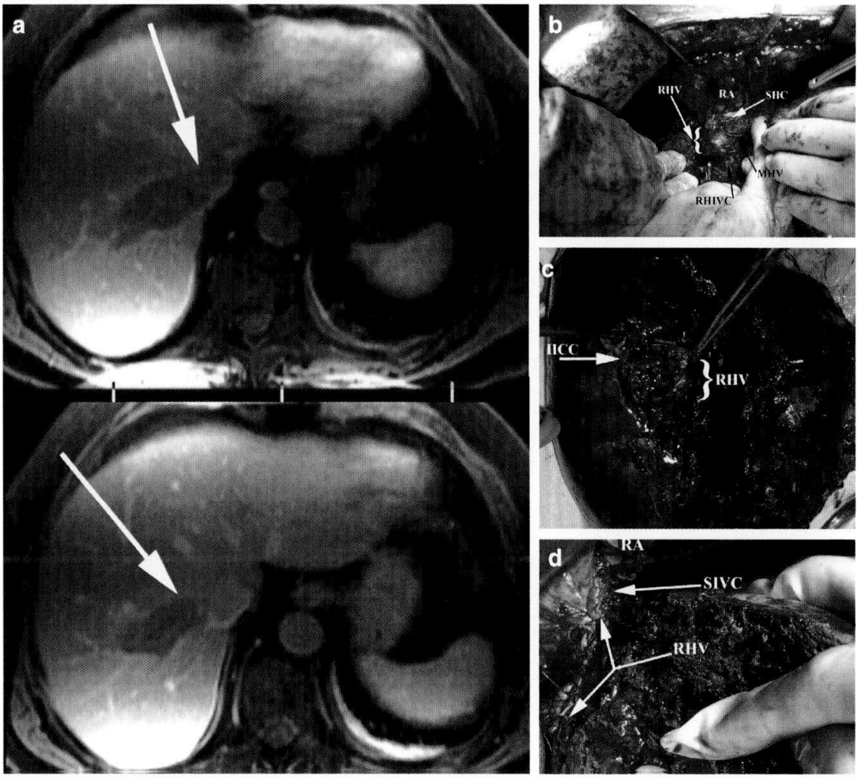

Fig. 15.4 (**a**) MR imaging of HCC with tumor thrombus in the right hepatic vein extending into the IVC. (**b**) Intraoperative picture of resection of patient in Fig. 15.4a. The liver has been divided centrally back to the retrohepatic inferior vena cava (RHIVC). The suprahepatic cava (SHC) has been controlled above the tumor extension by opening the pericardium from below and encircling the intrapericardial inferior vena cava at its junction with the right atrium(RA). The middle hepatic vein (MHV) has been divided at its origin using a vascular stapler. Notice the right hepatic vein (RHV) is distended and is enlarged much more than usual. (**c**) The resection specimen from 4b. Notice the right hepatic vein (RHV) is filled with loosely adherent tumor (HCC) and that the right hepatic vein orifice has been distended with tumor. (**d**) The completed resection from 4b. The right hepatic vein (RHV) orifice was enlarged further at the time of tumor removal and extended down the IVC requiring closure and tangential repair of the inferior vena cava. SIVC = suprahepatic inferior vena cava, RA = right atrium

saphenous, left renal, or gonadal veins [41, 42]. For longer reconstructions of hepatic veins cadaveric vein grafts may be used. For broad defects of the IVC, cadaveric vein or bovine pericardium patches may be used [43]. Replacement of the IVC has been described using woven Dacron [44]; however, expanded PTFE [45–48] has become the synthetic graft of choice (Fig. 15.5a–c).

A number of recent case series have been published regarding combined liver and hepatic vein/vena cava resections for HCC. The number of cases ranged from 2 to 29 per report, with a total of 59 patients who underwent resections of the IVC. More

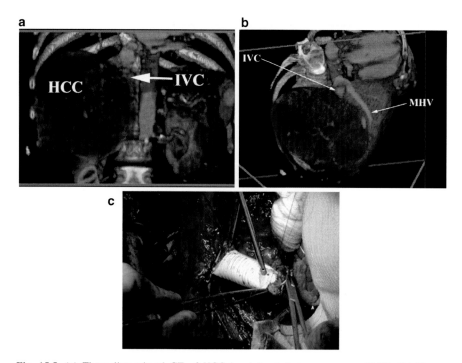

Fig. 15.5 (a) Three-dimensional CT of HCC involving inferior vena cava (IVC). (b) Three-dimensional CT of HCC from Fig. 15.5a that demonstrates that there is enough space below the hepatic veins to allow clamp placement on the inferior vena cava (IVC) but maintain outflow through the hepatic veins during caval flow interruption. (c) Ringed Gortex graft being sewn in place in patient from Fig. 15.5b. Notice that the right lobe (plus middle vein) has been removed from the field with caval clamps placed below the left hepatic vein, allowing continued perfusion of the remnant liver while replacing the IVC. In this case the tumor was not truly invading the IVC wall but could not be separated from the IVC with risk of either tearing the IVC or rupturing the tumor

recent data suggest that HCC involving the hepatic veins or IVC rarely requires vascular resections to achieve complete tumor thrombectomy [49]. However, tumors centrally involving hepatic veins that also drain peripheral uninvolved segments may need reconstruction in order to maintain outflow in parenchyma preserving resections.

Strategies to Achieve Vascular Control During Complex HCC Resections

Total Vascular Isolation

Tumors involving the retrohepatic IVC or the hepatic veins as they enter the IVC require a variety of techniques to establish inflow and outflow control to minimize blood loss. In total vascular isolation, control of the portal hepatic (inflow) and the suprahepatic and infrahepatic IVC (outflow) is established to minimize bleeding from the hepatic artery, portal vein, and hepatic veins. Some evidence suggests that hepatic venous back-diffusion may minimize ischemic injury and that total vascular isolation increases the degree of ischemic liver injury [50]. However, the majority of the hepatic parenchymal division can usually be performed without total vascular isolation, and IVC clamping can be reserved for the relatively short time period that is required to resect and reconstruct the inferior vena cava or hepatic veins. In one series of five patients with HCC extending into the IVC which required combined liver and IVC resections, total vascular isolation was used with ischemic times ranging from 40 to 90 min, the IVC exclusion time ranged from 25 to 90 min, and the average blood loss was $6,500 \pm 1,732$ mL [43].

For total vascular isolation as much mobilization of the liver off of the vena cava is performed as possible without encroaching on tumor planes prior to hepatic parenchymal transection. In some cases, however, the bulky nature of the tumor inhibits the ability to rotate the liver safely and a primary anterior approach to the IVC can be taken with little or no mobilization of the liver off of the IVC.

The approach to vena caval resection depends on the extent and location of tumor involvement. If the portion of vena cava involved with tumor is below the hepatic veins then the parenchyma of the liver can be divided exposing the retro-hepatic IVC. The parenchymal transection can be performed with inflow occlusion (Pringle maneuver); however, if possible the parenchymal division is done maintaining hepatic perfusion. Central venous pressure is kept at or below 5 cm H_2O during parenchymal transection to minimize blood loss. Once the IVC is exposed, portal inflow occlusion is released if utilized, the patient volume loaded, and clamps placed above and below the area of tumor involvement. The portion of liver and involved IVC is then removed allowing improved access for reconstruction of the IVC. The placing of clamps on the IVC below the hepatic veins allows continued perfusion of the liver and minimizes the hepatic ischemic time.

In cases where tumor involvement does not allow placement of clamps below the hepatic veins there were two different approaches. If there is only IVC and/or hepatic vein involvement the hepatic parenchyma can be divided back to the IVC, the patient volume loaded and then clamps are placed sequentially on the infrahepatic IVC, the porta hepatis and then above the hepatic veins with the liver and IVC removed en bloc. If hepatic vein repair or reconstruction is required, the remaining in situ portion of the liver is rotated up out of the patient allowing repair or reimplantation of the hepatic veins to be done under excellent visualization. This can be done under normothermic conditions if expected reconstruction time is short or the remnant liver can be cold perfused using the in situ technique (described below).

In patients with involvement of IVC, hepatic veins, and portal structures and it may be the only possibility of obtaining tumor-free margins would be to use ex vivo resection techniques. In these patients minimal mobilization of the liver off of the IVC is attempted in situ. The suprahepatic IVC is mobilized with the phrenic veins divided and the intrapericardial portion of the IVC lowered. It is frequently necessary to open the pericardium from below to obtain adequate length on the IVC for clamp placement. The portal structures are exposed with adequate length dissected for resection and reimplantation. The infrahepatic IVC is clamped and patients placed on the caval portion of veno-venous bypass. The liver is removed, flushed with University of Wisconsin solution, and placed in an ice bath for back table or ex vivo resection. The ex vivo procedure is further described below.

Whether normothermic or hypothermic, in situ or ex vivo, in general the superior anastomosis of the graft is performed first with clamps subsequently repositioned on the graft below the hepatic veins if necessary to allow release of portal inflow occlusion and reperfusion of the liver to minimize ischemic time.

Cold Perfusion and Ex Vivo Approach for Liver Resections with Vascular Reconstruction

Standard liver resection techniques are sufficient for almost every liver resection, without the use of hypothermic perfusion. However, tumors that are centrally placed and involve all three main hepatic veins, with or without involvement of the retrohepatic inferior vena cava, are essentially unresectable using standard liver resection techniques. Those few patients that require complex reconstruction of hepatic venous outflow may benefit from either ex vivo or in situ hypothermic perfusion of the liver with subsequent hepatic resection and vascular reconstruction.

In 1974, Fortner first described the use of hypothermic perfusion during liver resection to protect the liver from ischemic injury [51]. In an attempt to offer surgical cure to patients with tumors that were unresectable by conventional means and also inappropriate for liver transplantation, Pichlmayr developed hypothermic perfusion with ex vivo liver resection [52]. During ex vivo liver resection, the liver is completely removed from the body and perfused with cold preservation solution on the back table. The liver resection is then performed on the back table in a bloodless field, allowing reconstruction of hepatic venous outflow to be performed under ideal conditions. The development of in situ hypothermic perfusion techniques followed including the so-called in situ and *ante situm* procedures. In situ hypothermic perfusion uses standard liver mobilization techniques, but the liver is cold perfused via the portal vein. In the *ante situm* procedure the liver is cold perfused via the portal vein and the hilar structures are left otherwise intact. The suprahepatic IVC is divided and the liver is rotated forward, allowing improved access to the area of the liver and centered around the hepatic vein confluence. The procedure and role for each technique will be described below.

In Situ Hypothermic Perfusion

A limited in situ cold perfusion technique can be used when a single hepatic vein or the IVC requires reconstruction. In this technique, the majority of the parenchymal transection can be performed without inflow occlusion, and total vascular isolation is then applied to divide and reconstruct the vascular structures only. The portal vein dissection is carried high to gain control of the right and left branches and perfusion tubing placed into the portal vein side ipsilateral to the tumor but directed into the liver remnant. The cannulated portal vein branch is then divided above the cannula while maintaining portal flow to the remnant side. The patient is volume loaded, and clamps placed sequentially on the infrahepatic cava, the portal vein, hepatic artery, and then the suprahepatic IVC. If only the hepatic vein requires reconstruction, IVC flow can be maintained by clamping the trunk of the target hepatic vein tangentially and parallel to and only partially narrowing to the IVC. If a tumor thrombus is extending into the IVC, intraoperative ultrasound and gentle traction on the liver may insure that the thrombus is not truncated. The anterior wall of the IVC or hepatic vein is incised and cold perfusion of the liver with organ perfused. The hepatic vein trunk is transected and the specimen removed. The hepatic vein and/or IVC can then be reconstructed in a bloodless field, without time pressure. Prior to completing the anastomosis the liver is flushed with cold 5% albumin. At completion of the vascular anastomosis, portal and hepatic arterial flow is reestablished. With the majority of the parenchymal transection being done without vascular isolation and with shorter ischemic times with this technique, the author does not use veno-venous bypass [53, 54].

Standard in situ cold perfusion is considered for liver resections that require total vascular isolation for periods exceeding 1 h [32, 55]. This technique is used for tumors involving the hepatic veins and/or retrohepatic IVC where longer periods of vascular isolation will be required either due to vascular involvement or due to the need for dissection of long stretches of intrahepatic vasculature that may result in excessive blood loss.

In standard in situ cold perfusion the liver is mobilized as for total vascular isolation, with control of supra and infrahepatic IVC and the portal structures. The portal vein (3–4 cm) is exposed to place a perfusion catheter and a portal venous cannula for veno-venous bypass if utilized. Although most patients tolerate total vascular isolation without veno-venous bypass, bypass reduces the time pressure and gut edema associated with prolonged portal clamping. The infrahepatic IVC is clamped and the patient placed on the caval portion of veno-venous bypass. A portal clamp is placed high on the portal vein with bypass instituted below. The portal cannula can be inserted down toward the superior mesenteric vein, and full veno-venous bypass is started. The liver side of the portal vein is cannulated for cold preservation and the hepatic artery clamped. The suprahepatic IVC is clamped and a transverse venotomy created in the infrahepatic IVC just above the clamp. Cold perfusion of the liver is begun with preservation solution and the effluent suctioned from the venotomy in the infrahepatic IVC. Preservation solution is either histidine-tryptophan-ketoglutarate (HTK) [56] or University of Wisconsin solution (UW) [57] The liver resection and hepatic vein resection/reconstruction then proceeds in a bloodless field with excellent visualization of intrahepatic structures. At completion of the liver resection, the liver is flushed of cold preservation solution through the portal vein with cold 5% albumin prior to restoring flow to the liver. The portal bypass cannula is removed and the portal vein is repaired or reanastomosed if divided. The infrahepatic venting IVC venotomy is closed and the suprahepatic caval clamp is removed to assess the integrity of the hepatic vein reconstruction and the presence of cut surface bleeding. Portal and hepatic arterial inflow is then reestablished. The patient is then de-cannulated from caval bypass.

Ante Situm Procedure

The ante situm technique of liver resection can be utilized in cases where resection of the IVC and hepatic veins is expected to be difficult, and where improved access to the hepatic veins and IVC is required. The ante situm technique employs the same technique as in situ cold perfusion with some key differences. The suprahepatic IVC requires circumferential control and cephalad length in order to place a clamp, divide, and then reanastomose it. Greater exposure of the suprahepatic IVC is obtained by dividing the phrenic veins and gently pushing the diaphragm away from the IVC circumferentially. The pericardium may be opened anteriorly to control the intrapericardial IVC/right atrium. As much of the liver transection is performed without inflow occlusion and prior to cold perfusion, veno-venous bypass is recommended for this procedure, although many patients tolerate IVC clamping for short limited periods with volume loading. The steps for cold perfusion follow those described for in situ perfusion, but the venotomy to vent the perfusate is in the suprahepatic IVC where it will eventually be transected. Dividing the suprahepatic IVC allows the liver to be rotated forward and upward, allowing greater access to the area immediately around the IVC- hepatic vein junction. If further access is required, the infrahepatic IVC can also be divided allowing the liver to be completely rotated up onto the abdominal wall. With this technique continuous slow cold portal perfusion prevents excessive warming of the liver. The liver transection is completed, dividing the hepatic vein within the liver and then resecting the origin of the junction of the IVC and hepatic vein en bloc with the tumor. If extension grafts are required, vascular reconstruction is then performed with the hepatic vein anastomoses while the liver is rotated onto the abdominal wall. The liver is then replaced and the IVC anastomosis(es) performed. The liver is flushed with 5% albumin prior to reperfusion. There is no doubt that the ante situm approach gives better access to the caval-hepatic vein junction than does simple in situ cold perfusion. It does not, however, give as good exposure as a complete ex vivo approach. The advantages to the ante situm over the ex vivo approach are that biliary and hepatic arterial anastomoses are not required, reducing the ischemic time to the liver and reducing the potential anastomotic complications. Currently we will use the ante situm approach when combined IVC and hepatic vein reconstructions are required, where a single hepatic vein orifice will require reimplantation into the IVC. If the reconstruction is expected to be more complex we will use a complete ex vivo approach.

Ex Vivo Liver Resection

In practice almost all liver resections can be performed without the ex vivo approach. However, patients who have tumors that involve the IVC and hepatic veins that will require complex venous repair or patients with combined hepatic vein and hilar involvement may be candidates for ex vivo resection. During ex vivo resection the liver is completely removed from the patient and perfused with cold preservation solution on the back table. The hepatic resection and vascular reconstructions are performed on the back table prior to reimplanting the remnant liver into the patient.

One of the benefits of planning the ex vivo approach is tumors that are initially considered unresectable may be resected. General assessment of the patient is similar to that for liver transplantation, with particular assessment of cardiac risk factors. In patients over 50 years of age or with any cardiac abnormalities a functional stress test such as dobutamine stress echocardiogram is performed, and any significant cardiac abnormalities would preclude proceeding. Even mild renal dysfunction has been shown to increase the risk of standard extended hepatectomy [58] and a creatinine of over 1.3 mg/dl would be a contraindication. Ex vivo liver resection should only be attempted in otherwise healthy, well-selected patients.

The role of such an extensive procedure in what are clearly advanced malignancies is open for discussion. Relatively few surgeons have attempted ex vivo resections since Pichylmayr first description of the technique [52], and the largest reported series from Pichylmayr's group consists of only 22 patients [59]. There are several reasons behind the lack of adoption of this technique. The technique requires a surgeon that is familiar with advanced techniques in both liver resection and liver transplantation, which restricts the procedure to relatively few individuals. Perhaps the most compelling reason for the lack of adoption of this technique, however, is the relatively high risk to benefit ratio that the procedure offers. The majority of the literature on ex vivo liver resections has been case reports that describe aspects of technique, and long-term follow-up is not available. It is clear, however, that perioperative mortality even in well-selected patients is between 10 and 30%. At best the 5-year survival for ex vivo resections for malignancy is between 15 and 30%. In Oldhafer's series the six patients that underwent ex vivo resection for colorectal metastases had a median survival of 21 months [59]. While the benefits to ex vivo liver resection may be limited, there are patients cured by this aggressive procedure. One of our own patients undergoing ex vivo resection for HCC is alive and disease free at 7 years. Another benefit is that when assessed for an ex vivo liver resection, the experienced surgeon may find a less aggressive technique such as in situ cold perfusion or even standard vascular reconstruction. Currently it would appear reasonable to consider highly selected patients for ex vivo liver resection on a case-by-case basis; however, it must be clearly realized by the surgeon and the patient that for HCC actual cures with this approach remain few and far between. Risks involved with this procedure must be carefully weighed against perceived benefits.

Outcomes of Resection of HCC with Vascular Involvement

Due to both technical and physiologic limitations, a only 20–40% of patients with HCC with vascular involvement are surgical candidates [60, 61], with even a smaller percentage undergoing vascular resection and reconstruction. Recurrent HCC occurs in 50–80% of patients at 5 years after resection, with the majority occurring within 2 years [20, 62, 63]. However, for HCC with vascular invasion, the recurrence rate following resection has been reported to be as high as 60% at a mean of 233 days in the liver, lungs, and diaphragm. Recurrence may be a complication of resection of tumors with hepatic vein or IVC involvement due to tumor emboli. In one series, HCC cells were recovered from the right atrium in three of five patients only after resection [64]. Even without resection, HCC pulmonary emboli were found in 59% of 41 autopsy cases [39]. Patients die of their recurrence in 50–90% of deaths [61, 63], and recurrence shortens 5-year survival from 70 to 30% [65]. Both macrovascular [63, 66] and microvascular invasion are significant risk factors for recurrence [62, 65].

In the ideal patient with a single lesion and preserved liver function, resection is curative with 5-year survival rates of 50–70% [14]. However, patients with tumors with vascular involvement requiring extensive resections have poorer results [10]. In one multicenter review of 591 patients who underwent complete resections and were analyzed based on the AJCC classification, the respective 5-year survival rates for T2, T3 and T4 were 56, 31, and 21%, respectively, where T2 and T3 have vascular invasion [67]. Despite the negative impact of vascular involvement on survival following resection for HCC, most series show a significant survival advantage as compared to non-surgical management. In one series comparing patients who underwent HCC resections with portal vein tumor thrombectomy compared to medical management, the mean survivals were 3.42 ± 2.67 vs 0.36 ± 0.26 years, respectively [61].

The survival data for resection of HCC and major vessels are less robust as it is based on small case series from a few, highly specialized centers. In the one large series, 29 patients underwent resection HCC with IVC resection, with overall 1-, 3-, and 5-year survival rates of 90, 67, and 45%, respectively [10]. Another series of 29 patients who underwent HCC and portal vein resection, the 5-year overall and disease-free survivals were 41% and 18%, respectively [6]. In yet another series of 12 patients with HCC and various vascular resections (eight portal veins, three IVCs, and one hepatic artery) showed 1-year disease-free survival of 50% [68].

Conclusions

Combined liver and vascular resections and reconstruction are uncommonly performed for hepatocellular cancer. The surgical team that is experienced in both liver transplantation and hepatobiliary surgical techniques is best equipped technically to perform these resections. More importantly, such surgeons should understand the risks, benefits and limitations of these highly aggressive procedures and that they should be applied to a highly selected group of patients. An even smaller subset of patients with tumors involving major vasculature may be considered for resections utilizing cold preservations techniques. These extreme resections, performed by a handful of surgeons, offer the only hope for patients who would otherwise succumb to their liver cancers. The utility of these "extreme operations" must be carefully considered on a case-by-case basis.

References

1. Llovet JM, Burroughs A, Bruix J (2003) Hepatocellular carcinoma. Lancet 362(9399): 1907–1917
2. Tsai TJ, Chau GY, Lui WY, Tsay SH, King KL, Loong CC, Hsia CY, Wu CW (2000) Clinical significance of microscopic tumor venous invasion in patients with resectable hepatocellular carcinoma. Surgery 127:603–608
3. Sugino T, Yamaguchi T, Hoshi N, Kusakabe T, Ogura G, Goodison S, Suzuki T (2008) Sinusoidal tumor angiogenesis is a key component in hepatocellular carcinoma metastasis. Clin Exp Metastasis 25:835–841
4. Al-Mehdi AB, Tozawa K, Fisher AB, Shientag L, Lee A, Muschel RJ (2000) Intravascular origin of metastasis from the proliferation of endothelium-attached tumor cells: a new model for metastasis. Nat Med 6:100–102
5. Mitsunobu M, Toyosaka A, Oriyama T, Okamoto E, Nakao N (1996) Intrahepatic metastases in hepatocellular carcinoma: the role of the portal vein as an efferent vessel. Clin Exp Metastasis 14:520–529
6. Inoue Y, Hasegawa K, Ishizawa T, Aoki T, Sano K, Beck Y, Imamura H, Sugawara Y, Kokudo N, Makuuchi M (2009) Is there any difference in survival according to the portal tumor thrombectomy method in patients with hepatocellular carcinoma? Surgery 145: 9–19
7. Liotta LA, Saidel MG, Kleinerman J (1976) The significance of hematogenous tumor cell clumps in the metastatic process. Cancer Res 36:889–894
8. Weiss L, Orr FW, Honn KV (1989) Interactions between cancer cells and the microvasculature: a rate-regulator for metastasis Clin Exp Metastasis 7:127–167
9. Kim BK, Han KH, Park YN, Park MS, Kim KS, Choi JS, Moon BS, Chon CY, Moon YM, Ahn SH (2008) Prediction of microvascular invasion before curative resection of hepatocellular carcinoma. J Surg Oncol 97:246–252
10. Matsuda M, Suzuki T, Kono H, Fujii H (2007) Predictors of hepatic venous trunk invasion and prognostic factors in patients with hepatocellular carcinomas that had come into contact with the trunk of major hepatic veins. J Hepatobiliary Pancreat Surg 14:289–296
11. Hagiwara S, Kudo M, Kawasaki T, Nagashima M, Minami Y, Chung H, Fukunaga T, Kitano M, Nakatani T (2006) Prognostic factors for portal venous invasion in patients with hepatocellular carcinoma. J Gastroenterol 41:1214–1219
12. Adachi E, Maeda T, Kajiyama K, Kinukawa N, Matsumata T, Sugimachi K, Tsuneyoshi M (1996) Factors correlated with portal venous invasion by hepatocellular carcinoma: univariate and multivariate analyses of 232 resected cases without preoperative treatments. Cancer 77:2022–2031
13. Poon RT, Fan ST, Lo CM, Liu CL, Lam CM, Yuen WK, Yeung C, Wong J (2004) Improving perioperative outcome expands the role of hepatectomy in management of benign and malignant hepatobiliary diseases: analysis of 1222 consecutive patients from a prospective database. Ann Surg 240:698–708

14. Llovet JM, Schwartz M, Mazzaferro V (2005) Resection and liver transplantation for hepatocellular carcinoma. Semin Liver Dis 25:181–200
15. Farges O, Belghiti J, Kianmanesh R, Regimbeau JM, Santoro R, Vilgrain V, Denys A, Sauvanet A (2003) Portal vein embolization before right hepatectomy: prospective clinical trial. Ann Surg 237:208–217
16. Azoulay D, Castaing D, Krissat J, Smail A, Hargreaves GM, Lemoine A, Emile JF, Bismuth H (2000) Percutaneous portal vein embolization increases the feasibility and safety of major liver resection for hepatocellular carcinoma in injured liver. Ann Surg 232: 665–672
17. Hemming AW, Reed AI, Howard RJ, Fujita S, Hochwald SN, Caridi JG, Hawkins IF, Vauthey JN (2003) Preoperative portal vein embolization for extended hepatectomy. Ann Surg 237:686–691
18. Palavecino M, Chun YS, Madoff DC, Zorzi D, Kishi Y, Kaseb AO, Curley SA, Abdalla EK, Vauthey JN (2009) Major hepatic resection for hepatocellular carcinoma with or without portal vein embolization: Perioperative outcome and survival. Surgery 145: 399–405
19. Bruix J, Castells A, Bosch J, Feu F, Fuster J, Garcia-Pagan JC, Visa J, Bru C, Rodes J (1996) Surgical resection of hepatocellular carcinoma in cirrhotic patients: prognostic value of preoperative portal pressure. Gastroenterology 111:1018–1022
20. Llovet JM (2005) Updated treatment approach to hepatocellular carcinoma. J Gastroenterol 40:225–235
21. Noun R, Jagot P, Farges O, Sauvanet A, Belghiti J (1997) High preoperative serum alanine transferase levels: effect on the risk of liver resection in Child grade A cirrhotic patients. World J Surg 21:390–394
22. Eguchi H, Umeshita K, Sakon M, Nagano H, Ito Y, Kishimoto SI, Dono K, Nakamori S, Takeda T, Gotoh M, Wakasa K, Matsuura N, Monden M (2000) Presence of active hepatitis associated with liver cirrhosis is a risk factor for mortality caused by posthepatectomy liver failure. Dig Dis Sci 45:383–388
23. Lang H, Radtke A, Liu C, Fruhauf NR, Peitgen HO, Broelsch CE (2004) Extended left hepatectomy – modified operation planning based on three-dimensional visualization of liver anatomy. Langenbecks Arch Surg 389:306–310
24. Rossi S, Ghittoni G, Ravetta V, Torello VF, Rosa L, Serassi M, Scabini M, Vercelli A, Tinelli C, Dal BB, Burns PN, Calliada F (2008) Contrast-enhanced ultrasonography and spiral computed tomography in the detection and characterization of portal vein thrombosis complicating hepatocellular carcinoma. Eur Radiol 18:1749–1756
25. Miyata R, Tanimoto A, Wakabayashi G, Shimazu M, Nakatsuka S, Mukai M, Kitajima M (2006) Accuracy of preoperative prediction of microinvasion of portal vein in hepatocellular carcinoma using superparamagnetic iron oxide-enhanced magnetic resonance imaging and computed tomography during hepatic angiography. J Gastroenterol 41: 987–995
26. Togo S, Shimada H, Kanemura E, Shizawa R, Endo I, Takahashi T, Tanaka K (1998) Usefulness of three-dimensional computed tomography for anatomic liver resection: subsubsegmentectomy. Surgery 123:73–78
27. Yamanaka J, Saito S, Fujimoto J (2007) Impact of preoperative planning using virtual segmental volumetry on liver resection for hepatocellular carcinoma. World J Surg 31: 1249–1255
28. Lang H, Radtke A, Hindennach M, Schroeder T, Fruhauf NR, Malago M, Bourquain H, Peitgen HO, Oldhafer KJ, Broelsch CE (2005) Impact of virtual tumor resection and computer-assisted risk analysis on operation planning and intraoperative strategy in major hepatic resection. Arch Surg 140:629–638
29. Chen H, Merchant NB, Didolkar MS (2000) Hepatic resection using intermittent vascular inflow occlusion and low central venous pressure anesthesia improves morbidity and mortality. J Gastrointest Surg 4:162–167

30. Soonawalla ZF, Stratopoulos C, Stoneham M, Wilkinson D, Britton BJ, Friend PJ (2008) Role of the reverse-Trendelenberg patient position in maintaining low-CVP anaesthesia during liver resections. Langenbecks Arch Surg 393:195–198
31. Huguet C, Gavelli A, Bona S (1994) Hepatic resection with ischemia of the liver exceeding one hour. J Am Coll Surg 178:454–458
32. Hannoun L, Delriviere L, Gibbs P, Borie D, Vaillant JC, Delva E (1996) Major extended hepatic resections in diseased livers using hypothermic protection: preliminary results from the first 12 patients treated with this new technique. J Am Coll Surg 183:597–605
33. Man K, Fan ST, Ng IO, Lo CM, Liu CL, Wong J (1997) Prospective evaluation of Pringle maneuver in hepatectomy for liver tumors by a randomized study. Ann Surg 226:704–711
34. Clavien PA, Selzner M, Rudiger HA, Graf R, Kadry Z, Rousson V, Jochum W (2003) A prospective randomized study in 100 consecutive patients undergoing major liver resection with versus without ischemic preconditioning. Ann Surg 238:843–850
35. Serafin A, Fernandez-Zabalegui L, Prats N, Wu ZY, Rosello-Catafau J, Peralta C (2004) Ischemic preconditioning: tolerance to hepatic ischemia-reperfusion injury. Histol Histopathol 19:281–289
36. Gurusamy KS, Kumar Y, Pamecha V, Sharma D, Davidson BR (2009) Ischaemic preconditioning for elective liver resections performed under vascular occlusion. Cochrane Database Syst Rev Jan 21(1):CD007629
37. Nakashima T, Okuda K, Kojiro M, Jimi A, Yamaguchi R, Sakamoto K, Ikari T (1983) Pathology of hepatocellular carcinoma in Japan. 232 Consecutive cases autopsied in ten years. Cancer 51:863–877
38. Anthony PP (1973) Primary carcinoma of the liver: a study of 282 cases in Ugandan Africans. J Pathol 110:37–48
39. Sung AD, Cheng S, Moslehi J, Scully EP, Prior JM, Loscalzo J (2008) Hepatocellular carcinoma with intracavitary cardiac involvement: a case report and review of the literature. Am J Cardiol 102:643–645
40. Agelopoulou P, Kapatais A, Varounis C, Grassos C, Kalkandi E, Kouris N, Pierakeas N, Babalis D (2007) Hepatocellular carcinoma with invasion into the right atrium. Report of two cases and review of the literature. Hepatogastroenterology 54:2106–2108
41. Kubota K, Makuuchi M, Kobayashi T, Sakamoto Y, Inoue K, Torzilli G, Takayama T (1997) Reconstruction of the inferior vena cava using a hepatic venous patch obtained from resected liver. Hepatogastroenterology 44:378–379
42. Miyazaki M, Ito H, Kimura F, Shimizu H, Togawa A, Ohtsuka M, Yoshidome H, Kato A, Yoshitomi H, Sawada S, Ambiru S (2004) Hepatic vein reconstruction using autologous vein graft for resection of advanced hepatobiliary malignancy. Hepatogastroenterology 51:1581–1585
43. Ohwada S, Ogawa T, Kawashima Y, Ohya T, Kobayashi I, Tomizawa N, Otaki A, Takeyoshi I, Nakamura S, Morishita Y (1999) Concomitant major hepatectomy and inferior vena cava reconstruction. J Am Coll Surg 188:63–71
44. Iwatsuki S, Todo S, Starzl TE (1988) Right trisegmentectomy with a synthetic vena cava graft. Arch Surg 123:1021–1022
45. Kumada K, Shimahara Y, Fukui K, Itoh K, Morikawa S, Ozawa K (1988) Extended right hepatic lobectomy: combined resection of inferior vena cava and its reconstruction by EPTFE graft (Gore-Tex). Case report. Acta Chir Scand 154:481–483
46. Bower TC, Nagorney DM, Cherry KJ, Jr., Toomey BJ, Hallett JW, Panneton JM, Gloviczki P (2000) Replacement of the inferior vena cava for malignancy: an update. J Vasc Surg 31:270–281
47. Risher WH, Arensman RM, Ochsner JL, Hollier LH (1990) Retrohepatic vena cava reconstruction with polytetrafluoroethylene graft. J Vasc Surg 12:367–370
48. Miller CM, Schwartz ME, Nishizaki T (1991) Combined hepatic and vena caval resection with autogenous caval graft replacement. Arch Surg 126:106–108

49. Hashimoto T, Minagawa M, Aoki T, Hasegawa K, Sano K, Imamura H, Sugawara Y, Makuuchi M, Kokudo N (2008) Caval invasion by liver tumor is limited. J Am Coll Surg 207:383–392
50. Smyrniotis V, Kostopanagiotou G, Lolis E, Theodoraki K, Farantos C, Andreadou I, Polymeneas G, Genatas C, Contis J (2003) Effects of hepatovenous back flow on ischemic-reperfusion injuries in liver resections with the pringle maneuver. J Am Coll Surg 197: 949–954
51. Fortner JG, Shiu MH, Kinne DW, Kim DK, Castro EB, Watson RC, Howland WS, Beattie EJ Jr (1974) Major hepatic resection using vascular isolation and hypothermic perfusion. Ann Surg 180:644–652
52. Pichlmayr R, Bretschneider HJ, Kirchner E, Ringe B, Lamesch P, Gubernatis G, Hauss J, Niehaus KJ, Kaukemuller J (1988) [Ex situ operation on the liver. A new possibility in liver surgery]. Langenbecks Arch Chir 373:122–126
53. Hemming AW, Nelson DR, Reed AI (2002) Liver transplantation for hepatocellular carcinoma. Minerva Chir 57:575–585
54. Hemming AW, Reed AI, Langham MR, Jr., Fujita S, Howard RJ (2004) Combined resection of the liver and inferior vena cava for hepatic malignancy. Ann Surg 239:712–719
55. Azoulay D, Eshkenazy R, Andreani P, Castaing D, Adam R, Ichai P, Naili S, Vinet E, Saliba F, Lemoine A, Gillon MC, Bismuth H (2005) In situ hypothermic perfusion of the liver versus standard total vascular exclusion for complex liver resection. Ann Surg 241:277–285
56. Gubernatis G, Pichlmayr R, Lamesch P, Grosse H, Bornscheuer A, Meyer HJ, Ringe B, Farle M, Bretschneider HJ (1990) HTK-solution (Bretschneider) for human liver transplantation. First clinical experiences. Langenbecks Arch Chir 375:66–70
57. Kalayoglu M, Sollinger HW, Stratta RJ, D'Alessandro AM, Hoffmann RM, Pirsch JD, Belzer FO (1988) Extended preservation of the liver for clinical transplantation. Lancet 1(8586): 617–619
58. Melendez J, Ferri E, Zwillman M, Fischer M, DeMatteo R, Leung D, Jarnagin W, Fong Y, Blumgart LH (2001) Extended hepatic resection: a 6-year retrospective study of risk factors for perioperative mortality. J Am Coll Surg 192:47–53
59. Oldhafer KJ, Lang H, Schlitt HJ, Hauss J, Raab R, Klempnauer J, Pichlmayr R (2000) Long-term experience after ex situ liver surgery. Surgery 127:520–527
60. Gotohda N, Kinoshita T, Konishi M, Nakagohri T, Takahashi S, Furuse J, Ishii H, Yoshino M (2006) New indication for reduction surgery in patients with advanced hepatocellular carcinoma with major vascular involvement. World J Surg 30:431–438
61. Minagawa M, Makuuchi M, Takayama T, Ohtomo K (2001) Selection criteria for hepatectomy in patients with hepatocellular carcinoma and portal vein tumor thrombus. Ann Surg 233: 379–384
62. Imamura H, Matsuyama Y, Tanaka E, Ohkubo T, Hasegawa K, Miyagawa S, Sugawara Y, Minagawa M, Takayama T, Kawasaki S, Makuuchi M (2003) Risk factors contributing to early and late phase intrahepatic recurrence of hepatocellular carcinoma after hepatectomy. J Hepatol 38:200–207
63. Ercolani G, Grazi GL, Ravaioli M, Del Gaudio M, Gardini A, Cescon M, Varotti G, Cetta F, Cavallari A (2003) Liver resection for hepatocellular carcinoma on cirrhosis: univariate and multivariate analysis of risk factors for intrahepatic recurrence. Ann Surg 237:536–543
64. Koo J, Fung K, Siu KF, Lee NW, Lett Z, Ho J, Wong J, Ong GB (1983) Recovery of malignant tumor cells from the right atrium during hepatic resection for hepatocellular carcinoma. Cancer 52:1952–1956
65. Portolani N, Coniglio A, Ghidoni S, Giovanelli M, Benetti A, Tiberio GA, Giulini SM (2006) Early and late recurrence after liver resection for hepatocellular carcinoma: prognostic and therapeutic implications. Ann Surg 243:229–235
66. Shirabe K, Kanematsu T, Matsumata T, Adachi E, Akazawa K, Sugimachi K (1991) Factors linked to early recurrence of small hepatocellular carcinoma after hepatectomy: univariate and multivariate analyses. Hepatology 14:802–805

67. Vauthey JN, Lauwers GY, Esnaola NF, Do KA, Belghiti J, Mirza N, Curley SA, Ellis LM, Regimbeau JM, Rashid A, Cleary KR, Nagorney DM (2002) Simplified staging for hepatocellular carcinoma. J Clin Oncol 20:1527–1536
68. Nanashima A, Sumida Y, Abo T, Nagasaki T, Ohba K, Kinoshita H, Tobinaga S, Kenji T, Takeshita H, Hidaka S, Sawai T, Yasutake T, Nagayasu T (2008) Surgical treatment and adjuvant chemotherapy in hepatocellular carcinoma patients with advanced vascular involvement. Hepatogastroenterology 55:627–632

Chapter 16
Radiofrequency Ablation for Hepatocellular Carcinoma

E. Ramsay Camp, Nestor F. Esnaola, and Steven A. Curley

Keywords Radiofrequency ablation · HCC treatment strategy · Open RFA laparoscopic RFA · RFA outcomes HCC

Hepatocellular carcinoma (HCC) is the most frequent primary hepatic tumor and the fifth most common cancer worldwide. The incidence continues to rise worldwide due to its association with hepatitis B and C viral infections. Cirrhosis is present concurrently with HCC in approximately 90% of the identified cases [1, 2]. Furthermore, the incidence of HCC increases with the severity of cirrhosis. Follow-up studies have identified HCC as one of the most common causes of death in the cirrhotic patient [3, 4]. The management of HCC, therefore, is based both on the stage of the malignancy and on the underlying functional status of the liver. Local tumor ablative techniques remain a reasonable treatment consideration for patients with disease confined to the liver who are not candidates for resection or transplantation.

Radiofrequency Ablation

Surgical resection or orthotopic transplantation should still be considered the gold standard for patients with hepatocellular carcinoma (HCC), with reported 5-year survival rates exceeding 70% in appropriately selected patients [5, 6]. However, surgical resection is only possible in the minority of patients with HCC confined to the liver due to the degree of cirrhosis, the tumor burden, and/or the anatomical location of the tumors. Transplantation is limited by the paucity of donor organs. For non-surgical candidates with no evidence of extra-hepatic disease, radiofrequency ablation (RFA) should be considered as a viable treatment option. RFA may be delivered from a percutaneous, laparoscopic, or by an open approach based on multiple patient and technical factors. The ideal patients for RFA are cirrhotic patients

E.R. Camp (✉)
Department of Surgery, Medical University of South Carolina, Charleston, SC, USA

K.M. McMasters, J.-N. Vauthey (eds.), *Hepatocellular Carcinoma*,
DOI 10.1007/978-1-60327-522-4_16, © Springer Science+Business Media, LLC 2011

with small tumors who are not surgical candidates based on their underlying hepatic function. RFA in appropriate selected patients can produce durable long-term survival with minimal procedure-related complications.

Combination of RFA with other treatment strategies, particularly transarterial chemoembolization (TACE), can be effectively used to treat patients with advanced multifocal HCC or as a bridge to liver transplantation [7–9]. As the technique and experience improves, the indications for RFA to treat patients with HCC will likely continue to increase.

Technical Considerations for Radiofrequency Ablation

Radiofrequency ablation (RFA) may be considered as a treatment strategy for HCC patients who are not appropriate surgical resection candidates. RFA produces thermal tissue damage through the use of high-frequency alternating currents moving from the tip of an intra-tumoral electrode into the targeted surrounding tissue. The patient is part of a closed loop circuit that includes the RF generator, electrode needle, and grounding pads placed on the patient. Frictional heating of the targeted tissue results from the movement of ions within the tissue following the alternating currents. As temperatures rise above 60°C surrounding the electrode, tissue coagulative necrosis is achieved in the tumor and surrounding hepatic parenchyma. The region of necrosis is relatively consistent with a zone of ablation within the first few millimeters of the electrode–tissue interface. The final size of the ablative region is proportional to the square of the radiofrequency current referred to as the radiofrequency power density. Early RFA probes were simple straight unipolar needles, limiting the size of the tumor ablated to less than 2 cm in diameter. These unipolar probes have been replaced with multi-array probes that create a larger region of necrosis. These modern expandable probes have multiple tines that are deployed once the needle electrode is inserted within the tumor. The curved electrodes are then deployed to a desired distance based on the size of the tumor. Reliable tissue destruction can only be expected 5–10 mm away from the multiple array hook electrodes.

RFA can be successfully performed via either a percutaneous, laparoscopic, or open approach [10]. Using image guidance from either transcutaneous or intraoperative ultrasonography visualization, the RFA needle electrode is inserted into the targeted tissue and the needle tines are deployed. RF energy is then applied following an established algorithm [11]. Generally, small lesions (<2.5 cm) can be treated with a single deployment targeted at the center of the tumor (Fig. 16.1). Larger tumors (>2.5 cm) generally require multiple deployments to achieve complete tumor necrosis. Strategic deployment of the electrodes is planned so the regions of necrosis overlap to ensure complete tumor destruction. Typically, the most posterior portion is treated first followed by reapplication more anteriorly at 2–2.5 cm intervals within the tumor.

The appropriate technique for RFA whether percutaneous, laparoscopic, or open approach depends on multiple variables. A percutaneous approach should be considered for cirrhotic patients with small (<3 cm), early staged HCC tumors especially

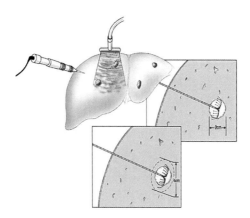

Fig. 16.1 The upper left image demonstrates the use of intra-operative ultrasound (IOUS) on the surface of the liver to visualize tumors within the hepatic parenchyma. The radiofrequency needle electrodes are placed within the tumor under IOUS guidance. The upper right image demonstrates deployment of the multiple array secondary electrodes within the tumor. For tumors 2 cm in diameter or smaller, a single placement of the multiple array electrode is usually adequate to produce a 4–5 cm diameter zone of coagulative necrosis completely destroying the targeted tumor (*lower inset illustration*) [10]

in the periphery of the liver. Lesions in the dome of the liver are often not accessible from a percutaneous approach. Patients undergoing a percutaneous approach usually require monitored sedation and are discharged from the hospital within 24 hours of the procedure.

A laparoscopic approach utilizes laparoscopic ultrasonography which has the advantage of improved resolution relative to transcutaneous visualization. Intra-operative ultrasound may better define the location of the tumors and allow more precise positioning of the RFA probes close to major vasculature near a given tumor. This approach is appropriate for patients with no prior history of abdominal surgery and centrally located tumors less than 4.0 cm in size.

Open RFA should be considered for larger tumors (>4.0 cm), multiple tumors, if the tumor is close to major hepatic blood vessels, or if dense adhesions prevent a laparoscopic approach. One major advantage of open RFA is that it allows for temporary hepatic inflow occlusion. This technique may improve the effectiveness in RFA of large hypervascular tumors and tumors in close proximity to major blood vessels by improving the RFA temperature response. Increased blood flow in the targeted RFA region leads to heat loss or a cooling effect limiting the degree of tissue necrosis and, therefore, the effectiveness of RFA. Hepatic inflow occlusion minimizes this cooling effect during RFA application. A second advantage of the open RFA approach is the ability to combine RFA with hepatic resection strategies to address multiple tumors.

Tumor position can impact treatment decisions regarding RFA. Tumor not amenable to a margin-negative resection such as tumors abutting the junction of the inferior vena cava and the hepatic veins can often be treated with RFA (Fig. 16.2).

Fig. 16.2 (**a**) CT scan image of a hepatocellular tumor abutting the inferior vena cava (*open arrows*) and the hepatic veins (*closed arrows*). For adequate ablation, serial deployments of the multiple array electrode probes are necessary beginning just outside of the inferior vena cava, and then sequentially withdrawn to treat the more anterior portions of the tumor. Blood flow through the inferior vena cava and hepatic veins prevents thermal damage of these major vessels. (**b**) CT scan 6 months after radiofrequency ablation reveals a larger necrotic cavity than the original tumor with patent hepatic veins (*closed arrows*) [10]

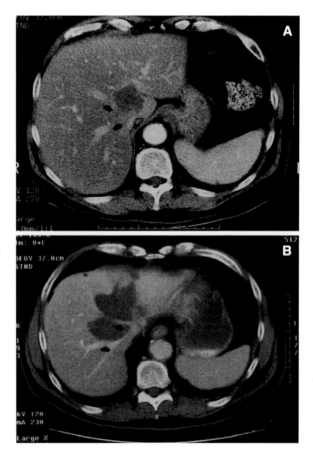

Conversely, tumors located in the region of the hilar plate where the portal vein and hepatic artery branches enter the liver should not be treated with RFA. The large bile ducts in this region are susceptible to thermal injury resulting in secondary biliary strictures or fistulas.

Imaging Considerations

A critical component to the effective use of RFA is preoperative planning and tumor surveillance with appropriate imaging studies [12]. Typically, serial dynamic MRI or multiphasic helical CT scans are used to plan RFA treatment and evaluate response. The goal of RFA is to produce a necrotic cavitary lesion greater in size than the pretreatment HCC lesion when compared by CT/MRI. This comparison is both to assess complete tumor ablation and to evaluate for tumor recurrence.

Dynamic MRI or multiphasic helical CT performed during the first 3 months following RFA often demonstrates a hypervascular enhancing rim of inflammatory tissue.
This inflammatory response can be difficult to distinguish from tumor recurrence
but typically resolves and is usually not evident by scans obtained after the first
6 months.

Identifying a local recurrence following RFA can be problematic. Early follow-
up scans may not be able to differentiate between a recurrence and an inflammatory
response. A local recurrence may be detected as progressive local ingrowth of vascularized tissue into the necrotic cavity or as vascularized outgrowth away from the
RFA cavity. The arterial phase of a dynamic imaging study is best to identify recurrences because the tumor tissue may appear otherwise isodense with the normal
parenchyma.

In small pilot studies, positron emission tomography (PET) scans have been used
effectively to identify local recurrence following RFA. In one study of 24 patients
who were treated by RFA for 33 lesions, PET scans were compared with CT scans
for tumor surveillance [13]. The overall detection rate was 92% for PET scan compared with 75% for CT scans. Early detection was also improved with the use of PET
scans. Other small studies in patients with metastatic hepatic tumors have supported
the role of PET scans in surveillance post-RFA [14–16].

Indications for RFA of Hepatocellular Carcinoma

The US Food and Drug Administration approved RFA for general tissue ablation in 1996 and for ablation of unresectable liver tumors in 2001. Generally, the
goal of RFA in HCC patients is treatment with curative intent. Therefore, patients
with preoperative or intra-operative evidence of extra-hepatic disease should not be
considered for RFA.

Recently, long-term outcomes were reported from a prospective collaboration
between the M.D. Anderson Cancer Center and the G. Pascale National Cancer
Institute in Naples, Italy [17, 18]. The initial study of 110 prospectively treated
patients was reported in 2000. In this investigation, 149 HCC tumors were treated
with RFA. Laparoscopic RFA was performed in 3 cases, open RFA in 31 cases,
and percutaneous RFA in 78 cases. Median diameter of tumors treated percutaneously (2.8 cm) was smaller than tumors treated open (4.6 cm). With a median
follow-up of 19 months, only four patients (3.6%) had evidence of local recurrence.
All recurrences occurred in patients with tumors larger than 4.0 cm in diameter. Complications occurred in 12.7% of the patients with no treatment-related
deaths. Complications included symptomatic pleural effusion, subcutaneous and
subcapsular hematoma, and ventricular fibrillation. One patient with Child's class B
cirrhosis developed intra-tumoral bleeding requiring transfusion and hepatic arterial
embolization. No patients developed hepatic or renal failure or sustained thermal
injury to the surrounding organs. This initial experience with RFA for cirrhotic

patients with HCC demonstrated this to be a safe and feasible alternative treatment strategy for early-stage tumors.

The follow-up experience in an extended cohort of patients continued to support the use of RFA in cirrhotic patients with early-stage, unresectable HCC [18]. The authors analyzed 194 patients who underwent RFA for 289 tumors with a median follow-up of 34.8 months. Disease recurred in 103 patients (53%) with a local recurrence rate of only 4.6%. The overall survival rates at 1, 3, and 5 years were 84.5, 68.1, and 55.4%, respectively. In further analysis, 5-year survival rates were similar between the groups of patients treated by percutaneous RFA, open RFA, and in combination with hepatic resection. The patients treated with a combination of surgery and RFA had a lower short-term survival rate, likely related to the increased surgical morbidity observed in cirrhotic patients.

Similar long-term survival data have been demonstrated in large clinical series with institutions in the United States, Europe, and Asia reporting 5-year survival rates with RFA comparable to hepatic resection [19–23] (Table 16.1). An Italian prospective, intention-to-treat analysis of RFA in 206 patients with HCC reported a 5-year overall survival rate of 48%. Based on multivariable analysis, they determined Childs-Pugh class and the presence of multiple tumors as predictors of long-term survival [20]. These long-term analyses highlight the potential curative results when RFA is used in appropriately selected patients.

Table 16.1 Long-term survival and local recurrence results with the use of radiofrequency ablation for HCC

Authors	No. of patients	No. of tumors	Median tumor size (cm)	Median follow-up period (months)	Local recurrence (%)	Overall survival (%)
Raut et al. [18]	194	289	3.3	34.8	4.6	5 yr – 55.4
Lam et al. [19]	273	357	3.0	24	12.8	5 yr – 38
Lencioni et al. [20]	187	240	2.8	24	5.3	5 yr – 41
Montorsi et al. [21]	58	58	<5 cm	25.7	35	4 yr – 45
Chen et al. [22]	71	71	–	27.9	–	4 yr – 67.9
Choi et al. [23]	570	674	2.2	26	12.1	5 yr – 58

Although effective treatment of large (>4.0 cm) HCC is possible with RFA, the concern of increased local recurrence from incomplete tumor destruction in this patient population still remains a significant problem. A recent report from China evaluated the effectiveness of RFA for HCC tumors between 3.1 and 8.0 cm in largest diameter [24]. In a total of 35 patients with tumors larger than 3.0 cm with a median follow-up of 11 months, complete ablation was achieved in greater than 80% of the cases. Using this treatment strategy, complications occurred in 17% of the patients with a mortality rate of 3%. During this short-term follow-up period, local recurrence, distant intra-hepatic recurrence, and extra-hepatic recurrence occurred in only 3, 24, and 6% of the patients, respectively. The cumulative 6-, 12-, and 18-month survival rates were 85, 81, and 76%, respectively.

Other series reporting RFA to treat large HCC tumors have demonstrated higher local recurrence rates with longer follow-up times highlighting the inherent technical difficulties associated with producing complete thermal destruction of larger tumors [17, 25]. In 84 patients treated with hepatic tumor RFA at the John Wayne Cancer Center, local recurrences were identified in 15 patients [25]. Approximately one third of the patients with tumors larger than 3 cm in diameter recurred despite treating larger tumors with multiple overlapping ablations to include the tumor with a 1 cm margin.

Comparing RFA to Surgical Resection for HCC

Investigations comparing RFA to surgical resection continue to show equivalent long-term outcomes in patients with early-stage HCC. A prospective, randomized trial from China was recently reported comparing RFA to surgical resection in appropriate surgical candidates with a solitary HCC tumor less than 5 cm in diameter [22]. Complete tumor necrosis was achieved in 91.5% of the patients treated with RFA. Major procedure-related complications were significantly greater in the surgical group (55%) compared with RFA treatment (4%). In this intention-to-treat trial of 180 patients, the RFA and surgical resection groups had similar overall survival rates (67.9% vs. 64%, respectively) as well as disease-free survival (46.4% vs. 51.6%, respectively).

Retrospective series have demonstrated equivalent survival outcomes between surgery and RFA for HCC tumors. Montorsi et al. compared laparoscopic RFA with surgery in patients with solitary HCC tumors smaller than 5 cm [21]. The 4-year survival rates were equivalent between surgical resection and RFA. In contrast, local recurrence was significantly higher in the RFA subset compared with surgery (53% vs. 30%). In a second prospective study from Italy, RFA at one specialized institution was compared to resection performed at a second institution for the treatment of HCC [26]. The overall 3-year survival rates and disease-free survival results heavily favored resection for Child's class A patients. The 3-year survival rates for RFA and resection were 33 and 65%, respectively. Similarly, the 3-year disease-free survival rates for RFA and resection were 20 and 50%, respectively. For Child's class B patients, the results were equivalent for the two treatment groups. Although this was a prospective study, the treatment groups were not comparable due to selection bias. The RFA group had a greater number of tumors per patient and worse hepatic function based on Child-Pugh class than the patients treated with surgical resection. These differences should be considered when interpreting the results. So while there were significant differences in outcomes between the two groups – RFA and surgery, the results might reflect the underlying disease rather than treatment effect.

RFA in Combination with Surgical Resection

RFA has been combined with surgical resection for the treatment of multiple HCC tumors. This combined approach is ideal for patients with bilobar tumors. Using a combined approach, surgical resection can be used for the largest lesion or for segments with the majority of the tumor burden reserving RFA for the preserved liver and smaller residual tumors. The experience from M.D. Anderson and the G. Pascale National Cancer Institute described this strategy for complex cases [18]. Of the 54 patients treated by open RFA, 22 (41%) patients underwent partial hepatic resection. Major hepatectomy was performed in only five patients. Procedure-related mortality (20%) and morbidity were increased when a combined approach was used. Open RFA with or without resection resulted in high local recurrence rates compared to the percutaneous approach, likely due to selection bias. Early survival rates were significantly worse in the combined resection and RFA group directly related to the high procedure-related mortality, increased tumor burden, and the morbidity associated with hepatic resection in cirrhotic patients. Long-term survival rates were equivalent among all patients highlighting the potential utility of aggressive liver-directed therapy even for patients with extensive bilobar disease. Five-year median survival rates for percutaneous RFA, open RFA without hepatic resection, and open RFA with hepatic resection were 57.5, 45.9, 44.8%, respectively.

Choi et al. reported a series of 53 patients with a total of 148 HCC tumors treated with a combined RFA and surgical resection approach [27]. Child-Pugh class A or B patients were considered candidates for a combined approach if (1) the indocyanine green dye retention rate at 15 min was less than 10%, (2) only one to three tumors <4 cm were left for RFA following resection, and (3) no extra-hepatic malignancy was present. There were no procedure-related deaths and an 8% morbidity rate was observed. Of the 66 tumors ablated, complete tumor ablation was achieved in 98% based on the 1-month follow-up CT scan. With a 22 month median follow-up period, local tumor progression occurred in two patients (3%) with, previously, completely ablated tumors. The 5-year survival rate for the entire group of patients was 55%. The only independent predictor of survival on multivariable analysis was resected tumor size. The estimated 1, 3, and 5-year cancer-free survival rates were 41, 28, and 0%, respectively. In addition to tumor size, the presence of microvascular invasion also increased the likelihood for recurrence based on multivariable analysis. These studies highlight an opportunity to impact survival in patients with multifocal HCC with a combination of surgical resection and RFA. Clearly, the patients must be carefully evaluated preoperatively for assessment of appropriate residual liver function before electing to pursue this strategy.

Comparing RFA to Other Ablative Techniques

In addition to RFA, other ablative techniques such as percutaneous ethanol injection (PEI), acetic acid injection, and cryoablation therapy have been used to treat patients with HCC. PEI is commonly delivered with ultrasound guidance for monitoring similar to RFA. As opposed to RFA which usually requires one procedure, PEI usually requires multiple injections performed over weeks to achieve adequate tumor necrosis. The number of treatments and quantity of alcohol injected depends on the size of the tumor. A similar treatment plan is used for delivery of acetic acid. Cryoablation creates a region of subzero temperatures to destroy tumors. Using the cryoprobe, an iceball with rapid tissue freezing is created. Like RFA, cryoablation may be delivered by percutaneous, laparoscopic and open approaches. Typically, two freeze-thaw cycles are used with the goal of achieving 5–10 mm ablation margin of normal tissue around the tumor. Cryoablation is associated with a high morbidity rate (50%) as well as a treatment-related mortality rate of 1.6% [28].

PEI and RFA are the most widely used local tumor destruction techniques for HCC and have been compared in several recent investigations [29–31] (Table 16.2). Two randomized studies have recently compared RFA and PEI in the treatment of early-stage HCC and both trials favored RFA as the superior technique. Lencioni et al. randomized HCC patients with a solitary tumor less than 5 cm in diameter or multiple tumors all less than 3 cm to either RFA or PEI. The schedule of PEI delivery was determined based on the tumor burden [29]. Complete tumor ablation was achieved in 91% of the patients with an average of 1.1 treatments using RFA compared to 82% complete ablation with an average of 5.4 treatments using PEI. A trend toward improved survival was observed in the RFA group, although the short observation period limited this analysis. However, local recurrence was significantly less in the RFA group compared with PEI. A Taiwan trial recently compared RFA, standard PEI, and high-dose PEI for HCC smaller than 4 cm in a total of 157 patients [30]. Similar to the previous study, the investigators observed improved tumor ablation requiring fewer sessions with RFA. Survival and local recurrence rates were significantly improved with RFA treatment compared with either PEI schedule. Multivariate analysis revealed tumor size and treatment strategy were significant factors determining outcomes. In summary, these trials suggest that RFA requires less treatment sessions and is associated with improved outcomes compared with PEI.

Table 16.2 Comparison of percutaneous ethanol injection with radiofrequency ablation for HCC

			PEI		RFA	
Authors	No. of patients PEI/RFA	Median follow-up period (months)	Local recurrence (%)	Overall survival (%)	Local recurrence (%)	Overall survival (%)
Lencioni et al. [29]	50/52	23	38	2 yr–88	4	2 yr – 98
Lin et al. [30]	52/52	24	34.6	3 yr–50	14	3 yr – 74
Shiina et al. [31]	114/118	36	11.4	4 yr–57	1.7	4 yr – 74

RFA in Combination with Other Liver-Directed Therapies

More recently, RFA has been combined with transarterial chemoembolization (TACE) for the treatment of unresectable HCC tumors. TACE embolizes the hepatic arterial branches supplying the tumor with a combination of chemotherapeutic agents and an oily contrast agent (lipiodol) followed by an occluding agent such as polyvinyl alcohol beads. Performing TACE prior to RFA may decrease the heat loss due to hepatic arterial perfusion enhancing the ablative effects. Reducing heat loss during RFA may allow more effective therapy for larger HCC tumors. In a phase 3 randomized investigation from China, the combination of TACE/RFA was compared with either therapy alone in 291 patients with HCC tumors >3 cm [3]. During a median follow-up period of 28.5 months, median survival for the combination group was 37 months, which was significantly longer than TACE (24 months) or RFA (22 months) alone. For patients with solitary tumors less than 3 cm in diameter, TACE/RFA demonstrated a survival benefit compared with RFA alone. Procedure-related complications were comparably low between treatment groups with five-related deaths (two deaths in the TACE/RFA group and three deaths in the TACE alone group). The investigators attributed the improved results to the altered tumor microenvironment following TACE which enhanced and improved the efficacy of RFA.

RFA as a Bridge Therapy to Transplantation

Based on the Milan criteria, appropriately selected patients with either a solitary HCC nodule <5 cm or no more than three tumors each <3 cm in diameter may achieve durable long-term outcomes with liver transplantation [32]. The landmark investigation from Milan, Italy reported 4-year overall and recurrence-free survival rates of 85 and 92% in this subset of patients with HCC [32]. These excellent results have been confirmed by various other institutions [33, 34].

Unfortunately, the demand for donor livers far exceeds the supply and, in the case of HCC candidates, many patients either die or become ineligible due to progression of disease before a donor liver is available. Bridging strategies have recently been incorporated to slow the progression of HCC allowing more time for donor organs to become available. The successful use of RFA as a bridging strategy to transplantation for HCC has been reported by various institutions [35–37]. In small series, RFA as a bridging therapy has decreased the dropout rate to less than 15% [36, 37]. Based on a historical control dropout rate of 30%, the use of RFA as a bridging therapy appears advantageous [38, 39]. Although the early experience with RFA as a bridging therapy to liver transplantation appears promising, these results need confirmation in randomized or larger non-randomized trials.

Conclusions

The ideal HCC patient population for RFA consists of cirrhotic patients with small tumors who are not surgical candidates based on their underlying hepatic function. RFA in appropriately selected patients can produce durable long-term survival with minimal procedure-related complications. Similarly, RFA may be used as a bridging therapy for patients who are candidates for liver transplantation to allow more time for available donor livers. As the technique and experience improves, the indications for RFA will likely continue to evolve. Combination of RFA with other treatment strategies can be effectively used to treat selected patients with advanced multifocal HCC.

References

1. Bruix J, Boix L, Sala M, Llovet JM (2004) Focus on hepatocellular carcinoma. Cancer Cell 5:215–219
2. Fattovich G, Stroffolini T, Zagni I, Donato F (2004) Hepatocellular carcinoma in cirrhosis: incidence and risk factors. Gastroenterology 127(5 Suppl 1):S35–S50
3. Degos F, Christidis C, Ganne-Carrie N et al Hepatitis C virus related cirrhosis: time to occurrence of hepatocellular carcinoma and death. Gut 47:131–136.
4. Benvegnu L, Gios M, Boccato S, Alberti A (2004) Natural history of compensated viral cirrhosis: a prospective study on the incidence and hierarchy of major complications. Gut 53:744–749
5. Mazzaferro V, Llovet JM, Miceli R et al (2009) Predicting survival after liver transplantation in patients with hepatocellular carcinoma beyond the Milan criteria: a retrospective, exploratory analysis. Lancet Oncol 10:35–43
6. Duffy JP, Vardanian A, Benjamin E et al (2007) Liver transplantation criteria for hepatocellular carcinoma should be expanded: a 22-year experience with 467 patients at UCLA. Ann Surg 246:502–509
7. Cheng BQ, Jia CQ, Liu CT et al (2008) Chemoembolization combined with radiofrequency ablation for patients with hepatocellular carcinoma larger than 3 cm: a randomized controlled trial. JAMA 299:1669–1677
8. Taketomi A, Soejima Y, Yoshizumi T, Uchiyama H, Yamashita Y, Maehara Y (2008) Liver transplantation for hepatocellular carcinoma. J Hepatobiliary Pancreat Surg 15:124–130
9. Georgiades CS, Hong K, Geschwind JF (2008) Radiofrequency ablation and chemoembolization for hepatocellular carcinoma. Cancer J 14:117–122
10. Curley SA (2003) Radiofrequency ablation of malignant liver tumors. Ann Surg Oncol 10:338–347
11. Curley SA, Izzo F, Delrio P et al (1999) Radiofrequency ablation of unresectable primary and metastatic hepatic malignancies: results in 123 patients. Ann Surg 230:1–8
12. Choi H, Loyer EM, DuBrow RA et al (2001) Radio-frequency ablation of liver tumors: assessment of therapeutic response and complications. Radiographics 21 Spec No:S41–S54
13. Paudyal B, Oriuchi N, Paudyal P et al (2007) Early diagnosis of recurrent hepatocellular carcinoma with 18F-FDG PET after radiofrequency ablation therapy. Oncol Rep 18: 1469–1473
14. Langenhoff BS, Oyen WJ, Jager GJ et al (2002) Efficacy of fluorine-18-deoxyglucose positron emission tomography in detecting tumor recurrence after local ablative therapy for liver metastases: a prospective study. J Clin Oncol 20:4453–4458

15. Barker DW, Zagoria RJ, Morton KA, Kavanagh PV, Shen P (2005) Evaluation of liver metastases after radiofrequency ablation: utility of 18F-FDG PET and PET/CT. AJR Am J Roentgenol 184:1096–1102
16. Travaini LL, Trifiro G, Ravasi L et al (2008) Role of [18F]FDG-PET/CT after radiofrequency ablation of liver metastases: preliminary results. Eur J Nucl Med Mol Imaging 35:1316–1322
17. Curley SA, Izzo F, Ellis LM, Nicolas Vauthey J, Vallone P (2000) Radiofrequency ablation of hepatocellular cancer in 110 patients with cirrhosis. Ann Surg 232:381–391
18. Raut CP, Izzo F, Marra P et al (2005) Significant long-term survival after radiofrequency ablation of unresectable hepatocellular carcinoma in patients with cirrhosis. Ann Surg Oncol 12:616–628
19. Lam VW, Ng KK, Chok KS et al (2008) Risk factors and prognostic factors of local recurrence after radiofrequency ablation of hepatocellular carcinoma. J Am Coll Surg 207:20–29
20. Lencioni R, Cioni D, Crocetti L et al (2005) Early-stage hepatocellular carcinoma in patients with cirrhosis: long-term results of percutaneous image-guided radiofrequency ablation. Radiology 234:961–967
21. Montorsi M, Santambrogio R, Bianchi P et al (2005) Survival and recurrences after hepatic resection or radiofrequency for hepatocellular carcinoma in cirrhotic patients: a multivariate analysis. J Gastrointest Surg 9:62–67
22. Chen MS, Li JQ, Zheng Y et al (2006) A prospective randomized trial comparing percutaneous local ablative therapy and partial hepatectomy for small hepatocellular carcinoma. Ann Surg 243:321–328
23. Choi D, Lim HK, Rhim H et al (2007) Percutaneous radiofrequency ablation for early-stage hepatocellular carcinoma as a first-line treatment: long-term results and prognostic factors in a large single-institution series. Eur Radiol 17:684–692
24. Poon RT, Ng KK, Lam CM, Ai V, Yuen J, Fan ST (2004) Effectiveness of radiofrequency ablation for hepatocellular carcinomas larger than 3 cm in diameter. Arch Surg 139:281–287
25. Wood TF, Rose DM, Chung M, Allegra DP, Foshag LJ, Bilchik AJ (2000) Radiofrequency ablation of 231 unresectable hepatic tumors: indications, limitations, and complications. Ann Surg Oncol 7:593–600
26. Vivarelli M, Guglielmi A, Ruzzenente A et al (2004) Surgical resection versus percutaneous radiofrequency ablation in the treatment of hepatocellular carcinoma on cirrhotic liver. Ann Surg 240:102–107
27. Choi D, Lim HK, Joh JW et al (2007) Combined hepatectomy and radiofrequency ablation for multifocal hepatocellular carcinomas: long-term follow-up results and prognostic factors. Ann Surg Oncol 14:3510–3518
28. Onik GM, Atkinson D, Zemel R, Weaver ML (1993) Cryosurgery of liver cancer. Semin Surg Oncol 9:309–317
29. Lencioni RA, Allgaier HP, Cioni D et al (2003) Small hepatocellular carcinoma in cirrhosis: randomized comparison of radio-frequency thermal ablation versus percutaneous ethanol injection. Radiology 228:235–240
30. Lin SM, Lin CJ, Lin CC, Hsu CW, Chen YC (2004) Radiofrequency ablation improves prognosis compared with ethanol injection for hepatocellular carcinoma < or =4 cm. Gastroenterology 127:1714–1723
31. Shiina S, Teratani T, Obi S et al (2005) A randomized controlled trial of radiofrequency ablation with ethanol injection for small hepatocellular carcinoma. Gastroenterology 129:122–130
32. Mazzaferro V, Regalia E, Doci R et al (1996) Liver transplantation for the treatment of small hepatocellular carcinomas in patients with cirrhosis. N Engl J Med 334:693–699
33. Llovet JM, Fuster J, Bruix J (1999) Intention-to-treat analysis of surgical treatment for early hepatocellular carcinoma: resection versus transplantation. Hepatology 30:1434–1440
34. Figueras J, Ibanez L, Ramos E et al (2001) Selection criteria for liver transplantation in early-stage hepatocellular carcinoma with cirrhosis: results of a multicenter study. Liver Transpl 7:877–883

35. Mazzaferro V, Battiston C, Perrone S et al (2004) Radiofrequency ablation of small hepatocel-
    lular carcinoma in cirrhotic patients awaiting liver transplantation: a prospective study. Ann
    Surg 240:900–909
36. Brillet PY, Paradis V, Brancatelli G et al (2006) Percutaneous radiofrequency ablation for hep-
    atocellular carcinoma before liver transplantation: a prospective study with histopathologic
    comparison. AJR Am J Roentgenol 186(5 Suppl):S296–S305
37. Lu DS, Yu NC, Raman SS et al (2005) Percutaneous radiofrequency ablation of hepatocellular
    carcinoma as a bridge to liver transplantation. Hepatology 41:1130–1137
38. Fisher RA, Maluf D, Cotterell AH et al (2004) Non-resective ablation therapy for hepatocellu-
    lar carcinoma: effectiveness measured by intention-to-treat and dropout from liver transplant
    waiting list. Clin Transplant 18:502–512
39. Mazzaferro V, Chun YS, Poon RT et al (2008) Liver transplantation for hepatocellular
    carcinoma. Ann Surg Oncol 15:1001–1007

Chapter 17
Microwave Ablation and Hepatocellular Carcinoma

Robert C.G. Martin

Keywords Microwave ablation · Hepatocellular cancer

Introduction

Hepatocellular carcinoma remains one of the most common malignant neoplasms and is responsible for greater than one million deaths per year [1]. Prognosis of HCC is exceedingly poor because of the high malignancy biology, high recurrence, and overall resistance to current therapies [2]. Partial hepatectomy remains the first option for the treatment of HCC; however, it is only suitable for 9–27% of all patients diagnosed [3]. The reasons for this are the severe underlying cirrhosis and the multifocality of the hepatic disease, which often precludes liver resection in most patients with hepatocellular carcinoma. Moreover, tumor recurrence is common after curative resection, and thus, few patients are candidates for further hepatectomy after undergoing their initial curative hepatectomy [4]. Therefore, minimally invasive yet effective therapeutic options are essential to improve the overall quality of lifetime in patients with hepatocellular carcinoma. Microwave energy is an effective local thermal ablation technique for the treatment of hepatocellular carcinoma which exhibits many of the advantages over alternative ablation and resection techniques [5–8]. In recent years microwave ablation technology has undergone tremendous progress due to the better understanding of the energy delivery and technological advances that are currently now commercially available.

R.C.G. Martin (✉)
Division of Surgical Oncology, Department of Surgery, University of Louisville School of Medicine, Louisville, KY, USA

K.M. McMasters, J.-N. Vauthey (eds.), *Hepatocellular Carcinoma*,
DOI 10.1007/978-1-60327-522-4_17, © Springer Science+Business Media, LLC 2011

Mechanism and Theoretical Benefits

Microwave ablation refers to the electromagnetic method of inducing tumor destruction by using devices with frequency greater than or equal to a 900 MHz [9]. The rotation of the dipole molecules accounts for the efficient amount of heat generated during microwave ablation [10]. One or more molecules are dipoles with unequal electrical charge distribution and as they attempt to continuously re-orient at the same rate in the microwave's oscillating electric field. As a result of the microwave transmission the water molecules flip back and forth at a billion times per second, leading to this vigorous movement to produce friction and heat which leads to cellular death via coagulation necrosis. An additional mechanism responsible for heat generation in microwave ablation is ionic polarization which occurs when ions move in response to the applied electric field of the microwave. The displaced ions cause collisions with other ions converting this kinetic energy into heat. However, this is the lesser of the two mechanisms that generate the efficient heat from microwave ablation.

The current frequencies of the commercially available microwave ablation devices are at either 915 or 2450 MHz (Fig. 17.1). The 2450 MHz is the most commonly adopted microwave ablation device which is the frequency used in the conventional microwave ovens giving the reported most optimal heating profiles. The benefit of the 915 MHz microwave is that it can penetrate deeper than the 2450 MHz microwave which may theoretically yield larger ablation zones. However, the energy deposition is also influenced by the dielectric properties of the antenna design; thus, there are specific antenna design limitations that do not necessarily translate into the 915 MHz generator leading to larger ablations (Fig. 17.2).

The theoretical advantage of microwave ablation over the more established and more published radiofrequency ablation is predominantly that microwave ablation

MW Spectrum
-Approved microwave frequency bands are at 915 and 2450 mHZ (regulated by FCC)
-Cell phone, cordless phones

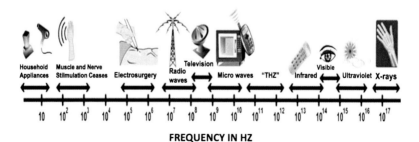

Fig. 17.1 Current frequencies of the two types of microwave ablation devices and corresponding frequencies

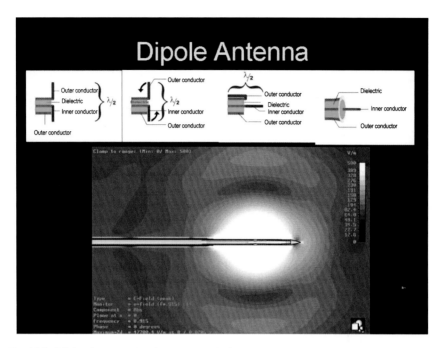

Fig. 17.2 Dielectric properties of the antenna design and the feed point of energy deposition

heating is primarily active while RFA heating is primarily passive. Microwave, thus, has a much broader zone of active heating and does not rely on the conduction of electricity into the tissue, and thus, the transmission of this energy is not limited by tissue desiccation and charring [11]. Therefore, intratumoral temperatures can consistently be driven higher leading to theoretically a larger zone of ablation over a more efficient treatment time and a more complete coagulative necrosis and tumor kill [12]. Second is the resistance of the heat sink effect, that being the cooling effect of blood flow from the tumor during this heating. Given the fact that microwave ablation is an active heating process, it is less affected by this perfusion-mediated effect which may allow for more uniform tumor necrosis within the target zone as well as in proximity to large vessels. Third, the simultaneous application of multiple microwave energy sources is allowed since there is no need to create a circuit as in RFA. Thus, multiple microwave ablations can be performed simultaneously leading to a more efficient ablation time when dealing with multiple tumors as well as the capability of ablating larger tumors in conjunction with multiple probes [13].

Microwave ablation therapy was initially developed in the 1980s to achieve hemostasis along the plane of transection during hepatic resection [14]. At that time, microwave coagulation was slower than electric cautery units and produced a much deeper area of necrosis and thus was not widely utilized for hemostasis during hepatic transection. This area of extended necrosis, however, did lead to an investigation of microwave coagulation therapy (MCT) to be another form of ablative technique.

Table 17.1 The Current Microwave Generator Systems that have been used and reported in Peer Review Literature

MW companies	Covidien	Microsulis	Microtaze	UMC-I (Institute 207 of Aerospace Industry – Beijing, China)
Generator frequency	915 MHz	2450 MHz	2450 MHz	2450 MHz
Power output	45 W	100 W	110 W	10–80 W
Antennas	3.7 cm active length 3 lengths, 12, 17, and 22 cm 13 gauge diameter	5.7 mm active diameter	15 and 25 cm length, 1.6–2 mm active diameter	24.7 cm length, 1.6 mm in diameter, 2.7 cm exposed antenna
Information:	– A single probe 45 W for 10 min produces 4 cm – 3 probes spaced 1.5 cm 45 W for 10 min produces 6 cm	– A single 100 W probe application for 8 min resulted in lesions consistently >5 cm – Unlike RF energy, microwave energy does not appear to be limited by charring and tissue desiccation	– Has been uniquely employed in liver surgery for more than 20 years.	– Local recurrence rates were 11.8% for MWA vs. 20.9% for RFA, without significant differences rates between the two groups ($P = 0.12$).

The initial microwave generators developed produced a microwave frequency of 2450 MHz and a wavelength of 12 cm (Table 17.1).

Equipment

The current microwave generators available have an output between 30 and 100 W. All of the commercially available reported microwave systems are composed of the three basic elements of generating microwave energy: microwave generator, low-loss flexible coaxial cable, and microwave antenna. The microwave energy is generated by a magnetron which contains spaces called resonance cavities which act as tuned circuits to generate an electrical field. The microwave output frequency is also determined by these cavities, which are connected to the antenna via a low-loss coaxial cable to transmit the microwaves from the magnetron to the tissue. The design of the antenna is crucial for the ability to deliver effective and efficient energy to create therapeutic efficacy [15]. This is one of its greatest advantages and limitations in that the length and diameter of the antenna is limited based on the energy available and low-loss flexible coaxial cables. Effective antennas have to be specifically tuned to the dielectric properties of the tissue and, thus, optimized for each solid organ that is to be ablative keeping the power of feedback to a minimum to ensure localized power deposition around the feed point and active tip of the antenna. To adequately destroy an entire tumor, the tumor ablation zone should extend at least 1.0–3.0 cm beyond the tumor. Therefore, antennas with larger coagulation diameter have the potential advantage over sources of energy deposition.

Microwave ablation for unresectable hepatocellular carcinoma was first reported in Japan with the use of the microwave coagulator developed by Tabuse in 1979 to achieve hemostasis during hepatic transaction [14]. Using the same device, Saitsu reported intraoperative and laparoscopic microwave ablation for small hepatocellular carcinomas in 1991 [16]. This first microwave system was used for percutaneous microwave and was the Microtaze system which had a needle antenna of 1.6 mm in diameter and a 2450 MHz generator with ablation performed at 60 W for 120 s demonstrating a coagulation zone of 2.4 × 1.6 cm in normal liver [17]. Since the coagulation diameters were not large enough, it was predominantly used to treat tumors less than 2.0 cm in size. A competing microwave generator system, the UMC-I microwave system, has been mainstay of microwave generators in China (Table 17.1) [18]. This antenna has a diameter of 1.4 mm, an active tip of 27.0 mm which also operates at 2450 MHz. It relies on a 14 gauge needle to facilitate antenna insertion and after 60 W of generator power for 300 s a 3.7 × 2.6 cm coagulation zone was obtained in the porcine livers [18]. Because of the ability to obtain larger zones of ablation, this antenna has been utilized to treat larger hepatocellular carcinomas and has so far been reported to obtain satisfactory therapeutic outcomes [7, 8]. However, this system has been plagued by higher power feedback enabling the temperature of the antenna shaft to rise very quickly and has led to severe adverse events including skin burns and potentially extrahepatic damage to surrounding tissues. Consequently, a protective cooling of the skin has to be performed during percutaneous ablation when the application of the energy is utilized for a certain duration of time. A third system in 2003 was released in the United States by Vivant Medical, capable of producing 60 W of power at a lower 915 MHz generator [19]. It was subsequently purchased by Covidien and is now called the Evident[TM] Microwave Ablation System. This antenna initially was a 13 gauge in diameter, 15.0 cm in length, and a 3.6 cm active tip with specific dielectric properties tuned for liver tumors thus reducing power feedback and increasing the amount of energy deposited to the tissue. In vivo experiments with a porcine liver using a triple antenna produced synergistically larger ablation lesions than used with a single antenna ablation. After initial animal experiments and recently reported phase II data, it currently is one of the two microwave ablation systems that are approved for use in the United States [19]. A maximum mean ablation diameter of 5.5 cm has been reported with the use of utilizing three antennas spaced at 2.0 cm apart. The fourth system that has been reported in the literature which is currently in use in Europe is the Microsulis system.

Indications

In general, similar to radiofrequency ablation the indication for microwave ablation should be applied to patients who are not candidates for the more definitive
and effective surgical resection. The definition of resectability for hepatocellular
carcinoma is quite complex, because in addition to taking into consideration the
underlying tumor biology (multiplicity of tumors). The treating physician must take
into consideration the health of the non-tumorous liver to ensure that a potential
curative resection may be an option. Unfortunately, given the fact that a majority of
patients with hepatocellular carcinoma have underlying cirrhosis from either hepatitis B or C, alcohol, or other sources, most patients who have potentially resectable
lesions based on the number and location are not surgical resectable candidates
based on the lack of health of the non-tumorous liver and the ability of that liver
to withstand that type of resection. Given those limitations, microwave ablation is
indicated currently to treat lesions approximately 5.0–7.0 cm in maximum size or
less [7, 8, 19]. Most treating physicians would agree that microwave ablation should
be utilized in a "curative" indication. These indications or criteria are predominantly
defined as a single hepatocellular carcinoma lesion of 6.0 cm or smaller, three or
fewer hepatocellular carcinoma lesions with a maximum diameter of 4.0 cm or less
and the absence of significant extrahepatic disease, and an expected life expectancy
greater than 6 months of survival. Patients in consideration for hepatic ablation must
undergo these same extensive pre-evaluations as would patients undergoing hemihepatectomy which should include high-quality dynamic cross-sectional imaging of
the liver as well as abdomen and chest, both for ablation planning and for staging of
the patients.

Choice of Approach

Microwave ablation has been reported to be effectively delivered through an open
laparotomy [19, 20], laparoscopically [21], percutaneously [8], and even thoraco-
scopically [22] in the appropriate patients. Each approach offers its advantages and
disadvantages. The current advantages of the percutaneous approach are that it is
less invasive and does not require an operation theater to perform the ablation. The
potential disadvantage of percutaneous ablation is the inability to evaluate the surface of the liver and inability to evaluate the abdomen for extrahepatic disease. As
has been demonstrated in metastatic colorectal cancer, percutaneous ablation has the
limitation of understaging patients when relying just on cross-sectional imaging.
The potential advantages of laparoscopic approach are the ability to truly evaluate the hepatic parenchyma, surface of the liver, as well as the intra-abdominal
peritoneum for more precise staging. The limitation is that this requires general
endotracheal anesthesia as well as an intra-abdominal access which has the potential
to be a greater risk for patients with marginal hepatic function. Microwave ablation
through an open technique has been reported to be effective also with the ability to

combine that technique with radical resection. Use of a combined hepatic resection and ablation technique has been found to be effective and safe in the management of patients with multifocal hepatocellular carcinoma. The ablation technique for microwave ablation is a complex technique requiring the treating physician to have extensive knowledge of the hepatic anatomy, knowledge of the histology of the tumor being treated, extensive knowledge of intra-ablation imaging, and appropriate knowledge for adequate follow-up. Ultrasound is currently the most commonly employed imaging technique because of its convenience and ability to continually allow for real-time evaluation of the ablation. However, ultrasound of the liver is a learned technique that must be optimized in order to appropriately and effectively treat patients utilizing microwave energy. Even with the advantages of microwave energy in comparison to radiofrequency ablation, microwave energy will not make a treating physician a better ablator of hepatocellular carcinoma if that treating physician does not have extensive knowledge in imaging guidance and image acquisition during the ablation process. Accurate pre-ablation imaging with ultrasound using either B-mode or combination B-mode and harmonic contrast-enhanced ultrasound leads to precise lesion size estimation as well as defining potential moderate-to-large heat sink vessels from either inflow or outflow structures. This then allows for a more precise antenna placement strategy leading to a greater incidence of overall ablation success and significantly reduced ablation recurrence. Given the rapidity of the heat generated using microwave ablation, the size of the ablation zone can be more precisely judged by the expanding hyperechoic area during the ablation especially in the first 3–5 min. Thermocoupling evaluation has also been reported to be utilized. Placed at 0.5 cm outside of the tumor margin, and once target temperature of 60°C is reached or 54°C for at least 3 min is reached, then successful ablation has occurred [23]. Post-ablation contrast-enhanced ultrasound has also been found to further enhance the accuracy of ablation using microwave and if there is any residual tumor, then focal ablations can be performed in those certain areas.

Assessing the efficacy of microwave ablation is of utmost importance and needs to be further standardized in order to avoid the wide ranging results that have plagued radiofrequency ablation. It has been recommended that an immediate follow-up CT (defined as within 1 month of ablation) be performed in order to accurately determine ablation success. Repeat imaging at 3-month intervals for the first year and then at 6-month intervals following is needed to accurately define ablation recurrence (recurrent disease within 1.0 cm of the ablation defect) as well as non-ablation hepatic recurrence and, lastly, extrahepatic recurrence. Defining ablation success utilizing these four criteria is of utmost importance.

Clinical Use

The initial result of MCT has come from Japan where the technique was first utilized in 1988. MCT in Japan has primarily been utilized to treat the cirrhotic hepatocellular carcinoma patient. The majority of these patients had small, less than 3 cm tumors and were not candidates for resection because of the underlying severe hepatic cirrhosis [17]. The initial MCT technology produced a reproducible and reliable zone of complete coagulation necrosis; however, because of the rapid development of this necrosis, the heat is quickly dissipated producing ablations of only 10 mm at maximum diameter. More recent evaluation of MCT therapy is based on a similar principle but improvements in probe, shape, and conduction have allowed for significantly greater size of ablation.

Currently, the overwhelming majority of reports utilizing microwave ablation in hepatocellular carcinoma have come from Japan and China. The initial report from Seki et al. of 18 patients with solitary, small hepatocellular carcinoma (less than or equal to 2.0 cm) demonstrated 100% complete ablation but very short follow-up following the ablation [17]. The smaller report from Murakami used the similar system as Seki et al. in evaluation of nine patients with hepatocellular carcinoma greater than 3.0 in size, which again demonstrated 100% complete ablation; however, local recurrence occurred in four of these nine tumors within 6 months of treatment [24]. When you compare these results using the UMC-1 system to the Microtaze system, the current UMC-1 system appears to yield larger ablations and potentially longer term durable control. The largest reported system using the UMC-1 microwave ablation system for HCC in a single institution evaluated 288 patients with 477 tumors [25]. The UMC-1 microwave system used in this study yielded 1-, 2-, 3-, 4-, and 5-year cumulative survival of 93, 82, 72, 63, and 51%, respectively with local tumor recurrence or ablation site recurrence in 8% of patients [23]. They demonstrated that single tumors measuring 4.0 cm and less had a far better overall predictor of ablation control. Izumi analyzed the risk factors for distal recurrence after complete percutaneous microwave ablation in 92 patients with three tumors or less, less than 3.0 cm in size [26]. His report found that two HCC nodules and a hepatitis C infection were associated with a higher incidence of recurrence.

Similar results have been reported in the use of microwave ablation for hepatocellular carcinoma through a laparoscopic as well as open technique. Yamanaka et al. evaluated the therapeutic effects of microwave ablation in 27 patients with that of 23 patients undergoing hepatectomy [27]. They demonstrated that microwave ablation achieved long-term survivals equivalent to that obtained with hepatectomy with significantly lower complications rates. Abe et al. also reported on 43 hepatocellular carcinoma patients treated with microwave ablation and demonstrated a complete ablation rate of 93% for tumors measuring 4.0 cm or less, but only 38.5% ablation success for tumors larger than 4.0 cm [21].

The complications of microwave ablation mirror those reported with radiofrequency ablation, similar to the fact that both energy systems generate significant amounts of heat. Because of that, bile duct stenosis, colon perforation, and skin burn have also been reported with microwave ablation [8, 25]. Similarly, liver abscess and tumor seeding have also been reported based on the type of technique utilized in performing ablation [28].

Side effects of microwave ablation do include postoperative pain as well as potential asymptomatic pleural effusions when ablating lesions high in the dome of the liver [19]. Similarly, the degree of postoperative pain and underlying fatigue is directly related to the volume of necrosis induced by the microwave ablation therapy [29]. There has also been an evaluation of combining therapies, especially in trying to manage hepatocellular carcinoma lesions greater than 5.0 cm in size [30]. The most common combined technique that has been evaluated is the use of transarterial chemoembolization prior to ablation. Transarterial chemoembolization is an effective method of reducing blood supply to the hepatocellular carcinoma and, thus, reducing any type of heat sink effect that could occur potentially improving the microwave ablation efficacy for lesions that are larger than 5.0 cm in size. Seki et al. has reported the use of microwave ablation 1–2 days after transarterial chemoembolization with good results as well as good long-term ablation control [31].

The use of microwave ablation in hepatocellular carcinoma has been reported in two US centers, predominantly using the Valley Lab Evident-based system. The initial report from Martin et al. demonstrated the use of the 915 MHz system on five patients with HCC with median lesion size of 3.3 cm (range 2.7–3.6 cm). They demonstrated 100% ablation success with ablation times ranging from 15 to 20 min in total, with initial 12-month follow-up demonstrating no evidence of ablation recurrence and a 50% hepatic non-ablation recurrence. These data have been further strengthened by a collaborative report from Iannitti et al. with a report of 23 HCC tumors ablated ranging in size from 3.6 to 5.5 cm [29]. All ablations were again performed using the Covidien Evident 915 MHz system.

Our current experience now includes the treatment of 20 hepatocellular carcinoma patients with a majority of them men, all but one of Caucasian descent with a median age of 66 years (range 45–83). The median number of tumors ablated was one with the median largest lesion being 4.0 cm (range 2.0–5.9 cm). Median ablation time was 15 min and the median OR time of 100 min, with an even distribution of access through either a laparoscopic incision or an open incision since a small minority of these patients underwent a concomitant hepatectomy at the time as microwave ablation. Four patients sustained six complications with the median highest grade being II, and the length of stay in these patients was 3 days (range 1–10 days). Post-ablation median volumes were 125.75 cm^3 (range 21.2–243.6). Median disease-free survival of 18 months and overall survival of 41 months has been seen in this patient cohort.

Despite its encouraging experimental and clinical results, microwave ablation, like other ablative techniques, is still in its evolutionary phase and needs to be standardized. The utility of microwave ablation, as with radiofrequency ablation, is strongly influenced by appropriate patient selection, anatomic location of the tumor(s), physician experience and training, and standardization of ablation techniques. There still remains a demand for minimum standards for defining ablation success, ablation recurrence, non-ablation site hepatic recurrence, as well as extrahepatic recurrence in order to establish true quality control in this technology.

With ever-increasing treatment options available now in the management of hepatocellular carcinoma, microwave ablation needs to be held to the highest standards in order to demonstrate where it is most effective in the treatment algorithm of patients with unresectable hepatocellular carcinoma.

References

1. Bosch FX, Ribes J, Cleries R et al (2005) Epidemiology of hepatocellular carcinoma. Clin Liver Dis 9:191–211, v
2. Jemal A, Siegel R, Ward F et al (2008) Cancer statistics, 2008. CA Cancer J Clin 58:71–96
3. Adam R, Azoulay D, Castaing D et al (2003) Liver resection as a bridge to transplantation for hepatocellular carcinoma on cirrhosis: a reasonable strategy? Ann Surg 238:508–518
4. Fong Y, Sun RL, Jarnagin W et al (1999) An analysis of 412 cases of hepatocellular carcinoma at a Western center. Ann Surg 229:790–799
5. Ohmoto K, Miyake I, Tsuduki M et al (1999) Percutaneous microwave coagulation therapy for unresectable hepatocellular carcinoma. Hepatogastroenterology 46:2894–2900
6. Shibata T, Iimuro Y, Yamamoto Y et al (2002) Small hepatocellular carcinoma: comparison of radio-frequency ablation and percutaneous microwave coagulation therapy. Radiology 223:331–337
7. Lu MD, Chen JW, Xie XY et al (2001) Hepatocellular carcinoma: US-guided percutaneous microwave coagulation therapy. Radiology 221:167–172
8. Lu MD, Xu HX, Xie XY et al (2005) Percutaneous microwave and radiofrequency ablation for hepatocellular carcinoma: a retrospective comparative study. J Gastroenterol 40:1054–1060
9. Goldberg SN, Charboneau JW, Dodd GD, III et al (2003) Image-guided tumor ablation: proposal for standardization of terms and reporting criteria. Radiology 228:335–345
10. Diederich CJ (2005) Thermal ablation and high-temperature thermal therapy: overview of technology and clinical implementation. Int J Hyperthermia 21:745–753
11. Skinner MG, Iizuka MN, Kolios MC et al (1998) A theoretical comparison of energy sources—microwave, ultrasound and laser–for interstitial thermal therapy. Phys Med Biol 43:3535–3547
12. Wright AS, Sampson LA, Warner TF et al (2005) Radiofrequency versus microwave ablation in a hepatic porcine model. Radiology 236:132–139
13. Wright AS, Lee FT, Jr., Mahvi DM (2003) Hepatic microwave ablation with multiple antennae results in synergistically larger zones of coagulation necrosis. Ann Surg Oncol 10:275–283
14. Tabuse K, Katsumi M, Kobayashi Y et al (1985) Microwave surgery: hepatectomy using a microwave tissue coagulator. World J Surg 9:136–143
15. Bertram JM, Yang D, Converse MC et al (2006) A review of coaxial-based interstitial antennas for hepatic microwave ablation. Crit Rev Biomed Eng 34:187–213
16. Saitsu H, Yoshida M, Taniwaki S et al (1991) [Laparoscopic coagulo-necrotic therapy using microtase for small hepatocellular carcinoma]. Nippon Shokakibyo Gakkai Zasshi 88:2727
17. Seki T, Wakabayashi M, Nakagawa T et al (1994) Ultrasonically guided percutaneous microwave coagulation therapy for small hepatocellular carcinoma. Cancer 74:817–825
18. Dong BW, Liang P, Yu XL et al (1998) Sonographically guided microwave coagulation treatment of liver cancer: an experimental and clinical study. AJR Am J Roentgenol 171:449–454
19. Martin RC, Scoggins CR, McMasters KM (2007) Microwave hepatic ablation: initial experience of safety and efficacy. J Surg Oncol 96:481–486
20. Sato M, Watanabe Y, Ueda S et al (1996) Microwave coagulation therapy for hepatocellular carcinoma. Gastroenterology 110:1507–1514
21. Abe T, Shinzawa H, Wakabayashi H et al (2000) Value of laparoscopic microwave coagulation therapy for hepatocellular carcinoma in relation to tumor size and location. Endoscopy 32:598–603
22. Aramaki M, Kawano K, Ohno T et al (2004) Microwave coagulation therapy for unresectable hepatocellular carcinoma. Hepatogastroenterology 51:1784–1787
23. Liang P, Wang Y (2007) Microwave ablation of hepatocellular carcinoma. Oncology 72(Suppl 1):124–131
24. Murakami R, Yoshimatsu S, Yamashita Y et al (1995) Treatment of hepatocellular carcinoma: value of percutaneous microwave coagulation. AJR Am J Roentgenol 164:1159–1164

25. Kuang M, Lu MD, Xie XY et al (2007) Liver cancer: increased microwave delivery to ablation zone with cooled-shaft antenna–experimental and clinical studies. Radiology 242:914–924
26. Izumi N, Asahina Y, Noguchi O et al (2001) Risk factors for distant recurrence of hepatocellular carcinoma in the liver after complete coagulation by microwave or radiofrequency ablation. Cancer 91:949–956
27. Yamanaka N, Tanaka T, Oriyama T et al (1996) Microwave coagulonecrotic therapy for hepatocellular carcinoma. World J Surg 20, 1076–1081
28. Liang P, Wang Y (2007) Microwave ablation of hepatocellular carcinoma. Oncology 72(Suppl 1):124–131
29. Iannitti DA, Martin RC, Simon CJ et al (2007) Hepatic tumor ablation with clustered microwave antennae: the US Phase II Trial. HPB (Oxford) 9:120–124
30. Shibata T, Murakami T, Ogata N (2000) Percutaneous microwave coagulation therapy for patients with primary and metastatic hepatic tumors during interruption of hepatic blood flow. Cancer 88:302–311
31. Seki T, Tamai T, Nakagawa T et al (2000) Combination therapy with transcatheter arterial chemoembolization and percutaneous microwave coagulation therapy for hepatocellular carcinoma. Cancer 89:1245–1251

Chapter 18
Transarterial Chemoembolization

Christos Georgiades and Jean-Francois Geschwind

Keywords Chemoembolization · TACE · Hepatocellular carcinoma · Drug eluting beads

This chapter discusses transarterial chemoembolization (TACE), which has become the mainstay of treatment for unresectable hepatocellular carcinoma (HCC). Its success is attributable to the ability to deliver high-dose chemotherapy into the tumor vascular bed. The addition of emulsifying agents (i.e., lipiodol) and/or particles to the chemotherapy slows down the blood flow through the tumor blood supply and increases the chemotherapy residence time. Recent technological advances such as drug eluting beads further increase the intra-tumoral drug concentration and residence time, while limiting the plasma concentration. This results in increased tumoricidal effect and less systemic toxicity related to TACE. The survival benefit from TACE has been repeatedly shown to be more than double that of supportive care or systemic chemotherapy alone, with less toxicity. The approval of targeted agents for the treatment of unresectable HCC, such as Sorafenib, can have synergistic effect with TACE on survival. Combination treatments that include TACE, ablation, and systemic maintenance chemotherapy will soon become the standard of care for patients with unresectable HCC. These treatments will also likely result in downsizing of many previously unresectable or non-transplantable patients, a likely benefit but also a challenge to ensure such treatment course is appropriate. Whatever the new standard treatment protocol is for HCC is undoubtedly TACE will play the central role.

Many risk factors have been implicated in the development of HCC, including chronic active infection by the hepatotropic viruses, Wilson's disease, chronic alcoholism, hemochromatosis, and α-1 antitrypsin deficiency. None of these conditions, however, has been proven to be directly carcinogenic. Rather, the increased risk of cancer is thought to result from the inflammation-related increased turnover

J.-F. Geschwind (✉)
Department of Radiology, Johns Hopkins University School of Medicine, Baltimore, MD, USA

of hepatocytes and consequently the increased rate of mutagenesis. The hepatotropic viruses include the DNA hepatitis B (Hep. B) and the RNA hepatitis C (Hep. C). The latter has also been implicated in certain lymphoproliferative disorders, especially non-Hodgkin's lymphoma, adding circumstantial evidence to a direct carcinogenic effect which has nonetheless not been proven. Aflatoxin B1 is the only chemical that has been shown to be directly carcinogenic to hepatocytes, while smoking, diabetes, and obesity appear to be synergistic factors that enhance the risk of HCC development [1]. Whatever the cause of HCC, the growing, viable tumor exhibits certain ubiquitous characteristics, one of which is increased vascularity compared to the surrounding, non-neoplastic liver parenchyma. This is the result of the strong pro-angiogenic effect exerted not only by the neoplastic cells themselves but also by the surrounding microenvironment and cell/chemical signaling cascades seen in chronic inflammatory states (cirrhosis in this case) and/or initiated directly by the hepatotropic viruses (i.e., increased concentration of matrix metalloproteinases [MMPs]). The importance of tumor angiogenesis for the survival and growth of HCC is further underlined by the recent positive outcomes in clinical trials where HCC patients were treated with Sorafenib (Bayer HealthCare, Leverkusen, Germany), a multi-kinase inhibitor with strong predilection for VEGF receptor kinases [1, 2]. The increased vascularity of HCC compared to the surrounding liver parenchyma provides an opportunity for intra-arterial locoregional treatment.

Vascular Anatomy of HCC

A number of different cell types are the target of tumor angiogenesis signals, but the final common denominator is the recruitment of vascular endothelial cells resulting in arteriolar and venular angiogenesis and lymphangiogenesis. The increased vascularity is more pronounced on the inflow side of the HCC, which manifests as large, tortuous, and disorganized hepatic arterioles (Fig. 18.1). The increased tumor blood supply can on occasion be so pronounced that results in shunting of blood from the rest of the liver ("sump" effect) or even an angiographically visible shunt between the arterial and the hepatic venous side of the tumor. Interestingly, the pro-angiogenic effect associated with HCC has only a weak effect on the portal venous side leaving the hepatic artery as the main HCC supplier (Fig. 18.2). This phenomenon has therapeutic implications in the field of Interventional Radiology. Transarterial Chemoembolization (TACE) has become the mainstay of treatment for unresectable HCC. During TACE, a catheter is placed in the branch of the hepatic artery supplying the tumor, and high-dose chemotherapy emulsified with ethiodol (Savage Laboratories, Melville, NY, USA) is infused to near occlusion aided by variable size particle embolization. Since the tumor receives most of its blood supply from the hepatic artery and the normal liver parenchyma from the portal vein, TACE selectively delivers chemotherapy to the tumor while mostly sparing normal liver. In addition, it has long been known based on empirical observations that

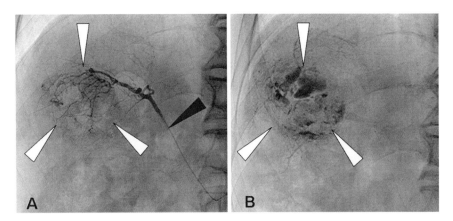

Fig. 18.1 Vascular supply of HCC. Angiogram just prior to TACE (**a**) performed via a selective microcatheter placed in a branch of the right hepatic artery (*black arrowhead*) shows the disorganized nature of the hepatic arterioles supplying the tumor (*white arrowheads*). Post-TACE image (**b**) shows pooling of the lipiodol–chemotherapy mixture in the abnormal vascular bed of the tumor (*arrowheads*)

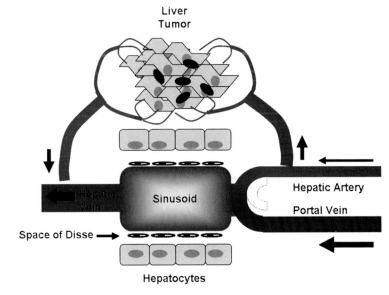

Fig. 18.2 Schematic of the vascular supply of HCC. The majority of the hepatic parenchyma blood supply (~70–80%) is via the portal vein. Tumor-induced angiogenesis recruits mostly hepatic arterial branches thus HCC supply is almost exclusively by the hepatic artery. Therefore, TACE will preferentially treat the HCC and mostly spare normal liver parenchyma

ethiodol selectively embolizes in the abnormal vascularity of tumors, further increasing the chemotherapy concentration and tumor residence time. The reasons for the tropism of ethiodol toward the tumor vascularity have not been clarified yet. Figure 18.3 shows the chemoembolization procedure. Figures 18.4 and 18.5

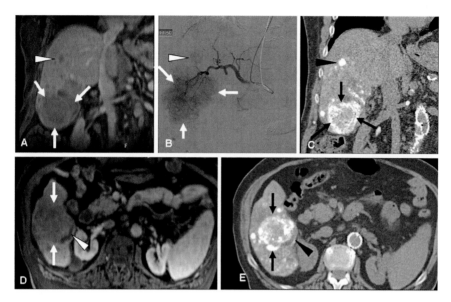

Fig. 18.3 Transarterial chemoembolization in a patient with unresectable HCC. Coronal T1-weighted, contrast-enhanced MRI image of the liver (**a**) shows a mass in the lower part of the right lobe of the liver (*arrows*) and a smaller lesion (*arrowhead*) more cranially. Digitally subtracted, selective, right hepatic arteriogram (**b**) shows the two masses, indicated by *arrows* (*larger*) and *arrowhead* (*smaller*) to enhance. Post-TACE, coronal, non-enhanced CT image of the liver (**c**) shows the distribution of the lipiodol–chemotherapy mixture to correspond to the larger (*arrows*) and smaller (*arrowhead*) masses. Axial, T-1 weighted, contrast-enhanced MRI prior to TACE (**d**) and axial non-enhanced CT of the liver post-TACE show distribution of the lipiodol–chemotherapy mixture within the vascular portions of the tumor (*arrows*) while sparing the necrotic (devascularized) portions (*arrowheads*)

showcase varied responses to treatment which include both Response Evaluation Criteria in Solid Tumors (RECIST) and European Association for the Study of Liver (EASL) responses. In reality, most HCCs will show both types of response to TACE; however, usually EASL criteria response is more pronounced than RECIST response.

Clinical Trials and Current Evidence

At the time of diagnosis the majority of HCC patients (approximately 85%) are not candidates for transplantation or resection, the two choices offering the best chance for cure. The lack of effective chemotherapy and the poor response of HCC to radiation treatment left TACE as the only realistic treatment option. Because of the lack of competing therapies, researchers were not compelled to seriously study the efficacy of TACE until the early 2000s, a source of frequent criticism. In 2002, Llovet et al [3] published results from a randomized controlled trial, which was

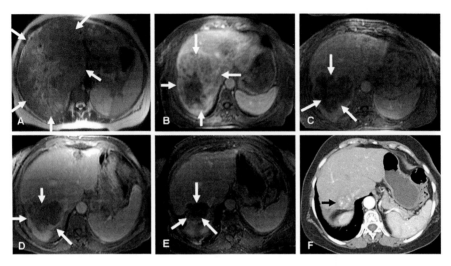

Fig. 18.4 50-year-old female with unresectable HCC. Three-month, sequential MRI (**a, b, c, d, e**) axial images of the liver after TACE. The initially large tumor replacing the entire right lobe of the liver shows gradual response based on RECIST criteria. At last follow-up, 5 years after initial TACE, the residual tumor is a 3 cm calcified nodule in the posterior right lobe of the liver (F)

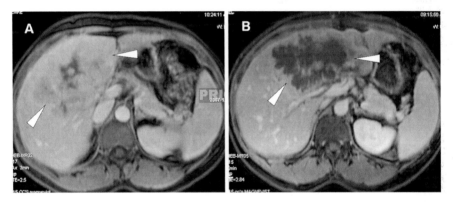

Fig. 18.5 34-year-old female with unresectable HCC. Pre- (**a**) and post-TACE (**b**), axial, contrast-enhanced, MRI images show the tumor (*arrows*) with mild RECIST response but significant EASL-based response, indicated by significant necrosis

stopped early because TACE provided a statistically significant survival benefit in the treatment group (1- and 2-year survival of 82% and 63% for TACE vs 63% and 27% for the supportive care) (Fig. 18.6). A meta-analysis of five randomized controlled trials published in the same year also concluded that TACE reduced the 2-year mortality of patients with unresectable HCC (odds ratio 0.54, CI 95%, 0.33–0.89, $p = 0.015$) [4]. The benefits of TACE were cemented after a study by Lo et al [5] showed statistically significant survival benefit in patients with unresectable HCC treated with lipiodol–cisplatin chemoembolization. The 1-, 2-, and

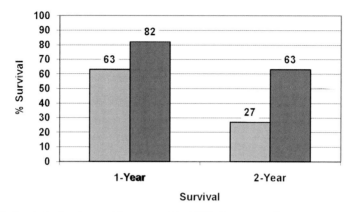

Fig. 18.6 Survival of patients with unresectable HCC. The 1- and 2-year survival of patients treated with TACE (*dark gray*) is significantly better than those receiving supportive care alone (*light gray*)

3-year survival in TACE-treated patients was reported by Lo et al to be 57, 31, and 26%, compared to 32, 11, and 3%, respectively, in the control group. Finally, in a meta-analysis of randomized controlled trials, Llovet and Bruix [6] showed significantly decreased 2-year mortality in patients treated with chemoembolization with an odds ratio of 0.53 (CI 95%, 0.32–0.89, $p = 0.017$). Recent evidence has emerged that compares resection vs. locoregional treatments for HCC with favorable conclusions for TACE. Yamagiwa et al [7], for example, have shown that combination treatment using radiofrequency ablation (RFA) and TACE resulted in significantly longer overall 5-year survival compared to hepatic resection (72% vs 59%), albeit a shorter disease-free survival (14 vs 32 months). Combination locoregional treatment using RFA and TACE were also compared to hepatic resection for small HCCs (≤3 cm) by Yamakado et al [8]. The 1-, 3-, and 5-year survival was identical between the two groups at 98%, 94%, 75% and 97%, 93%, 81% for locoregional treatment and resection, respectively (Fig. 18.7). Also identical was the cancer recurrence rate at 36 and 37% for locoregional and surgical treatments, respectively.

Fig. 18.7 Survival for patients with resectable HCC. Overall, 5-year survival is identical between patients treated with resection (*light gray*) and those treated with combination RFA+TACE (*dark gray*). The comparison was for patients with HCC ≤ 3 cm

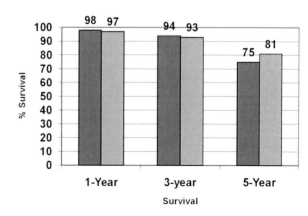

One of the lingering criticisms of TACE is that the protocol has not been standardized yet. While most physicians will use a triple chemotherapy cocktail that includes cisplatin, mitomycin C, and doxorubicin, others will use double or monotherapy regimens while still a minority will only embolize the feeding vessel without chemotherapy. To date, there has not been a prospective, randomized trial comparing the efficacy of different chemotherapy regimens. Cisplatin causes DNA intrastrand crosslinks, mitomycin C is an alkylating agent that causes DNA interstrand crosslinking and inhibits DNA-dependent RNA polymerase, and doxorubicin intercalates DNA and inhibits proliferation-specific DNA polymerases. The choice of triple-regimen TACE rests on the theory that a multi-pronged attack on the neoplastic cell DNA is more effective and can overcome possible tumor drug resistance.

TACE as a Bridge to Transplantation

Recently there has been considerable interest regarding the role of TACE as a bridge to liver transplantation. It has been postulated that TACE shrinks and/or slows the progression of HCC thus possibly minimizing waiting list drop-off rates. This would theoretically be the case especially for those patients who are barely within Milan or San Francisco transplantation criteria. There is a lack of well-designed, prospective, randomized studies however, and the published ones have thus far been equivocal. One prospective (but not randomized) study showed a 1-, 2-, and 5-year survival after TACE and orthotopic liver transplantation (OLT) of 98, 98, and 93%, respectively [9], which is better than historical controls, suggesting that pretransplantation TACE does improve survival. The same study, however, concluded that downstaging of patients to within Milan criteria using TACE did not result in any survival benefit. Two other studies [10, 11] have correlated the degree of necrosis with outcome after OLT. One concluded that a high percent of lesion necrosis after TACE predicts lower tumor recurrence rates after OLT, whereas the other concluded that low necrosis rates after TACE "facilitate tumor recurrence." The latter is unlikely, as there is no teleological effect for TACE. The results above, rather, suggest that good response to TACE indicates favorable disease biology. Overall, the current literature suggests (but is not definitive) that (1) pretransplantation TACE for patients within but close to falling out of criteria may be beneficial and (2) response to TACE may be predictive of disease biology and by extension, survival after liver transplantation. Further studies are needed in order to define TACE's role as a bridge to liver transplant.

Quality of Life/Toxicity Profile

HCC and cirrhosis are frequent comorbid conditions that have a significant impact on the patients' quality of life. Pain from the expanding tumor, especially if it is in a subcapsular location is a common presenting symptom for HCC. Ascites, edema, fatigue are symptoms related to the cirrhosis. Under these circumstances any treatment (except transplantation) has a potential of worsening the symptoms, be it surgical resection, percutaneous ablation, systemic chemotherapy, or TACE. (Possible TACE-related complications are shown in Table 18.1.) Strong contraindications to TACE include Child-Pugh C liver cirrhosis and poor performance status, i.e., Eastern Cooperative Oncology Group (ECOG) $\geq$ 3 or Karnofsky status <60. Performing TACE in patients with minimal if any liver functional reserve increases the risk of hepatic failure and in any case is unlikely to prolong survival. When indicated, however, TACE has been shown to result in much lower plasma concentration and greater intra-tumoral chemotherapy concentration, compared to systemic treatment. Data from our group (pending publication) show a very favorable toxicity profile for TACE. The group recorded hematologic and non-hematologic toxicities related to TACE and categorized them based on the Common Terminology Criteria for Adverse Events (CTCAE). Grade 3–4 toxicities were found in about 20% of patients, a number much lower than reported for systemic chemotherapy [12]. This is an important consideration because TACE is usually reserved as salvage treatment in many patients with moderate cirrhosis. Furthermore, recent evidence suggests that the newer form of TACE – i.e., drug eluting beads – shows an even better pharmacokinetic profile than lipiodol-based TACE, including lower plasma chemotherapy levels and lower related systemic toxicity (Fig. 18.6) [13].

Table 18.1 Possible TACE-related complications. Third column shows the overall percent risk as reported in literature if the risk factor in column 2 is present. For example, patients who have Child-Pugh C liver cirrhosis (row 1, column 2) have a significant risk for liver failure (column 3) with TACE. If TACE can be performed in a superselective manner (column 4) thus sparing most of the liver then the chances of liver failure are minimized

Complication	Risk factor	% Risk	Risk mitigation action
Liver failure, death, encephalopathy	Child-Pugh C T. bilirubin $\geq$4 mg/dl Albumin $\leq$2 mg/dl Poor performance status	5–10% for Child-Pugh C	Superselective embolization
Liver abscess	Compromised Sphincter of Oddi	30–80% (else <5%)	Broad spectrum Abx/ GI preparation
Non-target embolization	Aberrant anatomy especially left or right gastric artery	<10%	Place catheter distal to origin of gastric artery/watch for chemo reflux
Pulmonary embolism	Tumor shunting	<1%	Gelfoam embolization of shunt
Upper GI bleeding	Gastroesophageal varices	Unknown (rare)	Pre-TACE banding?
Acute renal failure	Renal insufficiency, diabetes	0.05–5%	Hydration, renoprotection, minimize contrast

Future Directions/Conclusions

The excitement generated by the release of the SHARP trial results (systemic chemotherapy with Sorafenib) overshadowed reality. That is, the survival benefit seen by Child-Pugh A patients with unresectable HCC treated with Sorafenib was a modest 2.8 months. The initial enthusiasm, more than anything else, highlights the historical absence of measurable progress in the treatment of HCC among the medical oncology community. Therefore, and despite these modest advances in the treatment of HCC, TACE will likely remain the most important treatment option. That is not to say that TACE is an optimal treatment or that these advances have not shaped future clinical trials. While TACE occasionally results in complete and sustained tumor response, in the majority of patients there is eventual regrowth of the neoplasm, underlying TACE's inability to completely eradicate the disease or to permanently sustain its initial good response. Currently, many combination treatments are planned that aim to attack HCC's critical survival points. For example, a TACE-Avastin as well as a TACE-Sorafenib trial is underway, which aims to prevent HCC regrowth after TACE by inhibiting tumor angiogenesis. TACE technique is also evolving, in current trials. Porous particles loaded with chemotherapeutics (i.e., doxorubicin eluting beads – DEBs) are replacing simple drug-ethiodol infusions. Such particles further increase the residence time of chemotherapy within the tumor and have prolonged drug eluting characteristics, properties that further enhance tumoricidal effect and reduce systemic toxicities (Fig. 18.8). Whatever the new standard of care treatment is for unresectable HCC, transarterial chemoembolization is evolving and will undoubtedly remain one of the most important – if not the most important – component.

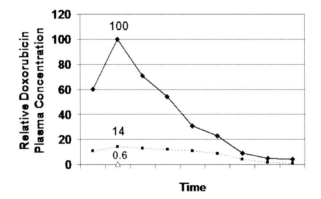

Fig. 18.8 Relative plasma doxorubicin concentrations. Intra-arterial infusion (*solid line*) via the hepatic artery shows the least optimum pharmacokinetic profile with an early spike in plasma concentration and the highest area-under-curve value. TACE with lipiodol (*dashed line*) decreases both the peak average plasma concentration of doxorubicin and the area-under-curve. Treatment with doxorubicin eluting beads (single value, peal plasma concentration) further decreases the peak plasma concentration of doxorubicin. Data are normalized to peak plasma concentration of doxorubicin after intra-arterial infusion

In conclusion, TACE has been shown to provide the longest survival benefit among all treatment options for unresectable HCC. Combination therapies that include TACE, ablation, and maintenance chemotherapy with newer, targeted agents are becoming the standard of care for such patients. Many challenges will be encountered in the future for HCC treatment. For example, what is the best combination treatment protocol and which chemotherapy should we use? Locoregional treatments and then follow-up with systemic chemotherapy or the reverse? What to do we need to use with those patients who respond to these new treatments? If they are downstaged into criteria for resection or transplantation, will it be beneficial? If a significant percent of patients is indeed downstaged to transplantation criteria, what will be the impact on liver availability?

References

1. Devita VT, Lawrence TS, Rosenberg SA, eds (2008) DeVita, Hellman & Rosenberg's Cancer: principles and practice of oncology, 8th ed. Wolters Kluwer and Lippincot Williams & Wilkins, Philadelphia, PA
2. Llovet JM, Ricci S, Mazzaferro V, Hilgard P, Raoul J, Zeuzem S, Poulin-Costello M, Moscovici M, Voliotis D, Bruix J, For the SHARP Investigators Study Group J Clin Oncol (2007) Sorafenib improves survival in advanced hepatocellular carcinoma (HCC): results of a phase III randomized placebo-controlled trial (SHARP trial). ASCO Annual Meeting Proceedings Part I 25(June 20 Supplement), LBA1
3. Llovet JM, Real MI, Montana X et al (2002) Arterial embolization or chemoembolization versus symptomatic treatment in patients with unresectable hepatocellular carcinoma: a randomized controlled trial. Lancet 1:1734–1739
4. Camma C, Schepis F, Orlando A et al (2002) Transarterial chemoembolization for unresectable hepatocellular carcinoma: meta-analysis of randomized controlled trials. Radiology 1:47–54
5. Lo CM, Ngan H, Tso WK et al (2002) Randomized control trial of transarterial lipiodol chemoembolization for unresectable hepatocellular carcinoma. Hepatology 1:1164–1171
6. Llovet JM, Bruix J (2003) Systematic review of randomized trials for unresectable hepatocellular carcinoma: chemoembolization improves survival. Hepatology 1:429–442
7. Yamagiwa K, Shiraki K, Yamakado K et al (2008) Survival rates according to the Cancer of the Liver Italian Program scores of 345 hepatocellular carcinoma patients after multimodality treatments during a 10-year period in a retrospective study. J Gastroenterol Hepatol 1: 482–490
8. Yamakado K, Nakatsuka A, Takaki H et al (2008) Early stage hepatocellular carcinoma: radiofrequency ablation combined with chemoembolization versus hepatectomy. Radiology 1:260–266
9. Graziadei IW, Sandmueller H, Waldenberger P et al (2003) Chemoembolization followed by liver transplantation for hepatocellular carcinoma impedes tumor progression while on the waiting list and leads to excellent outcome. Liver Transplant 1:557–563
10. Stockland HA, Walser EM, Paz-Fumagalli R, McKinney JM, May GR (2007) Preoperative chemoembolization in patients with hepatocellular carcinoma undergoing liver transplantation: influence of emergent versus elective procedures on patient survival and tumor recurrence rates. Cardiovasc Intervent Radiol 1:888–893
11. Ravaioli M, Grazi GL, Ercolani G et al (2004) Partial necrosis on hepatocellular carcinoma nodules facilitates tumor recurrence after liver transplantation. Transplantation 1:1780–1786

12. Buijs M, Vossen JA, Frangakis C, Hong K, Georgiades CS, Chen Y, Liapi E, Geschwind JF (2008) Nonresectable hepatocellular carcinoma: long-term to treated with transarterial chemoembolization: a single centre experience. Radiology 1:346–354
13. Poon RT, Tso WK, Pang RW et al (2007) A phase I/II trial of chemoembolization for hepatocellular carcinoma using a novel intra-arterial drug-eluting bead. Clin Gastroenterol Hepatol 5:1100–1108

Chapter 19
Chemoembolization with Drug-Eluting Beads

Robert C.G. Martin and Stewart Carter

Keywords Liver-directed therapy · Chemoembolization · Drug-eluting bead · Doxorubicin · Hepatocellular

Introduction

Primary hepatic carcinoma remains a relatively uncommon disease in North America and Western Europe (0.5–2.0% of all cancers) [1, 2]. However it remains a much larger fraction (20–40%) in developing countries and is the 5th–6th most common malignancy worldwide (approximately 5.6% of all cancers) [3, 4]. Hepatocellular carcinoma (HCC) is the most common primary malignancy of the liver (70–85%) with an estimated 500 thousand to 1 million new cases annually and an associated mortality of approximately 600,000 [3, 5]. Recent studies in the USA have shown that the incidence of HCC is increasing, most likely related to chronic HCV infection [6].

Unfortunately, many of these patients will have diffuse, multifocal disease rendering them unresectable, defined as the inability to remove or ablate all tumors and leave enough normal liver parenchyma to regain an acceptable quality of life. Additionally, many patients have significant comorbid conditions that preclude a major liver resection. Not long ago, most patients with unresectable liver cancers had few therapeutic options other than systemic chemotherapy. The last two decades have seen the development of several hepatic-directed treatment options that are expanding the therapeutic armamentarium of the clinician and lengthening the patient's survival.

It is for this very reason that other treatment modalities are being investigated for their roles in enhancing the results in the treatment of early, intermediate,

R.C.G. Martin (✉)
Division of Surgical Oncology, Department of Surgery, University of Louisville School of Medicine, Louisville, KY, USA

K.M. McMasters, J.-N. Vauthey (eds.), *Hepatocellular Carcinoma*,
DOI 10.1007/978-1-60327-522-4_19, © Springer Science+Business Media, LLC 2011

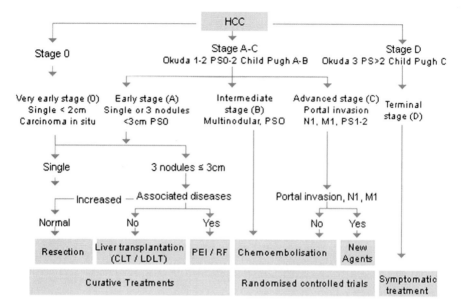

Fig. 19.1 Treatment algorithm according to the Barcelona Clinic Liver Cancer (BCLC) classification

and advanced stage HCC [7, 8] (Fig. 19.1). These include percutaneous ethanol injection (PEI), radiofrequency ablation (RFA), transarterial chemoembolization (TACE), and more recently, drug-eluting bead transarterial chemoembolization (DEB-TACE).

TACE involves the periodic injection of a chemotherapeutic agent, mixed with embolic material, administered selectively into the feeding arteries of the tumor resulting in higher intra-tumoral drug concentrations compared to intravenous therapy, with occlusion of the blood vessel causing infarction and necrosis [9]. In HCC patients, TACE achieved partial responses in up to 62% of patients, and significantly delayed tumor progression and vascular invasion [10–12]. Although survival benefit of TACE over symptomatic treatment or systematic chemotherapy was demonstrated in a meta-analysis of randomized controlled trials, overall survival at 3 years remain low (<30%) for intermediate HCC patients [13]. A further review failed to demonstrate a survival difference between TACE and embolization alone or superiority of one chemotherapeutic agent over another. Post-TACE complications, e.g., acute liver or renal failure, encephalopathy, ascites, and upper gastrointestinal bleeding, may be severe [14]. There is therefore a need for treatment regimens that improve response rates and survival, while reducing the risk of post-TACE complications.

DEB-TACE is a new drug delivery system that combines local embolization of vasculature with release of chemotherapy into adjacent tissue [15, 16]. Its intended use is for the treatment of hypervascular tumors such as HCC. The administration is

similar to conventional TACE, a minimally invasive procedure performed by interventional radiologists [15, 16]. Beads are composed of biocompatible polymers such
as polyvinyl alcohol (PVA) hydrogel that has been sulfonated in order for binding of chemotherapy (Fig. 19.2) [17]. The beads occlude distal vasculature causing
embolization, while the chemotherapy is delivered locally [18, 19].

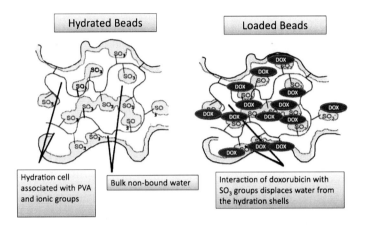

Fig. 19.2 Loading beads

In Vitro/In Vivo Data

Initial in vitro evaluation of the doxorubicin drug-eluting bead was performed by
Lewis et al. who performed a gravimetric analysis demonstrating the effect of drug
loading on bead water content and its consequent impact on bead compressibil-
ity was evaluated [16]. A T-cell apparatus was used to monitor the in vitro elution
of the drug from the beads over a period of 24 hours in various elution media. His
report determined DC bead™ spheres (Biocompatibles) could be easily loaded with
doxorubicin by immersion of the beads in the drug solution for 10–100 min depending on microsphere size. The maximum theoretic capacity of the DC bead™ was
45.0 mg/mL, but the most common commercial use is 37.5 mg/mL. Bead sizes
from 100 to 700 μm in size yielded somewhat similar kinetics in drug elution and
consistent drug delivery. This report confirmed that doxorubicin-loaded beads provide accurate dosage of drug per unit volume of beads. Drug elution is dependent
on ion exchange with the surrounding environment and this controlled and sustained
much more consistently than the rapid separation of the drug from historical lipiodol
use. An in vivo evaluation of the drug-eluting beads was again performed by Lewis
et al. evaluating both the 100300 and the 700–900 μm beads loaded at 37.5 mg of
doxorubicin per milliliter of hydrated beads [15]. Animals underwent embolization

with either gland beads or doxorubicin-loaded beads with serial systemic plasma levels of doxorubicin being measured during a 90-day follow-up period. Maximum plasma concentration of doxorubicin was seen at 650 ng/mL and 42.8 ng/mL for the 100–300 and 700–900 μm beads, respectively, observed at the 1-min time interval from infusion. They concluded that hepatic arterial embolization with drug-eluting beads was safe and well tolerated. In addition, they were able to demonstrate that the delivery of the doxorubicin drug-eluting bead caused consistent target tissue damage with minimal systemic impact based on the pharmacokinetic studies presented [19].

Phase I–II Studies

The initial pharmacokinetics of both conventional transarterial chemoembolization (cTACE) and DEB-TACE were reviewed in Varela et al. [20] and demonstrated that the DEB-TACE is an effective therapy with a favorable pharmacokinetic profile with significantly less systemic doxorubicin exposure when compared to cTACE. Doxorubicin maximum concentration and area under the curve were significantly lower in the DEB-TACE arm (78 ± 38 ng/ml and 662 ± 417 ng/ml min) than conventional TACE (2341 ± 3951 ng/ml and 1812 ± 1094 ng/ml min, $p = 0.0002$ and $p = 0.001$).

The Phase I/II study from Poon et al. [21] also demonstrated no dose-limiting toxicity for 150 mg per dose therapy, a low peak plasma doxorubicin concentration, and no evidence of doxorubicin-related toxicity. The results of these two

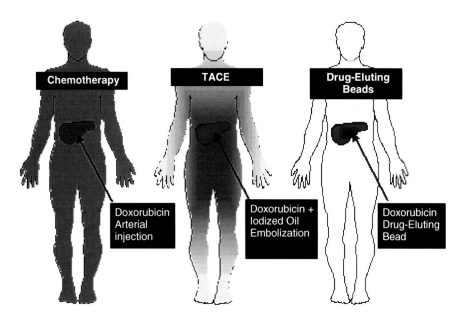

Fig. 19.3 Drug distribution

studies demonstrated the precise delivery of doxorubicin without systemic exposure and thus the theoretical advantage over systemic chemotherapy and conventional chemoembolization (Fig. 19.3).

Patient Selection

Chemotherapeutic options for DEB are DC/LC Beads loaded with doxorubicin (Adriblastin® and Adriamycin® RDF powder) at a maximum loaded dose of 75 mg/2 ml (one vial) with the total doses delivered at one setting should not exceed 150 mg.

DEB-TACE is indicated for the treatment of HCC who are not suitable for resection, liver transplantation, with confirmed diagnosis of HCC by clinical criteria (EASL) or confirmation by biopsy (Fig. 19.1).

Patient exclusion criteria for the treatment of HCC included bilirubin levels >3 mg/dL, advanced tumors including extensive vascular invasion and extrahepatic spread, and any contraindication for hepatic embolization procedures [portosystemic shunts, hepatofugal blood flow, impaired coagulation (platelet count <50,000/mm^3, prothrombin activity <50%)], renal insufficiency or failure (serum creatinine >3 mg/dL), and severe atheromatosis.

Delivery Technique

DEB administration is performed via angiography. After initial staging 3 Phase CT or dynamic MRI of the liver a planned two to three dose treatment schedule is needed before estimating true clinical response. After the initial treatment, additional treatments are given at 1–2 months, then again at 3–4 months based on patient's disease, tolerance, underlying hepatic dysfunction, and most importantly, physician assessment of the patient's overall condition. Treatment dosing and bead size is determined by the extent of the cancer within the liver, defined as either finite number of lesions or diffuse disease. For finite number of lesions, a minimum of two doses of 150 mg of doxorubicin loaded into two DC Bead^{TM} vials (100–300 μm given in a superselective catheter placement and 300–500 μm given in a lobar catheter placement) every 6–8 weeks (following toxicity and extending interval if toxicity seen) is administered. A repeat CT or MRI scan 1 month after the last treatment to evaluate response is recommended to decide on future treatments. For diffuse disease, a minimum of four doses of 150 mg doxorubicin loaded into two DC Bead^{TM} vials (100–300 μm and 300–500 μm both given in a lobar infusion) every 3–4 weeks (following toxicity and extending the interval if toxicity is seen). Repeat imaging 1 month after the last treatment to evaluate response is recommended to decide on future treatments.

Calculation of Tumor Response

Tumor response continues to be an Achilles' heel of hepatic intra-arterial therapy because of its lack of consistency in the literature and the current utilization of three different methods: RECIST [22], modified RECIST [23], and EASL [24]. Standards in measuring response are that no more than 5 "target lesions," defined as lesions >1 cm in size, should be identified in the liver. Tumor response can be calculated using either contrast-enhanced spiral computed tomography or MRI with quantification of tumor response according to either RECIST or EASL criteria.

Treatment response assessment using RECIST response criteria is defined as:

Complete Response (CR): CR is defined as the disappearance of measurable disease that persists for at least 4 weeks without the appearance of new measurable lesions.

Partial Response (PR): PR is defined as a ≥30% reduction in the sum of the products of the longest diameter (length) and the longest perpendicular diameter (width) of all measurable lesions compared to baseline, and no appearance of new measurable lesions.

Stable Disease (SD): Neither PR nor progressive disease (PD) criteria are met, taking as reference the smallest sum of the longest diameter recorded since the commencement of treatment.

Progressive Disease (PD): Occurs when one of the following conditions is met: [1] the sum of the cross products of all measurable lesions, including new lesions, increases by more than 50% compared to nadir or [2] new measurable lesions occur in any part of the body outside the liver.

The limitation of this system is the inability to take in account the lost of arterial enhancement. In other words, even though a lesion may go from completely solid to cystic, indicating tumor necrosis (Fig. 19.4), if it is the same size or even bigger this will be called SD or PD. Similarly there are no radiologic standards for reporting such responses, so it is incumbent on the treating physician to personally review the images in order to guide therapy decisions.

Recently some investigators have gone to using the another type of modified RECIST system described by Choi et al. in the reporting of response to therapy for gastrointestinal stromal tumors [25]. This system does take into account lack of enhancement, but only by measuring Hounsfield units. The challenge of using this system is that estimating Hounsfield units in a large heterogeneous mass can be difficult. These challenges can lead to a large amount of inter-observer and intra-observer variation in estimating response in HCC patients.

An additional modification to the RECSIT criteria was reported by Llovet et al., which keeps the core descriptions of the RECIST criteria but includes not just tumor size but the loss of arterial enhancement. These criteria include for a CR: loss of all arterial enhancement, PR: a 30% reduction in arterial enhancement, and PD: a new nodule greater than 1 cm in size [23].

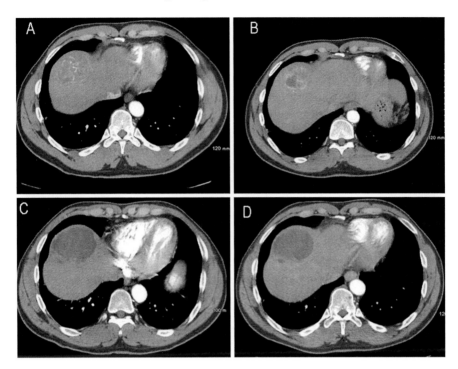

Fig. 19.4 Response. (**a**) Pre Drug Eluting Bead Therapy; (**b**) 6 weeks post therapy; (**c**) 6 months post therapy; (**d**) 12 months post therapy

The European Association for the Study of the Liver (EASL) Criteria measures local tumor response based on tumor progression with respect to change in necrosis. Since extensive tumor necrosis may not be paralleled by a reduction in the diameter of the tumor, in 2000, the EASL recommended a modification to the WHO criteria for use in HCC. The EASL Consensus Conference proposed that a reduction in viable tumor is more appropriate. The use of the EASL criteria is now accepted in assessment of treatment response in HCC particularly following the use of locoregional therapies such as chemoembolization; however, a guideline for measurement is not currently available. Local tumor response is measured as regression of treated lesions. New tumor development in a previously untreated area and extrahepatic disease is considered progressive disease.

The EASL criteria are applied for each target lesion as follows (see Fig. 19.5):

1) Record the longest diameter (as in RECIST measurements)
2) Estimate the percentage of the tumor volume that appears necrotic
3) Calculate the viable diameter by multiplying the longest diameter by (100% necrosed)/100.
4) Compare the viable diameter for each tumor to the baseline diameter

Tumor at Baseline   **Tumor at Follow-Up**
                                         (Necrosis shown as dark shading)

Diameter = 4.5 cm   Diameter = 3.8 cm
                                     Necrosis = 60%
                                     Viable diameter: 3.8 cm* (100–60)/100 = **1.5 cm**
                                     % Reduction: (4.5 –1.5)/4.5*100   = **67%**

Fig. 19.5 EASL example

Evaluation of Best Overall Response

The best overall response is defined as the best response from start of treatment through all follow-up visits or until disease progression/recurrence. In some circumstances, it may be difficult to distinguish residual disease from normal tissue. When the evaluation of complete response depends on this determination, it is recommended that the residual lesion be evaluated with dynamic imaging at two separate intervals (6–8 weeks apart) before confirming the complete response status.

Patients with a global deterioration of health status requiring discontinuation of treatment without objective evidence of disease progression at that time should be classified as having "symptomatic deterioration."

Clinical Use

Several studies have been published evaluating the safety and efficacy of DEB in HCC. The larger of the two studies by Malagari et al. evaluated 71 patients (60% men; 11% women; mean age 63; range 46–71 years) with documented unresectable HCC and a mean lesion size of 6.2 cm (range 3–10 cm) in diameter. Only patients with Child A or B cirrhosis were included in this study. The mean follow-up period was 23 months (range, 6–32 months). The total number of procedures was 196, with a median of 2.7 treatments per patient (range 1–4). Procedure-related mortality at 30 days was 0%. Eight patients (11.2%) completed only one embolization, 9 patients (12.8%) received 2 sessions, 54 patients (76%) received 3 sessions, and 8 (11.2%) received an additional fourth embolization. Further treatment was aborted in cases of cirrhosis decompensation (n = 5; 9.8%), progression of the disease in four patients (5.6%), or after a serious adverse event (one patient who developed liver abscess). Treatment was also discontinued when complete necrosis was observed.

Alphafetoprotein (AFP) levels decreased significantly in measurements 1 month post each procedure ($p < 0.001$). Bilirubin, c-GT, aspartate aminotransferase, alanine aminotransferase, and alkaline phosphatase (ALP) showed only transient increases observed during the study period. Severe procedure-related complications were seen in 4.2% (cholecystitis: $n = 1$; liver abscess: $n = 1$; pleural effusion: $n = 1$). Post-embolization syndrome (PES) was observed in all patients. Overall complete response (CR) according to EASL on an intention to treat basis was seen in 11 patients who developed complete necrosis (15.5%). Objective response (OR) ranged from 66.2 to 85.5% across the four treatments. Survival at 12 months was 97%. Sustained CR was observed in 11 (16%) and OR in 49 (72%). Sustained partial response was seen in 49 patients (72%). Survival at 18 months was 94%. At 24 months follow-up survival was 91%. Sustained OR was seen in 45 patients (66%) while sustained CR was 16% (11/68). At 30 months survival was 88%. One patient with CR developed multifocal HCC in areas that most likely were not embolized during the previous embolization sessions. In this patient recurrence-free survival was 28 months. The authors were able to conclude that DEB-TACE was an effective and safe procedure in the treatment of HCC patients not eligible for curative treatments, with high rates of response and high rates of mid-term survival.

The second study by Kettenback treated 30 patients with unresectable HCC in a single-center prospective trial using drug-eluting microspheres with the 500–700 μm beads were loaded with doxorubicin [26]. Interestingly, if required, additional unloaded beads were used to complete occlusion of the tumor feeding vessels in the belief that more ischemia would lead to greater response. Each patient was treated with up to four embolization cycles. According to RECIST criteria, at 6-month follow-up CR was obtained in 8 of 30 patients (27%), PR in 4 of 30 patients (13%), SD in 1 of 30 patients (3%), and PD in 12 of 30 patients (40%). Seven patients (23%) received one embolization cycle, 5 patients (17%) received two, 7 patients (23%) received three, and 11 patients (37%) received four cycles. The 30-day mortality of all embolization procedures performed was 1 of 82 (1%) and major adverse events were observed following 2 of 82 (2%) procedures (temporary liver failure and acute cholecystitis). The overall survival rate at 6 months was 93%. Interestingly, clinical symptoms were worse after the first cycle than in the subsequent cycles.

The last study is a prospective, single-blind, Phase II randomized controlled trial evaluating DEB-TACE against a control arm of conventional TACE (cTACE) in HCC, which was recently reported at the 10th Congress of the Cardiovascular and Interventional Radiological Society of Europe, Copenhagen, Sweden, on September 16, 2008 [27]. Two hundred and twelve patients were recruited at 23 European hospitals, with 201 patients receiving at least one treatment between November 25, 2005, and June 27, 2007. A total of 212 patients were randomized to DEB-TACE with DC Beads^{TM} ($n = 102$) or cTACE ($n = 110$). Due to dropouts prior to first treatment, the intention to treat population included 93 and 108 patients, of which 66 and 68, respectively, completed the study (Fig. 19.6). The majority of patients (66.7%) in both groups were considered more advanced as they met the higher

	DC Bead™ Group		cTACE Group
Visit 1	N=102*	Baseline Assessments/ Randomisation N=212*	N=110*
		↓	
Visit 2	N=93	First Chemoembolization: Procedure 1 and 1B‡ (Month 0)	N=108
		↓	
Visit 3		1-month MRI	
		↓	
Visit 4	N=76	Second Chemoembolization: Procedure 2 (Month 2)	N=88
		↓	
Visit 5		3-month MRI	
		↓	
Visit 6	N=57	Third Chemoembolization: Procedure 3 (Month 4)	N=61
		↓	
Visit 7	N=66†	6-month MRI & Study Completion†	N=68†
		↓	

* Causes for dropouts (DC Bead™ vs. cTACE) between randomisation and first chemoembolization were: post-consent ineligibility (4 vs. 1); patient or physician decision (3 vs. 0); surgical treatment (1 vs. 1); progression (1 vs. 0).

‡ For patients with bilobar disease who could not be treated superselectively in a single treatment, a second embolization was performed (Procedure 1B) for the alternative lobe within 3-weeks of the first procedure: DC Bead™ (n=8) vs. cTACE (n=5).

† Causes for dropouts between first chemoembolization and 6 months were (DC Bead™ vs. cTACE): AEs (12 vs. 14 patients), down staging (5 vs. 8), patient withdrawal (3 vs. 4), lack of efficacy (ie, extrahepatic progression of cancer, 2 vs. 8), lost to follow-up (2 vs. 1), patient death due to disease progression (0 vs. 3), and other (3 vs. 2).

Fig. 19.6 Flowchart of patients in the PRECISION V Trial

risk criteria for one or more of the four prognostic factors, i.e., Child–Pugh B, ECOG 1, bilobar, or recurrent disease (63/93 DEB-TACE and 72/108 cTACE patients). The mean total dose of doxorubicin administered was higher in the DEB-TACE group compared with the cTACE group (295 vs. 223 mg); this also applied to all subgroups.

Tumor response was measured by EASL Criteria. At 6 months, a CR was achieved in 25 (26.9%) vs. 24 (22.2%) patients, PR in 23 (24.7%) vs. 23 (21.3%) patients, and SD in 11 (11.8%) vs. 9 (8.3%) patients in the DEB-TACE vs. cTACE arms, respectively. Progressive disease (PD) was observed in 30 (32.3%) vs. 44 (40.7%) patients; data were missing or non-evaluable in 12 patients. Therefore, the objective response rate was 51.6% vs. 43.5% in the DEB-TACE vs. cTACE arms, respectively; the hypothesis of superiority was not met (one-sided $p = 0.11$) (Fig. 19.7).

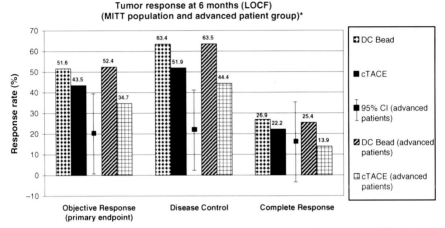

* More advanced disease was at least one of: Child-Pugh B, ECOG 1, undergone prior curative treatment (ie, recurrent disease), and presence of bilobar disease. In accordance with the EASL criteria: complete response (CR) - complete disappearance of all known viable tumour (assessed via uptake of contrast in the arterial phase of the MRI scan) and no new lesions; partial response (PR) - 50% reduction in viable tumour area of all measurable lesions; stable disease (SD) - all other cases; progressive disease (PD) - 25% increase in size of one or more measurable lesions or the appearance of new lesions. Objective Response was defined as CR + PR, and Disease Control as CR + PR + SD.

**Analysis of Advanced patient subgroup: Objective Response rate p=0.038, Disease Control rate p=0.026, Complete Response rate p=0.091 (Chi-square analysis).

Fig. 19.7 Tumor response at 6 months (LOCF) (MITT population and advanced patient group)*

Supplementary analyses showed that in the 67% of patients with more advanced disease, the incidence of objective response and disease control rates was statistically higher ($p = 0.038$ and $p = 0.026$, respectively) in the DEB-TACE group compared with the cTACE group (Fig. 19.7). The greatest difference in disease control rates between DEB-TACE vs. cTACE occurred in the ECOG 1 and Child–Pugh B subgroups (both 63% vs. 32%; Fig. 19.8).

There was no statistically significant difference ($p = 0.86$) between treatments for the primary safety endpoint (treatment-related SAEs within 30 days of a procedure): 19 (20.4%) DEB-TACE patients experienced 28 events and 21 (19.4%) cTACE patients experienced 24 events. Supplementary analysis indicated that the incidence of all serious adverse events (SAEs) within 30 days of procedure was consistently lower in the DEB-TACE group for the less advanced and more advanced patients based on the four stratification factors (Fig. 19.9).

The overall frequency of treatment-emergent adverse events (TEAEs) per 100 treatments was lower in the DEB-TACE compared with the cTACE group, as were

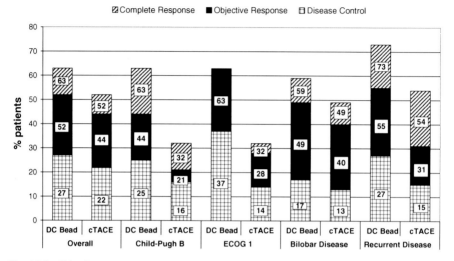

Fig. 19.8 Objective response rate and disease control rate of patients at 6 months by prognosis at baseline (MITT population)

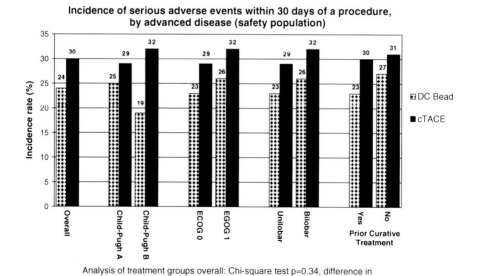

Fig. 19.9 Incidence of serious adverse events within 30 days of a procedure, by advanced disease (safety population)

treatment-related TEAEs, Southwestern Oncology Group (SWOG) toxicity Grade 3 or 4 TEAEs, Grade 3 or 4 treatment-related TEAEs and treatment-related SAEs.

The majority of TEAEs were mild or moderate in intensity with a lower frequency of severe events (20.4% vs. 30.6%) reported in DEB-TACE vs. cTACE patients. The only event with a difference in incidence of $\geq 10\%$ was alopecia, reported in 2.2% DEB-TACE and 19.4% cTACE patients. Serious liver toxicity post-chemoembolization was also lower in the DEB-TACE group. Cardiac function was maintained in the DEB-TACE group whereas there was a deterioration in left ventricular ejection fraction in the cTACE group (DEB-TACE $+2.7\pm10.1$ percentage points, cTACE -1.5 ± 7.6 percentage points, $p = 0.018$, Fig. 19.5). There were eight deaths in each arm of the study. Of these, two and six patients in the DEB-TACE and cTACE arms, respectively, died within 30 days of a procedure. Four patients died due to disease progression (one DEB-TACE and three cTACE).

Further analyses established a significant benefit (estimate of true incidence – 14.1%, 95% CI -24.7% to -3.5%, $p = 0.012$) in favor of DEB-TACE over cTACE in reducing the effects of systemic doxorubicin (alopecia, skin discoloration, mucositis, and marrow suppression): 12 events in 11 (11.8%) patients vs. 40 in 28 (25.9%). Alopecia, the most commonly occurring event, was almost completely absent in DEB-TACE patients (1 vs. 23 events). Using the assumption of independence of events, the difference in frequencies of doxorubicin-related events was also significant ($p = 0.0001$). The incidence and frequency of post-embolization syndrome events were comparable in the treatment groups: 35 events in 23 (24.7% DEB-TACE) and 43 events in 28 (25.9%) cTACE patients.

Additional studies in the earlier use of DEB-TACE have also been reported to evaluate the toxicity of the therapy and the sensitivity of the radiologic response rates [28, 29]. Two recent bridge to transplant studies demonstrated no evidence of procedure-related mortality in multiple treatments (median number 3) of potential transplant candidates. These studies also demonstrated a much higher rate of histologic complete necrosis (46%) when compared to the reported radiologic complete response (26%), demonstrating the insensitivity of current radiologic response criteria.

Response Rates

Using EASL criteria, publications following the treatment of HCC reported overall response (OR) of 65% at 1 month, 71% at 4 months, 75% at 6–7 months, and 88% at 10 months (Table 19.1). An investigation by Lencioni et al. involving combination therapy of RFA with DEB-TACE after incomplete ablation using EASL criteria reported OR of 75% in 20 patients with HCC after 12 months as well as SD and PD rates of 0 and 25%, respectively (Table 19.2) [30]. Using RECIST criteria, overall response was less based on the limitations of the criteria with 4 months 36% and 6 months 42%.

Table 19.1 Five published studies reviewed

Author	Date	Histology	Pt #	CT agent	Response rate reported?	Complications reported	Survival reported?
K. Malagari	Nov 2007	HCC	71	Doxorubicin	Yes	Yes	Yes
R. Lencioni	Aug 2008	HCC	20	Doxorubicin	Yes	Yes	Yes
R.T.P. Poon	Sep 2007	HCC	35	Doxorubicin	Yes	Yes	Yes
M. Varela	Mar 2007	HCC	27	Doxorubicin	Yes	Yes	Yes
J. Kettenbach	Jan 2007	HCC	30	Doxorubicin	Yes	Yes	Yes

Overall Safety

Two methods of calculating complications were reported in publications, by procedure and by patient. The most common DEB-TACE procedure-associated complications included fever (85% of patients, 46% of procedures), nausea and vomiting (93% of patients, 52% of procedures), abdominal pain (80% of patients, 44% of procedures), and liver abscess (2% of patients, 1% of procedures). Postembolic syndrome (PES), consisting of fever, abdominal pain, and nausea/vomiting, was reported instead of individual symptoms in two studies as 82% of patients (75/91). All studies reported length of hospital stay, averaging 2.3 days per procedure. Mortality was reported as 11 in 533 (2%) procedures (11 in 253 or 5% of patients). Causes of mortality included three myocardial infarctions, five cases of progressive liver disease, one pulmonary embolism, one case of postoperative sepsis, and one case of liver failure. Additional complications included eight cases of mild asthenia, seven cases of alopecia, two cases of acute cholecystitis, two hepatic infarctions, one pulmonary effusion, one gastric ulcer hemorrhage, a single case of variceal bleed, one case of spontaneous bacterial peritonitis, a single case of rash, and a single case of pancreatitis. Transient increase in liver function enzymes was reported in most studies [26, 31].

Summary

The current collective data on the use of DEB-TACE in HCC patients provides sufficient evidence to support the use of this treatment as a safe and effective chemoembolic treatment in HCC patients. In addition, with the recent completion of the randomized phase II study there is growing evidence to support the use of DEB-TACE therapy over conventional doxorubicin TACE. Lastly, patients who would benefit from tumor down-staging prior to surgery, transplant, or resection should be considered candidates for DEB-TACE treatment with the knowledge that early radiologic tumor necrosis rates may not correlate with tumor histological outcome.

However, problems still remain in evaluating hepatic arterial treatments. Lack of standardization of response and other criteria has made it difficult to compare studies utilizing various hepatic arterial therapies, including Yttrium-90, TACE, TAE,

Table 19.2 Response rate according to criteria and follow-up in HCC

Author	Criteria	F/U (month)	Pt#	OR	CR	PR	SD	PD	N/A
Malagari et al. (2007)	EASL	1	71	45(63%)	3(4%)	42(59%)	26(37%)	0(0%)	0(0%)
Poon et al. (2007)	EASL	1	30	21(70%)	2(7%)	19(63%)	2(7%)	7(23%)	0(0%)
Malagari et al. (2007)	EASL	4	63	53(84%)	4(6%)	49(78%)	8(13%)	2(3%)	0(0%)
Poon et al. (2007)	EASL	4	28	12(43%)	4(14%)	8(29%)	3(11%)	13(46%)	0(0%)
Malagari et al. (2007)	EASL	7	54	43(80%)	4(7%)	39(72%)	9(17%)	2(4%)	0(0%)
Varela et al. (2007)	EASL	6	27	18(67%)	7(26%)	11(41%)	1(4%)	5(19%)	3(11%)
Malagari et al. (2007)	EASL	10	8	7(88%)	2(25%)	5(63%)	1(13%)	0(0%)	0(0%)
Lencioni et al. (2008)[a]	EASL	12	20	15(75%)	10(50%)	5(25%)	0(0%)	5(25%)	0(0%)
Poon et al. (2007)	RECIST	1	30	15(50%)	0(0%)	15(50%)	8(27%)	7(23%)	0(0%)
Poon et al. (2007)	RECIST	4	28	10(36%)	0(0%)	10(36%)	5(18%)	13(46%)	0(0%)
Varela et al. (2007)	RECIST	6	27	12(44%)	0(0%)	12(44%)	7(26%)	5(19%)	3(11%)
Kettenbach et al. (2007)	RECIST	6	30	12(40%)	8(27%)	4(13%)	1(3%)	12(40%)	5(17%)

[a]Study utilized combined therapy with RFA followed by DEB-TACE

and DEB-TACE for treatment of hepatic malignancy. Future studies must specifically report the number of treatment cycles of DEB administered, total dose of chemotherapy given to patients, differences in inclusion and exclusion criteria, and criteria used to report responses.

Certain trends can be seen clearly, such as an increase in overall response as patients receive additional cycles of DEB-TACE and higher levels of chemotherapy. Patients who did not respond adequately to initial therapy and who did not have significant toxicity were candidates for additional treatments until either adequate response was achieved or they received the maximal dose of chemotherapy. It will be helpful to correlate these factors with response criteria in future studies in order to determine if overall response is significantly dependent on multiple treatments.

The difference in response reported by EASL criteria vs. RECIST criteria was notable as well. Among publications reporting both criteria (i.e., Poon et al.) [21], EASL had greater tumor response rates than measurements using RECIST criteria. RECIST criteria determine measurements based on extent of measurable disease and the presence of arterial phase on CT, not taking extent of necrosis into consideration. EASL criteria, in contrast, measures both tumor necrosis and viable tumor in order to determine extent of response. While results based on criteria varied, long-term response and survival should not consider that DEB-TACE administration was similarly independent of evaluation criteria.

Short-term follow-up provided valuable information concerning response rates. While short-term evaluation indicates that the procedure effectively embolizes and causes tumor necrosis, continued follow-up is essential in order to determine the long-term significance of DEB-TACE and its role as an alternative therapy or palliative measure in treating patients with hepatic malignancy.

DEB-TACE remains a relatively safe procedure, with few long-term, serious complications associated with its administration. While symptoms of PES, such as fever, nausea or vomiting, and abdominal pain, appear to occur in most patients, these symptoms are associated with short hospital stays averaging 2.3 days among publications, significantly less when compared to conventional TACE procedures. The most frequent major complication associated with this procedure is liver abscess, the rate of which has been reported as 0.29–1.6%. Other complications were infrequent although some were quite severe. Overall procedure-related mortality is potentially lower than the reported values (2.1–5.2%) because these studies included both procedure-related causes of death such as sepsis and hepatic failure and death secondary to progressive disease, cardiovascular disease, pulmonary embolism, and other causes. Patients selected for these studies have predispositions to comorbidities due to diminished hepatic function, and potentially other age-related, lifestyle-related conditions which should be taken into consideration [26].

Use of DEB-TACE in current publications seems to be restricted to patients with unresectable liver disease and reasonable hepatic function (Child–Pugh A or B). However future work is ongoing in treating patients with more severe disease, specifically Child–Pugh class C patients. In addition with the recent study by Lencioni et al. evaluating the use of DEB-TACE as combination therapy with radiofrequency ablation failures; further studies are needed to evaluate combination of DEB-TACE with other procedures. Lastly, with the recent United States Food and Drug Administration approval of Sorafenib for intermediate stage HCC, the current SPACE study will further answer the potential benefit of combination DEB and Sorafenib.

Conclusions

DEB-TACE is becoming a more widely utilized therapy in hepatocellular cancer. Expansion of success beyond response rates is needed since this is not a reliable surrogate of progression-free survival or overall survival. Ongoing clinical trials will further clarify the optimal timing and strategy of this technology.

The current results show DEB-TACE to produce beneficial tumor response and to low complication rates. DEB-TACE has the potential to become an effective alternate therapy or palliative measure in the treatment of hepatic malignancy, but standardization needs to be established in both delivery and data collection in order to clarify efficacy. It is a safe alternative in the treatment of unresectable hepatic malignancy, but is unproven as adjunctive therapy to other standard therapies such as resection and radiofrequency ablation. Further investigation is essential to better define its role as an adjunct in treating hepatic malignancy.

References

1. El Serag HB, Davila JA, Petersen NJ et al (2003) The continuing increase in the incidence of hepatocellular carcinoma in the United States: an update. Ann Intern Med 139:817–823
2. Davila JA, Morgan RO, Shaib Y et al (2004) Hepatitis C infection and the increasing incidence of hepatocellular carcinoma: a population-based study. Gastroenterology 127: 1372–1380
3. Parkin DM, Bray F, Ferlay J et al (2005) Global cancer statistics, 2002. CA Cancer J Clin 55:74–108
4. Bosch FX, Ribes J, Cleries R et al (2005) Epidemiology of hepatocellular carcinoma. Clin Liver Dis 9:191–211, v
5. Srivatanakul P, Sriplung H, Deerasamee S (2004) Epidemiology of liver cancer: an overview. Asian Pac J Cancer Prev 5:118–125
6. Ahmed F, Perz JF, Kwong S et al (2008) National trends and disparities in the incidence of hepatocellular carcinoma, 1998–2003. Prev Chronic Dis 5:A74
7. Bruix J, Sherman M (2005) Management of hepatocellular carcinoma. Hepatology 42: 1208–1236
8. Reuter NP, Woodall CE, Scoggins CR et al (2009) Radiofrequency Ablation vs. Resection for Hepatic Colorectal Metastasis: Therapeutically Equivalent? J Gastrointest Surg 13:486–491
9. Raoul JL, Heresbach D, Bretagne JF et al (1992) Chemoembolization of hepatocellular carcinomas. A study of the biodistribution and pharmacokinetics of doxorubicin. Cancer 70:585–590
10. Raoul JL, Guyader D, Bretagne JF et al (1994) Randomized controlled trial for hepatocellular carcinoma with portal vein thrombosis: intra-arterial iodine-131-iodized oil versus medical support. J Nucl Med 35:1782–1787

11. Raoul JL, Guyader D, Bretagne JF et al (1997) Prospective randomized trial of chemoembolization versus intra-arterial injection of 131I-labeled-iodized oil in the treatment of hepatocellular carcinoma. Hepatology 26:1156–1161

12. Bruix J, Llovet JM, Castells A et al (1998) Transarterial embolization versus symptomatic treatment in patients with advanced hepatocellular carcinoma: results of a randomized, controlled trial in a single institution. Hepatology 27:1578–1583

13. Llovet JM, Bruix J (2003) Systematic review of randomized trials for unresectable hepatocellular carcinoma: Chemoembolization improves survival. Hepatology 37:429–442

14. Marelli L, Stigliano R, Triantos C et al (2006) Treatment outcomes for hepatocellular carcinoma using chemoembolization in combination with other therapies. Cancer Treat Rev 32:594–606

15. Lewis AL, Taylor RR, Hall B et al (2006) Pharmacokinetic and safety study of doxorubicin-eluting beads in a porcine model of hepatic arterial embolization. J Vasc Interv Radiol 17:1335–1343

16. Lewis AL, Gonzalez MV, Lloyd AW et al (2006) DC bead: in vitro characterization of a drug-delivery device for transarterial chemoembolization. J Vasc Interv Radiol 17:335–342

17. Tang Y, Taylor RR, Gonzalez MV et al (2006) Evaluation of irinotecan drug-eluting beads: a new drug-device combination product for the chemoembolization of hepatic metastases. J Control Release 116:e55–e56

18. Taylor RR, Tang Y, Gonzalez MV et al (2007) Irinotecan drug eluting beads for use in chemoembolization: in vitro and in vivo evaluation of drug release properties. Eur J Pharm Sci 30:7–14

19. Lewis AL, Gonzalez MV, Leppard SW et al (2007) Doxorubicin eluting beads – 1: effects of drug loading on bead characteristics and drug distribution. J Mater Sci Mater Med 18:1691–1699

20. Varela M, Real MI, Burrel M et al (2007) Chemoembolization of hepatocellular carcinoma with drug eluting beads: efficacy and doxorubicin pharmacokinetics. J Hepatol 46:474–481

21. Poon RT, Tso WK, Pang RW et al (2007) A phase I/II trial of chemoembolization for hepatocellular carcinoma using a novel intra-arterial drug-eluting bead. Clin Gastroenterol Hepatol 5:1100–1108

22. Therasse P, Arbuck SG, Eisenhauer EA et al (2000) New guidelines to evaluate the response to treatment in solid tumors. European Organization for Research and Treatment of Cancer, National Cancer Institute of the United States, National Cancer Institute of Canada. J Natl Cancer Inst 92:205–216

23. Llovet JM, Di Bisceglie AM, Bruix J et al (2008) Design and endpoints of clinical trials in hepatocellular carcinoma. J Natl Cancer Inst 100:698–711

24. Bruix J, Sherman M, Llovet JM et al (2001) Clinical management of hepatocellular carcinoma. Conclusions of the Barcelona-2000 EASL conference. European Association for the Study of the Liver. J Hepatol 35:421–430

25. Choi H, Charnsangavej C, Faria SC et al (2007) Correlation of computed tomography and positron emission tomography in patients with metastatic gastrointestinal stromal tumor treated at a single institution with imatinib mesylate: proposal of new computed tomography response criteria. J Clin Oncol 25:1753–1759

26. Kettenbach J, Stadler A, Katzler IV et al (2008) Drug-loaded microspheres for the treatment of liver cancer: review of current results. Cardiovasc Intervent Radiol 31:468–476

27. Lammer J (2009) Evidence for Drug-Eluting Bead, initial data release from a 212 patient international, multicentre, prospective randomised controlled trial of doxorubicin in the treatment of hepatocellular carcinoma by drug-eluting bead embolisation. 2008. Oral presentation, Plenary session, Cardiovascular and Interventional Radiological Society of Europe annual meeting, 15th Sept 2009 Copenhagen

28. Nicolini A, Crespi S, Martinetti L (2007) TAE vs precision TACE in patients in the transplant waiting list. Cardiovascular and Interventional Radiological Society of Europe October 18th 2007 Milan

29. Goffette P (2008) Drug-eluting beads in the management of hepatocellular carcinoma prior to liver transplantation. European Conference of Interventional Oncology, Florence, Italy, April 12, 2008.
30. Lencioni R, Crocetti L, Petruzzi P et al (2008) Doxorubicin-eluting bead-enhanced radiofrequency ablation of hepatocellular carcinoma: a pilot clinical study. J Hepatol 49: 217–222
31. Malagari K (2008) Drug-eluting particles in the treatment of HCC: chemoembolization with doxorubicin-loaded DC bead. Expert Rev Anticancer Ther 8:1643–1650

Chapter 20
Yttrium-90 Radioembolotherapy for Hepatocellular Cancer

Ravi Murthy, Pritesh Mutha, and Sanjay Gupta

Keywords Hepatocellular cancer · Yttrium-90

Introduction

Hepatocellular carcinoma (HCC) accounts for between 85 and 90% of primary liver cancers. Over a million cases of hepatocellular cancer occur annually making it the fifth most common cancer worldwide and the third most common cause of cancer mortality. In the United States, the incidence of HCC has steadily increased over the past two decades, with an estimated 21,370 new cases having occurred in 2008 [1]. HCC-related mortality has increased in parallel with 18,410 estimated deaths during the same time period [1]. In addition, the incidence of HCC in patients with both known risks such as hepatitis C and unknown risk factors is increasing [2]. Additionally, at presentation most patients with HCC have limited treatment options because of their advanced and multifocal distribution. Compounding the problem in management, the majority of patients with HCC are not candidates for surgical intervention, with only 15–25% suitable for resection. Despite the improvement in survival following transplantation, the incidence of tumor recurrence and associated mortality is high [3]. Therefore, the vast majority of patients with unresectable or recurrent disease are eventually relegated for consideration of various forms of local-regional in-situ cytoreductive treatments. One such treatment modality is non-selective extracorporeal X-ray radiotherapy. While radiotherapy represents a very effective tumoricidal modality, it has limited applicability because intrinsic low radiation tolerance of the innocent bystander 'normal' hepatocytes. Experimental approaches for enhancing the selectivity are possible by employing a multi-dimensional approach. However, since the vast majority of patients possess

R. Murthy (✉)
Section of Interventional Radiology, Division of Diagnostic Imaging, The University of Texas MD Anderson Cancer Center, Houston, TX, USA

K.M. McMasters, J.-N. Vauthey (eds.), *Hepatocellular Carcinoma*,
DOI 10.1007/978-1-60327-522-4_20, © Springer Science+Business Media, LLC 2011

disease that is multifocal or irregular in morphology, the total dose that is administered to the liver parenchyma adjacent to the cancer curtails these approaches [4].
Therefore, techniques that circumvent this limitation of radiotherapy non-selectivity
are paramount to enhance clinical outcomes. One such method exploits the preferential arterial flow and enhanced microvascular density of hepatic neoplasia that is
central to the efficacy of other more common transarterial therapies such as hepatic
artery chemoembolization. Biocompatible microspheres acting as carriers can con-
ceptually deliver radiation preferentially to tumors following hepatic artery delivery
via embolization in the tumor-related vessels (Fig. 20.1). Furthermore, employing
high-energy beta radiation as opposed to a traditional gamma radiation would create an intense local radiotherapeutic effect that is proportional to the density of
microsphere distribution. Yttrium-90 (^{90}Y) incorporated on appropriately calibrated
microspheres fulfills these criteria as the prototypical device that has been used for
decades in the treatment of hepatic neoplasia including HCC.

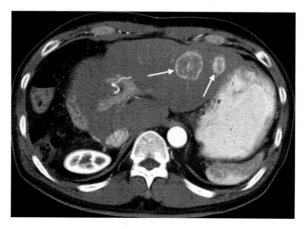

Fig. 20.1 A 64-year-old Asian male with chronic hepatitis B. Right hepatectomy had been performed for a pathology proven HCC. Seven months later the patient was developed new multifocal
HCC. Axial image from contrast-enhanced CT scan. Two discreet hypervascular foci (*white
arrows*) consistent with HCC are noted in the left lobe remnant. 39.2 mCi resin microspheres
were delivered via the left hepatic artery

Development of ^{90}Y Microsphere Embolotherapy for HCC

The added clinical benefit and potential toxicities of regional cancer therapy via
the introduction of therapeutic agents into their blood supply was investigated
by Kloop et al [5]. Since most of the therapeutic substance passed into the
systemic circulation the therapeutic index was narrow. The necessary advance
required provision of a carrier for the therapeutic agent that prevented the passage
through the tumor via vascular entrapment. This was investigated by Muller and
Rossier who administered radioactive zinc and gold adsorbed onto calibrated carbon

particles, whereby the particles were trapped in the lung precapillary arterioles via embolization [6]. Under similar conditions, Pochin et al. were also able to demonstrate liver radioisotope deposition secondary to the dissociation of the isotope from its carrier. They also suggested that the safety to the patient and personnel would be best served by using a beta as opposed to gamma radiation source that would allow compensation for non-uniform distribution [7]. Ya et al. suggested that ^{90}Y would be the ideal agent *(vide infra)* and was used to successfully treat two patients with metastatic liver adenocarcinoma [8]. Kim et al. published a model in which ^{90}Y was used to make experimental observations in humans and rabbits in which the principles of the delivery remain the same as utilized today. The ceramic microspheres $(60\mu +/- 5)$ used in these experiments were provided by 3M corporation (Minneapolis, MN). Seventeen patients with either primary or metastatic tumors were treated by either direct or blood stream infusion of ^{90}Y microspheres (range 27–380 mCi). Five patients who had objective improvement harbored vascular tumors [9]. Blanchard et al. demonstrated regression could be achieved using 15 μ +/- 3 ^{90}Y laden plastic microspheres in a VX_2 carcinoma in rabbit liver model [10]. The same group published their results of ^{90}Y microspheres delivered by direct injection and by local transvascular infusion in 31 patients in which objective regression was noted in 30% of tumors [11]. In a larger series 118 patients with liver cancer were randomly selected to receive chemotherapy alone, transhepatic arterial delivery of 10–20 μ plastic or ceramic ^{90}Y microspheres alone, and chemotherapy with ^{90}Y microspheres [12]. Scintigraphy was performed following the delivery documenting intra-abdominal distribution. The combination was well tolerated. Parallel research was performed by Grady et al. who used yttrium oxide particles to treat 76 patients and demonstrated objective tumor response that included HCC [13]. Subsequent publications have confirmed the observation of a survival benefit with hypervascular tumors [14]. In a pilot study, a whole-liver treatment was performed under fluoroscopy and planar secondary gamma emission scans (Bremsstrahlung) were successfully used to confirm the localization of radiation confined to the liver. The potential lethality of the therapy was noted when ^{90}Y inadvertently dissociated from the microspheres resulted in fatal bone marrow suppression. Wollner et al. performed two safety studies of non-radioactive and radioactive glass microspheres in a canine model [15] in which alterations of the central veins were noted in both groups but fibrosis was seen only with radioactive microspheres. They extrapolated that the optimal human dose would range between 50 and 100 Gy forming the basis of activity selection for human dose-escalation studies. Concurrent safety and toxicity data became available through brief reports [16–20]. The tolerability of the therapy was then re-assessed in separate phase I trials. Shepherd et al. conducted a phase I study in 10 patients with primary HCC [21] in which extrahepatic shunting was assessed scintigraphically using gamma emitting technetium-labeled macroaggregated albumin (^{99m}Tc MAA) and bremsstrahlung scans were obtained to assess distribution. The maximal dose delivered was 100 Gy dose; although the median tolerated dose was not achieved survival favored hypervascular tumors. This study also provided the initial safety data that served as the basis for patient selection and technique that enabled further studies with ^{90}Y in HCC. The role of arteriography in toxicity reduction via assessment of extrahepatic arteries that would preclude gastrointestinal dispersion of the microspheres was studied within a separate phase I study of 25 patients by Andrews et al. [22] in which 24 patients with HCC were treated with ^{90}Y microspheres with doses ranging between 50 and 150 Gy. The only complications were reversible gastritis/duodenitis. Partial response was noted in five patients (21%) with three long-term survivors exceeding 4 years. Yan et al. published similar data reporting a 50% reduction in tumor mass in 13 of 18 patients [17]. The recent commercial introduction of ^{90}Y microspheres worldwide has led to a renewed interest in this multidisciplinary therapy.

Characteristics of Yttrium-90

Yttrium-90 (^{90}Y) is a pure β-emitter with a physical half-life of 64.2 h, after which it decays into stable Zirconium. It is produced via neutron bombardment of Yttrium-89. The average energy of β-emission is 0.9367 MeV, with a mean tissue penetration of 2.5 mm and a maximum penetration of 10 mm. One gigabecquerel (27 mCi) of ^{90}Y per kilogram of tissue provides a dose of 50 Gy.

Commercially Available ^{90}Y Microspheres: SIR-Spheres and Therasphere

In the United States, two Food and Drug Administration (FDA)-approved ^{90}Y microsphere products are in current clinical use; TheraSphere® (MDS Nordion Inc., Kanata, Ontario, Canada), which are glass microspheres, and the resin-based SIR-Spheres® (SIRTeX Medical Ltd., Sydney, New South Wales, Australia) (Table 20.1).

The glass ^{90}Y microspheres are approved in the USA for use in radiation treatment or as a neoadjuvant to surgery or transplantation in patients with hepatocellular carcinoma (HCC) under the auspices of a humanitarian device exemption for orphan devices. Therasphere is supplied in a 0.5 mL of sterile, pyrogen-free water contained in a 0.3-mL V-bottom vial secured within a 12-mm clear acrylic shield. Therasphere

Table 20.1 Glass & Resin ^{90}Y microsphere device description

Parameter	Resin	Glass
Trade	SIR-Spheres	TheraSphere
Diameter	22 +/− 10 μ	32 +/− 10 μ
Specific gravity	1.6 g/dl	3.6 g/dl
Activity per particle	50 Bq	2500 Bq
Average number of microspheres per administered activity	40–80 million	1.2–8 million
Material	Resin with bound ^{90}Y	Glass with ^{90}Y in matrix

has been used for neoplasia other than HCC under compassionate circumstances adherence to FDA-related guidelines on such use are encouraged. Therasphere is available in six activity (GBq) sizes: 3, 5, 7, 10, 15, and 20. The corresponding number of microspheres per vial is 1.2, 2, 2.8, 4, 6, and 8 million.

The resin ^{90}Y microspheres have premarket approval for the treatment of hepatic metastasis from colorectal primary (mCRC), with adjuvant hepatic arterial infusion of floxuridine. However, globally the regulatory approval for both products is more generic with hepatic neoplasia being the most common. SIR-Spheres® are supplied in a vial that contains 3 GBq of the device. Use of resin microspheres outside of the FDA-specific labeling is considered off-label. Users should consult their institutional and regulatory agencies before such utilization and is beyond the scope of this chapter.

Patient Selection

Patients who are being considered for ^{90}Y radioembolotherapy (Fig. 20.2) should have good performance status (ECOG ≤2, Karnofsky performance status >60%), unresectable primary or metastatic hepatic disease with liver-dominant tumor burden, normal bone marrow function, and adequate pulmonary reserve. No contraindications for hepatic artery catheterization and expected survival ≥3 months. Patients should have measurable disease, and a triple phase CT contrast-enhanced scan is the preferred imaging modality of choice since it can accurately quantify the tumor, normal liver volume, and portal vein patency; however, MRI is becoming increasingly common. Serum chemistry should be obtained to evaluate for liver function tests, complete blood count, and renal function [23].

Absolute contraindications to ^{90}Y radioembolotherapy include pretherapy ^{99m}Tc MAA scan demonstrating the potential of 30 Gy radiation exposure to the lung

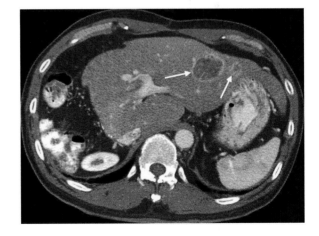

Fig. 20.2 Axial image from contrast-enhanced CT scan. Two months after therapy demonstrates lack of arterial enhancement and hypervascular rim highly suggestive of response to ^{90}Y radioembolotherapy

or flow to the gastrointestinal tract that cannot be corrected by catheter techniques. Relative contraindications include prior radiation therapy involving the liver, pregnant or pediatric patients [24].

Hepatic Arterial Supply and Gastrointestinal Ulceration

There is an increasing volume of technologies for transarterial liver-directed therapy for patients with inoperable HCC. All of these modalities require applied arteriographic knowledge of the liver, since only 60% of the population has a "classic" hepatic arterial anatomy. Readers are directed to a comprehensive review of this topic [25]. When hepatic arteries arise aberrantly they divide the liver into separate perfused segments. Extrahepatic occlusion of these vessels may facilitate delivery of the microspheres to the entire liver or to a tumor-bearing segment via a single efferent in most cases if necessary. The identification and characterization of arteries that supply the gastro-duodenum are paramount. High volume hepatic arteriography with delayed imaging can often identify these arteries that are usually the right gastric, gastroduodenal, retroduodenal, umbilical, accessory left gastric, and accessory phrenic. Once identified, they should be catheterized and occluded via fibered microcoils at their hepatic artery origins. Although historically ulceration has been reported to occur in up to 12% of the population, in most experienced centers the risk is currently less than 1% [26].

Unlike traditional brachytherapy sources that possess physical mass, ^{90}Y microspheres are unique. They share characteristics with radiopharmaceuticals as they require suspension in either sterile water or saline during delivery. Furthermore, the ^{90}Y microspheres are radiolucent and due to concerns of increased viscosity iodinated contrast cannot be used as the suspending agent thereby making the actual administration a 'blind' process. In the case of the low embolic load glass device, arterial occlusion of the parent vessel has not been reported [27]. However, with the higher embolic load SIR-Spheres, such embolic occlusion has been observed, therefore, the prescribed volume of ^{90}Y microspheres is delivered in divided aliquots alternating with contrast to assess for persistent arterial patency [28]. As a consequence of these unique problems associated with the delivery process, the prevention of non-target dispersion of the ^{90}Y microspheres can only be reliably achieved by blockade of all potential routes of extrahepatic flow before actual therapeutic ^{90}Y microsphere delivery. Compounding the problems of delivery, the catheters become radiation sources once delivery has commenced.

Hepatopulmonary Shunting

Pathological arteriovenous shunts are integral with the development of hepatic neoplasia. Non-radioactive microspheres used for hepatic embolotherapy are typically larger than 100 μ. These shunts allow particles to traverse the capillary plexus of the tumor without impeding their egress into the hepatic vein. Once in the hepatic venous side, these particles then travel via the venous circulation of the heart into the pulmonary artery and subsequently embolize in the arteriolar bed. ^{90}Y microspheres are considerably smaller, with a median diameter of 25μ. When these particles embed in the pulmonary interstitium, they irradiated in addition to causing vascular blockade. Therefore, inherent to the therapy is some element of pulmonary irradiation that is clinically silent until a threshold of 30 Gy is reached from a single or 50 Gy from cumulative exposure, but modern imaging techniques have called this threshold into question [29, 30]. Clinically apparent radiation pneumonitis is often fatal despite aggressive treatment with steroids.

The magnitude of hepatopulmonary shunting is estimated via the hepatic arterial injection of ^{99m}Tc MAA, acting as a microsphere surrogate in terms of both size and distribution. It is important that liver injection of MAA is delivered with flow rates and catheter position that mimic the anticipated ^{90}Y infusion rate and catheter position. The ratio of the lung to liver deposition corrected for background is expressed as a percentage of the injected activity. The factors that increase the likelihood of lung shunting are the histology of the primary tumor (HCC> neuroendocrine>colorectal), tumor burden, and prior ^{90}Y radioembolotherapy [31]. Hepatic venous occlusion has been observed to decrease the shunt fraction to allow for safe radioembolotherapy.

Dosimetry

Users are directed to the product insert provided for each device. Dosimetry improvements represent a current area of intense research for many groups. The dose calculation methodologies currently available assume uniform distribution of the ^{90}Y microspheres in the end organ, although with the resin ^{90}Y microsphere equations that integrate relative tumor burden and lung shunting allows for refinement in dosimetry. Although these assumptions of uniformity are intrinsically erroneous, in clinical practice objective benefits observed thus far with mild to minimal toxicity have created an atmosphere of optimism for the therapy.

The cumulative lung dose calculation is identical regardless of which device is utilized and is given by the following equation:

$$\text{Cumulative absorbed lung radiation dose} = 50$$

$$\times \text{ lung mass} \sum_{i=1}^{n} A_i \times LSF_i$$

where A_i = activity infused, LSF_i = lung shunt fraction, n = number of infusions with the assumption of approximately lung blood volume mass = 1 kg.

Activity reduction is allowed for resin microsphere using the following table.

Hepatopulmonary shunting %	Recommended dose reduction %
<10	0
10–15	20
15–20	40
>20	100

Therasphere activity can be calculated using the following equation:

$$A \text{ (Gbq) glass} = \frac{D(Gy) \times M \text{ (kg)}}{50}$$

When the hepatopulmonary shunting is taken into account, the dose is then calculated as

$$D(Gy) = [A(GBq) \times 50 \times (1 - LSF)]/M \text{ (kg)}$$

where A = Activity delivered to the liver, D = Absorbed dose to the target liver tumor, and M = Target liver mass. The mass is extrapolated from CT by using a conversion factor of 1.03 g/ml.

SIR-spheres® can be calculated as per the package insert by two methodologies. The "Empiric method" is a simplified method in which tumor burden is used.

Liver involvement by tumor %	Recommended activity (GBq)
<25	2.0
25–50	2.5
>50	3.0

Alternatively the activity can be calculated with the body surface area that factors the tumor burden in the liver

$$A = (BSA - 0.2)(\text{Tumor Volume})/(\text{Tumor Volume} + \text{Liver})$$

A resin is the activity of the ^{90}Y content of the resin microspheres (gigabecquerels).

Post-procedure Evaluation

Overall the treatment is associated with a favorable sub-acute and acute toxicity profile probably related to the low-level arterial occlusion following implantation. This allows for outpatient treatment. Empiric treatment with gastric mucosal-protectant agents is prescribed since small unmanned arteries that are undetectable with arteriography (resolution or reversal of flow) may supply extrahepatic structures.

Some clinicians prescribe a short, tapering course of methylprednisolone to minimize the edema and pain associated with capsular stretch due to the radiation.

It is advisable to give patients a detailed sheet that identifies them as having received the implantation and it is unnecessary to shield patients from bystanders due to the low level of radiation at skin surface (<1 mrem per hour); however, standard radiation safety precautions are advisable. Unlike the glass microspheres, due to the ionic dissociation of ^{90}Y from the resin microsphere the urine will be marginally radioactive for the first day after delivery [24].

The optimal interval for imaging after treatment is not defined; however, most clinicians agree that an interval between 60 and 90 days is optimal to allow for resolution of treatment-related edema. Both MRI and CT have been utilized as surrogates for response. Kamel et al. reported on patients who prospectively underwent MR imaging pre- and post-therapy. Targeted tumors demonstrated a decrease in arterial enhancement, a decrease in venous enhancement of 25%, and unchanged tumor size in both targeted and non-targeted tumors [32]. Keppke et al reported on the imaging findings of 42 patients using ^{90}Y glass microspheres [33]. The response rates according to WHO, RECIST, necrosis, and combined criteria (RECIST & necrosis) were 26, 23, 57, and 59%, respectively. Tumor response was also reported by Salem et al. for 43 consecutive patients with HCC treated with glass ^{90}Y microspheres. Based on percent reduction in tumor size, 47% had an objective tumor response. When necrosis was used as a composite measure of response, 34 patients (79%) had an objective tumor response [34]. The most accurate assessment of tumor response after ^{90}Y radiotherapy appears to be volumetric with necrosis.

Kennedy et al. analyzed four explanted livers previously treated with yttrium-90 microspheres. Two patients underwent orthotopic liver transplantation, and two patients had advanced metastatic colon cancer. A complete histopathological analysis was performed including an assessment of microsphere distribution. Histopathology from the tumor liver parenchyma interface was sectioned for three-dimensional radiation dosimetry analyses. Heterogeneous deposition of microspheres at the interface with non-tumorous liver compared with the central zones without evidence of RILD in the surrounding parenchyma was noted [35]. This appeared to correlate with a zone of rim enhancement that can be appreciated on MRI. Riaz et al. reported their results of radiological–pathological correlation after liver explantation in 35 patients who harbored 38 lesions. CT or MRI was used for imaging and the explants were examined for assessment of necrosis and the correlation of radiological and histological findings was analyzed. All lesions harbored some degree of necrosis. Twenty three (61%) of target lesions showed complete pathologic necrosis, the vast majority of which were <3 cm. Imaging findings of response by EASL and WHO criteria were predictive of the degree of pathologic necrosis. Complete necrosis was seen in 100, 78, and 93% of the lesions that were shown to have complete response by EASL necrosis criteria, partial response by WHO criteria, or thin rim enhancement on post-treatment imaging, respectively. In contrast, complete necrosis was seen in only 52 and 38% of the lesions that showed partial response by EASL criteria and peripheral nodular enhancement, respectively. Rim enhancement was a characteristic that correlated well with necrosis [36].

Toxicity

Fatigue is the most common toxicity occurring in the vast majority of patients and lasting for up to 2 weeks. Post-embolization syndrome (low-grade fever, abdominal pain) occurs in a minority of patients and is of significantly lower incidence than following chemoembolization. Goin et al. performed a historical comparison of chemoembolization to radioembolotherapy utilizing glass ^{90}Y microspheres for incidence of post-embolization syndrome (PES). While the median survival was similar for each group the incidence of PES was nearly four times higher in the TACE group ($p = 0.003$; 95% CI, 1.6–16.3), demonstrating a toxicity profile strongly favoring radioembolization [37]. It is often self-limiting and treated with narcotic analgesics. Radiation-induced gastrointestinal injury can be occult, present with abdominal pain, hematemesis, or melena. Pancreatitis has also been described. Radiation pneumonitis has not been reported in the USA following use of either product. Radiation-induced liver disease (RILD) is related to excessive radiation exposure of normal liver tissue to radiation. This is manifested as a clinical syndrome of anicteric hepatomegaly, ascites, and increased liver enzymes occurring weeks to months after therapy. While it is known that RILD will develop when the whole liver is exposed to more than 40–45 Gy of external beam radiation, ^{90}Y microspheres are point sources of radioactivity and the tolerance is thought to be much higher approximating 70–80 Gy. More recently a study by Gulec et al. concluded that doses up to 100 Gy to the uninvolved liver were tolerated without the development of veno-occlusive disease or liver failure [38]. It also appears that there is a low occurrence of toxicity even with cumulative radiation doses of 390 Gy and 196 Gy, respectively [39]. An analysis of the biochemical liver toxicities was studied by Goin et al. in 88 patients who harbored [40] multifocal HCC (50%), >50% of liver replaced with tumor (16%), and portal vein thrombosis or portal vein compromise (17%). The most frequent liver abnormalities included ascites, elevated bilirubin, increased aminotransferase levels, and the majority (78%) of liver toxicities resolved. In this patient population, RILD was not seen and other forms of liver dysfunction were only transient. Lymphopenia without sequelae of clinical immunosuppression has been described; the etiology remains unknown [41]. Bile ducts are exclusively supplied by the hepatic artery and ischemic injury can occur. These rare complications can manifest as biliary necrosis, biloma, abscess and cholecystitis [42, 43]. While the exact incidence of radiation induced gall bladder injury requiring cholecystectomy is unknown, some investigators advocate routine empiric embolization of the cystic artery.

Clinical Studies

The first published manuscript of the modern experience of ^{90}Y radioembolotherapy appeared in a phase II study involving 22 patients by Dancey et al. [44] to determine the duration and frequency of response and to gain a renewed understanding of the toxicities following treatment. Of the 20 evaluable patients, nine patients were Okuda Stage I/II. The median dose delivered was 104 Gy. Fourteen patients experienced serious adverse events; most of which were hepatocellular dysfunction and gastrointestinal ulceration. A 20% response rate was noted with one complete response. Median time to progression and survival were 44 and 54 weeks, respectively. Multivariate analysis suggested that a total dose $\geq$104 Gy, Okuda Stage I, and ^{99m}Tc MAA tumor to liver uptake ratio $\geq$2 were associated with prolonged survival. In separate studies, Lau et al. was able to demonstrate a dose–response and dose–survival relationship in a phase I/II and II trial involving 18 and 73 patients, respectively. Tumor regression and survival improved in patients receiving $\geq$120 Gy [45].The same group published a retrospective analysis of 82 patients treated over an 8-year period [24,46]. Patients were sub-classified as "short survivors" (mortality < 1 year; 62%) or "long survivors" (mortality > 1 year; 34%). Comparisons between groups suggested high ^{99m}Tc MAA tumor to liver uptake ratios favored longer survival.

Carr et al. [41] also reported the results of a single institutional study that supported both the safety and the efficacy of glass ^{90}Y microspheres for inoperable HCC. Sixty-five patients with biopsy-proven HCC received a median radiation dose of 134 Gy. Major toxicities included two episodes of cholecystitis and transient hepatocellular transaminase elevations in 25 patients. Interestingly, the majority of patients developed lymphopenia, a previously unreported finding, not associated with adverse clinical events such as opportunistic infections. Median survival was more than double compared with historical controls of 649 and 302 days for Okuda I and II patients, respectively, a finding common to other studies. Geschwind et al. in 2004 reported on 80 patients from a multi-institutional database of 121 patients who were treated with glass ^{90}Y microspheres using varied approaches [47]. Patients were staged using the Child-Pugh, Okuda, or Cancer of the Liver Italian Program (CLIP) scoring systems. Among the three systems, the pretreatment CLIP scores were found to be the best means of stratifying risk. Survival was found to be 628 and 324 days for Okuda I (68%) and II (32%) patients, respectively. In 2004, Liu et al. presented a retrospective review of 14 patients treated for unresectable HCC [48]. The response rate was 65% (Table 20.2).

Table 20.2 ^{90}Y microspheres: recent published experience in HCC

Investigator	Device	N	PR	Okuda	Survival Okuda I	Survival Okuda II
Carr [41]	TS	65	25	I – 65% II – 35%	649 d	302 d
Liu et al. [48]	TS	14	8	I – 64% II – 36%	11 m	7 m
Geschwind et al. [47]	TS	80	nr	I – 68% II – 32%	628 d	324 d
Salem et al. [34]	TS	43	51%	I – 49% II – 51%	24 m	13 m

Survival results were also reported by Salem et al. in 43 patients treated with glass ^{90}Y microspheres [36]. The median survival reported in this study was 20.8 months for a low-risk group, whereas high-risk patients with diffuse disease faired worse with a median survival from the first treatment of 11.1 months. There were no life-threatening adverse events related to the treatment [34]. Gulec et al. retrospectively analyzed the data from a heterogeneous cohort of 40 patients with liver malignancies who underwent single whole liver treatments using ^{90}Y resin microspheres. Tumor absorbed doses ranged from 40.1 to 494.8 Gy. Sixty-seven percent of the treated cohort responded to therapy again with responses favoring patients with higher ^{99m}Tc MAA tumor ratio [38].

Portal venous thrombosis is a uniformly poor prognostic variable and concerns over excessive toxicity following traditional embolotherapies exist. In 2004 a report on a series of 15 patients with unresectable HCC and portal vein thrombosis of at least the first order and related segmental portal venous branches received glass ^{90}Y microspheres. Two patients developed bilirubin toxicity and had evidence of disease progression. Eight patients continued to demonstrate stable or improved liver function after a second treatment cycle with no procedure-related complications. This clinical experience showed that in a select group of patients with compromised portal venous flow, glass ^{90}Y microspheres treatment is technically feasible and relatively safe [49]. Subsequently, Kulik et al. reported on the results of glass ^{90}Y microspheres in a 118 patient cohort, with a 37 patient subset analysis comparing patients with and without portal vein thrombosis [50]. Patients were stratified by Okuda, Child-Pugh, baseline bilirubin, ECOG, presence of cirrhosis, and location of portal vein thrombosis (none, branch, and main). The cumulative dose administered to those with and without portal vein thrombosis were 139.7 Gy and 131.9 Gy, respectively. Liver-related adverse events (bilirubin, ascites, and encephalopathy) were more in patients with cirrhosis versus no cirrhosis and the minimal embolic effect of ^{90}Y glass microspheres was not felt to have increased the risk of liver decompensation. Median survival from the date of first treatment for patients without portal vein thrombosis and cirrhosis was 27 months versus patients with branch portal vein thrombosis, survival was 10 months. Sangro et al. reported on 24 HCC patients with Child-Pugh A disease who underwent ^{90}Y radioembolization with resin microspheres. The overall response rate was 88% with a volume reduction noted in 19 patients. Two patients became jaundiced and two treatment-related deaths were noted. At median follow-up of 12.5 months none of the treated patients progressed [51]. Results of a recent pilot phase II study were presented by Ertle et al. A total of 60 patients predominantly with cirrhosis and preserved liver function (87% Childs A, 93% cirrhosis, 50% PVT) were treated with glass microspheres [52]. The volumetric response rate was 52% and this increased to 80% with the addition of necrosis. Median survival was 12.1 months.

Preliminary results have been reported recently by many authors. Romito et al. presented the results of glass microsphere therapy in 23 HCC patients, most with either main or branch portal vein thrombosis were treated with the glass microsphere. The response rate was 25 and 74% were alive at 9 months (57% with PVT, 100% no PVT) [53]. Iñarrairaegui et al. recently presented data with resin microsphere use in 62 patients (77% cirrhosis, 20% PVT). The median survival was 10 months favoring those patients with higher dose delivered (>3 GBq 15m versus <3 GBq 6 m and paucinodular disease; ≤5 nodules 23 m, >5 nodules 7 m) [54]. Additional results supporting the efficacy of resin microspheres for HCC was presented by D'Avola et al. The survival of 23 patients (72% cirrhosis, 32% PVT) was superior compared with a match-controlled cohort of 14 versus 8 months (p = <0.05) [55]. Similar survival benefit was noted by Carpenese et al. who treated 22 predominantly Childs A cirrhotics with resin microspheres. The response rate was 81% and the median survival for Childs A patients was 12 months [56]. Given the survival benefits, tumor response, and minimal toxicity profile, radioembolization should be considered as a viable therapy for patients with portal vein thrombosis and preserved liver function. It is a reasonable treatment option for disease stabilization in patients who were awaiting transplant.

In order to improve outcomes in patients with limited volume disease, Rhee et al. tested a procedure employing catheter-directed CT angiography. This technique delineates the arterial supply to HCC, which in turn allows for selective administration of supra-therapeutic radioactivity to segments/lobes of liver. This concept is referred to as radiation "segmentectomy" [57]. This allows for significantly greater radiation doses (range, 105–857 Gy) to small portions of liver parenchyma treating all viable neoplastic and non-neoplastic tissue without increased toxicity.

Kulik et al. reported on 21 patients from a large database of 251 patients who had undergone glass ^{90}Y microsphere therapy and subsequently bridged to transplantation [58]. Target tumor dose administered was 120 Gy with toxicities including fatigue in the majority of patients (42%). The authors reported a mean reduction in alpha fetoprotein (AFP) of 33% from pretreatment levels. The investigators noted complete necrosis by pathologic exam in 14 patients (66%). Four of 21 patients had disease recurrence, a finding not uncommon following transplantation.

Summary

[90]Y radioembolotherapy is a promising outpatient transarterial therapy for unresectable hepatocellular cancer. It is a unique form of brachytherapy that shares characteristics of radiopharmaceuticals and a radiation therapy source, requiring multidisciplinary involvement. Knowledge of technical aspects of embolization, hepatic artery anatomy, and flow characteristics are essential for safe and effective delivery of this new therapy. Published data from multiple independent sources support enhancement of survival in a distinct subset of patients with hypervascular tumors and intact liver function. Unlike other embolotherapies, portal vein thrombosis is not considered to be a major contraindication. [90]Y radioembolotherapy has served as an effective instrument to downstage to resection or as a bridge to transplantation. Compared to historical controls, the post-embolization syndrome following ^{90}Y radioembolotherapy is milder than chemoembolization while conferring a similar survival advantage.

Future Directions

Historically transarterial therapies have been utilized for unresectable lesions not amendable to thermal ablation. The advent of molecular targeted agents has brought new perspectives to cancer therapy especially HCC. The recent FDA approval of sorafenib for the treatment of unresectable HCC has created a regulatory benchmark and renewed interest for HCC therapies. Until such treatments become standard of clinical care, integration of these agents with local-regional therapies may maximize benefits to the patients and should be the focus of future endeavors with therapies such as ^{90}Y radioembolotherapy.

References

1. Jemal A, Siegel R, Ward E et al (2008) Cancer statistics, 2008. CA Cancer J Clin 58:71–96
2. El-Serag HB (2007) Epidemiology of hepatocellular carcinoma in USA. Hepatol Res 37(Suppl 2):S88–S94
3. Mazzaferro V, Regalia E, Doci R et al (1996) Liver transplantation for the treatment of small hepatocellular carcinomas in patients with cirrhosis. N Engl J Med 334:693–699
4. Dawson LA (2005) Hepatic arterial yttrium 90 microspheres: another treatment option for hepatocellular carcinoma. J Vasc Interv Radiol 16:161–164
5. Kloop CT, Alford TC, Bateman J, Berry GN, Winship T (1950) Fractionated Intraarterial cancer; chemotherapy with methyl bis amine hydrochloride; a preliminary report. Ann Surg 132:811–832
6. Muller JH, Rossier PH (1951) A new method for the treatment of cancer of the lung by means of artificial radioactivity. Act Radiol 35:449–468
7. Pochin EE CG, Cunningham RM, Hollman A, Hudswell F, Payne BR (1954) Localization of colloidal gold in the lungs. Proceedings of the Radioisotope Conference 1:30
8. Ya PM, Guzman T, Loken MK, Perry JF Jr (1961) Isotope localization with tagged microspheres. Surgery 49:644–650
9. Kim YS LaFave JW, MacLean LD (1962) The use of radiating microspheres in the treatment of experimental and human malignancy. Surgery 52:220–231
10. Blanchard RJ, Grotenhuis I, LaFave JW et al (1964) Treatment of experimental tumors: Utilization of radioactive microspheres. Arch Surg 89:406–410
11. Blanchard RJ, LaFave JW, Kim YS et al (1964) Treatment of patients with advanced cancer utilizing Y90 microspheres. Cancer 18:375–380
12. Ariel I, Pack G (1967) Treatment of inoperable cancer of the liver by intra-arterial radioactive isotopes and chemotherapy. Cancer 20:793–804
13. Grady E (1979) Internal radiation therapy of hepatic cancer. Dis Colon Rectum 22:371–375
14. Mantravadi R, Spigos D, Tan W, Felix E (1982) Intraarterial yttrium 90 in the treatment of hepatic malignancy. Radiology 142:783–786
15. Wollner I, Knutsen C, Smith P et al (1988) Effects of hepatic arterial yttrium 90 glass microspheres in dogs. Cancer 61:1336–1344
16. Yan ZP, Lin G, Zhao HY, Dong YH (1993) Yttrium-90 glass microspheres injected via the portal vein. An experimental study. Acta Radiol 34:395–398
17. Yan ZP, Lin G, Zhao HY, Dong YH (1993) An experimental study and clinical pilot trials on yttrium-90 glass microspheres through the hepatic artery for treatment of primary liver cancer. Cancer 72:3210–3215
18. Shen S, DeNardo GL, Yuan A, DeNardo DA, DeNardo SJ (1994) Planar gamma camera imaging and quantitation of yttrium-90 bremsstrahlung. J Nucl Med 35:1381–1389

19. Shen S, DeNardo GL, DeNardo SJ (1994) Quantitative bremsstrahlung imaging of yttrium-90 using a Wiener filter. Med Phys 21:1409–1417

20. Stabin MG, Eckerman KF, Ryman JC, Williams LE (1994) Bremsstrahlung radiation dose in yttrium-90 therapy applications. J Nucl Med 35:1377–1380

21. Shepherd F, Rotstein L, Houle S, Yip T, Paul K, Sniderman K (1992) A phase I dose escalation trial of yttrium-90 microspheres in the treatment of primary hepatocellular carcinoma. Cancer 70:2250–2254

22. Andrews J, Walker S, Ackermann R, Cotton L, Ensminger W, Shapiro B (1994) Hepatic radioembolization with yttrium-90 containing glass microspheres: preliminary results and clinical follow-up. J Nucl Med 35:1637–1644

23. Murthy R, Nunez R, Szklaruk J et al (2005) Yttrium-90 microsphere therapy for hepatic malignancy: devices, indications, technical considerations, and potential complications. Radiographics 25(Suppl 1):S41–S55

24. Kennedy A, Nag S, Salem R et al (2007) Recommendations for radioembolization of hepatic malignancies using yttrium-90 microsphere brachytherapy: a consensus panel report from the radioembolization brachytherapy oncology consortium. Int J Radiat Oncol Biol Phys 68: 13–23

25. Liu DM, Salem R, Bui JT et al (2005) Angiographic considerations in patients undergoing liver-directed therapy. J Vasc Interv Radiol 16:911–935

26. Murthy R, Brown DB, Salem R et al (2007) Gastrointestinal complications associated with hepatic arterial Yttrium-90 microsphere therapy. J Vasc Interv Radiol 18:553–561; quiz 562

27. Sato K, Lewandowski RJ, Bui JT et al (2006) Treatment of unresectable primary and metastatic liver cancer with yttrium-90 microspheres (TheraSphere): assessment of hepatic arterial embolization. Cardiovasc Intervent Radiol 29:522–529

28. Murthy R, Xiong H, Nunez R, et al (2005) Yttrium 90 resin microspheres for the treatment of unresectable colorectal hepatic metastases after failure of multiple chemotherapy regimens: preliminary results. J Vasc Interv Radiol 16:937–945

29. Leung T, Lau W, Ho S et al (1995) Radiation pneumonitis after selective internal radiation treatment with intraarterial 90yttrium-microspheres for inoperable hepatic tumors. Int J Radiat Oncol Biol Phys 33:919–924

30. Salem R, Parikh P, Atassi B et al (2008) Incidence of radiation pneumonitis after hepatic intra-arterial radiotherapy with yttrium-90 microspheres assuming uniform lung distribution. Am J Clin Oncol 31:431–438

31. Murthy R, Kennedy A, Line B, Lund G, Stainken B, Van Echo D (2002) Augmentation of hepatopulmonary shunting following trans-arterial hepatic brachytherapy (TAHB) with yttrium 90 25micron spheres: therasphere – Therapeutic implications. Radiology 225:307

32. Kamel IR, Reyes DK, Liapi E, Bluemke DA, Geschwind JF (2007) Functional MR imaging assessment of tumor response after 90Y microsphere treatment in patients with unresectable hepatocellular carcinoma. J Vasc Interv Radiol 18:49–56

33. Keppke AL, Salem R, Reddy D et al (2007) Imaging of hepatocellular carcinoma after treatment with yttrium-90 microspheres. AJR Am J Roentgenol 188:768–775

34. Salem R, Lewandowski R, Atassi B et al (2005) Treatment of unresectable hepatocellular carcinoma with use of 90Y microspheres (TheraSphere): safety, tumor response, and survival. J Vasc Interv Radiol 16:1627–1639

35. Kennedy A, Nutting C, Coldwell D, Gaiser J, Drachenberg C (2004) Pathologic response and microdosimetry of (90)Y microspheres in man: review of four explanted whole livers. Int J Radiat Oncol Biol Phys 60:1552–1563

36. Riaz A, Kulik L, Lewandowski RJ et al (2009) Radiologic-pathologic correlation of hepatocellular carcinoma treated with internal radiation using yttrium-90 microspheres. Hepatology 49:1185–1193

37. Goin J, Dancey JE, Roberts C et al (2004) Comparison of post-embolization syndrome in the treatment of patients with unresectable hepatocellular carcinoma: Trans-catheter arterial chemo-embolization versus yttrium-90 glass microspheres. World J Nucl Med 3:49–56

38. Gulec SA, Mesoloras G, Dezarn WA, McNeillie P, Kennedy AS (2007) Safety and efficacy of Y-90 microsphere treatment in patients with primary and metastatic liver cancer: The tumor selectivity of the treatment as a function of tumor to liver flow ratio. J Transl Med 5:15

39. Young JY, Rhee TK, Atassi B et al (2007) Radiation dose limits and liver toxicities resulting from multiple yttrium-90 radioembolization treatments for hepatocellular carcinoma. J Vasc Interv Radiol 18:1375–1382

40. Goin J, Salem R, Carr B et al (2005) Treatment of unresectable hepatocellular carcinoma with intrahepatic yttrium 90 microspheres: factors associated with liver toxicities. J Vasc Interv Radiol 16:205–213

41. Carr B (2004) Hepatic arterial ^{90}Yttrium glass microspheres (Therasphere) for unresectable hepatocellular carcinoma: interim safety and survival data on 65 patients. Liver Transpl 10:S107–S110

42. Atassi B, Bangash AK, Lewandowski RJ et al (2008) Biliary sequelae following radioembolization with Yttrium-90 microspheres. J Vasc Interv Radiol 19:691–697

43. Ng SS, Yu SC, Lai PB, Lau WY (2008) Biliary complications associated with selective internal radiation (SIR) therapy for unresectable liver malignancies. Dig Dis Sci 53:2813–2817

44. Dancey J, Shepherd F, Paul K et al (2000) Treatment of nonresectable hepatocellular carcinoma with intrahepatic 90Y-microspheres. J Nucl Med 41:1673–1681

45. Lau W, Leung W, Ho S et al (1994) Treatment of inoperable hepatocellular carcinoma with intrahepatic arterial yttrium-90 microspheres: a phase I and II study. Br J Cancer 70:994–999

46. Lau W, Ho S, Leung W, Chan M, Lee W, Johnson P (2001) What determines survival duration in hepatocellular carcinoma treated with intraarterial Yttrium-90 microspheres? Hepatogastroenterology 48:338–340

47. Geschwind J, Salem R, Carr B et al (2004) Yttrium-90 microspheres for the treatment of hepatocellular carcinoma. Gastroenterology 127:S194–S205

48. Liu MD, Uaje MB, Al-Ghazi MS et al (2004) Use of yttrium-90 TheraSphere for the treatment of unresectable hepatocellular carcinoma. Am Surg 70:947–953

49. Salem R, Lewandowski R, Roberts C et al (2004) Use of yttrium-90 glass microspheres (TheraSphere) for the treatment of unresectable hepatocellular carcinoma in patients with portal vein thrombosis. J Vasc Interv Radiol 15:335–345

50. Kulik LM, Carr BI, Mulcahy MF et al (2008) Safety and efficacy of 90Y radiotherapy for hepatocellular carcinoma with and without portal vein thrombosis. Hepatology 47:71–81

51. Sangro B, Bilbao JI, Boan J et al (2006) Radioembolization using 90Y-resin microspheres for patients with advanced hepatocellular carcinoma. Int J Radiat Oncol Biol Phys 66:792–800

52. Ertle J, Antoch G, Hamami M, Bockisch A, Ferken G, Hilgard P (2008) Radioembolization with therasphere yttrium-90 glass microspheres for advanced hepatocellular carcinoma: a European pilot phase II study. Presented at the Second Annual Meeting of the International Liver Cancer Association, Chicago, IL, September 2008, O-035

53. Romito R, Mazzaferro V, Spreafico C et al (2008) Intra-hepatic arterial radioembolization with 90Y-glass microspheres for hepatocellular carcinoma with macrovascular invasion: preliminary results. Presented at the Second Annual Meeting of the International Liver Cancer Association (ILCA), Chicago, IL, September 2008, p 142

54. Iñarrairaegui M, Thurston KG, Martinez-Cuesta A et al (2008) Radioembolization of hepatocellular carcinoma in patients presenting with portal vein occlusion: a safety analysis. Presented at the Second Annual Meeting of the International Liver Cancer Association (ILCA), Chicago, IL, September 2008, p 140

55. D'Avola DD, Iñarrairaegui M, Bilbao JI et al (2008) Extended survival in patients with unresectable advanced hepatocellular carcinoma treated using radioembolization. Presented at the Second Annual Meeting of the International Liver Cancer Association (ILCA), Chicago, IL, September 2008, p 139

56. Carpanese LPG, Vallati G et al (2008) Selective internal radiation therapy 90Y (SIRT) in multifocal HCC: clinical preliminary results in one year follow-up. World Conference on Interventional Oncology 2008, Poster P69

57. Rhee T, Omary R, Gates V et al (2005) The effect of catheter-directed CT angiography on yttrium-90 radioembolization treatment of hepatocellular carcinoma. J Vasc Interv Radiol 16:1085–1091
58. Kulik LM, Atassi B, van Holsbeeck L et al (2006) Yttrium-90 microspheres (TheraSphere) treatment of unresectable hepatocellular carcinoma: downstaging to resection, RFA and bridge to transplantation. J Surg Oncol 94:572–586

Chapter 21
Cytotoxic Chemotherapy and Endocrine Therapy for Hepatocellular Carcinoma

Daniel Palmer and Philip J. Johnson

Keywords Cytotoxic chemotherapy · Endocrine therapy · Doxorubicin · Tamoxifen · Somatostatin analogues · Drug resistance

For the minority of patients with hepatocellular carcinoma (HCC), surgical therapy, including transplantation, or local ablation may offer the prospect of cure (see Chapters 9–17). However, these treatments are typically constrained by size and/or number of tumours as well as liver dysfunction and other comorbidities. For other patients with preserved liver function and a patent portal venous system, chemoembolization may afford a modest survival benefit (see Chapters 19–21). For the remainder, providing liver function and performance status permit, systemic therapies are often used with palliative intent. Traditionally, this has taken the form of cytotoxic chemotherapy or endocrine manipulation, although recently molecular targeted therapies have been employed with some success.

This chapter aims to summarize the current status of chemotherapy and endocrine therapies, with reference to the limitations of these data and recommendations for future research directions. Novel molecular therapies are discussed in Chapter 22.

Cytotoxic Chemotherapy for Advanced Hepatocellular Carcinoma

A large number of (mostly uncontrolled) studies have been performed using the major classes of chemotherapeutic drugs as single agents or in combination. These are summarized in Tables 21.1 and 21.2.

Response rates for single-agent chemotherapy are low and durable remission is rare. The anthracycline, doxorubicin, has been the most studied agent, the first study reporting a response rate of 79% in a cohort of patients in Uganda [1]. Subsequent

P.J. Johnson (✉)
Clinical Trials Unit, CRUK Institute for Cancer Studies, The University of Birmingham, Birmingham, UK

K.M. McMasters, J.-N. Vauthey (eds.), *Hepatocellular Carcinoma*,
DOI 10.1007/978-1-60327-522-4_21, © Springer Science+Business Media, LLC 2011

Table 21.1 Phase II trials of single-agent chemotherapy in hepatocellular carcinoma

Drug	Dose (mg/m^2)	Patient number	Response rate (%)	Ref.
Doxorubicin	75	14	79	[1]
	20–75	41	11	[2]
	60	44	32	[3]
	40–60	31	10	[4]
	75	74	30	[5]
	60	63	35	[6]
	60	28	28	[7]
	75	52	11	[8]
	70	45	25	[9]
	40–60	51	10	[10]
	40–60	29	11	[11]
	60	34	21	[12]
	60	109	1	[13]
	60	29	11	[14]
	60–75	60	3	[15]
	60	30	18	[16]
Cisplatin		28	15	[22]
Epirubicin		18	17	[19]
		44	9	[20]
5-FU		25	28	[23]
Gemcitabine		28	18	[34]
Mitoxantrone		17	23	[21]
T-136		34	9	[25]
Nolatrexed		28	7	[27]

Table 21.2 Phase II trials of combination chemotherapy in hepatocellular carcinoma

Drugs	Patient number	Response rate (%)	Ref.
PIAF (Phase II)	50	26	[30]
(Phase III)	149	17	[31]
Epirubicin+etoposide	36	39	[32]
Cisplatin+5-FU	38	47	[33]
Gemcitabine+oxaliplatin	32	18	[35]

studies failed to corroborate this apparent activity and in 15 other trials the response rate ranged from 1 to 35% [2–14]. The overall response rate for more than 700 patients treated in these studies was 18%. The method of response assessment, particularly in earlier studies often in the form of clinical examination, is likely to have contributed to an over-estimation of response and the true objective radiological response rate is likely to be lower, as reflected in more recent trials. The small, non-randomized design and patient heterogeneity in these trials make it difficult to assess any effect of doxorubicin on overall survival. One small randomized trial has compared doxorubicin with symptom control. This study reported a statistically significant survival advantage in favour of doxorubicin. However, with median survival of 10.6 weeks vs. 7.5 weeks, it is clear that the absolute difference in survival was modest with very short survival in both arms, suggesting inclusion of patients with very advanced disease and/or poor liver function. Further, there was significant doxorubicin toxicity, notably cardiotoxicity, which may be accounted for by many patients receiving a cumulative dose exceeding 500 mg/m^2 [15].

The main toxicity for doxorubicin is myelosuppression and this correlates with serum bilirubin, which is particularly pertinent to patients with HCC, who usually have underlying chronic liver disease. This was demonstrated in a study in which 143 patients received doxorubicin. The response rate in patients with normal bilirubin was 46% compared with 10% in those with bilirubin elevated above the normal range. This is likely to be due to dose reductions to ameliorate toxicity in the elevated bilirubin group leading to sub-optimal dosing and emphasizes the need for careful patient selection for trials involving doxorubicin and further confounds the interpretation of trials to date [16]. Pegylation of doxorubicin prolongs its circulating half-life, reduces systemic toxicity and may promote drug accumulation in the liver. However, two trials indicate no advantage in the setting of HCC with response rates of 0 and 10% [17, 18].

Other anthracyclines have been investigated in HCC. In two phase II trials of epirubicin, a total of 62 patients were treated, with a combined response rate of 11% [19,20]. In five trials involving 118 patients treated with mitoxantrone, an anthracenedione, the response rate was 16%, with less toxicity and this became the first systemic agent to be licensed for use in HCC [21], although it was never widely adopted as a standard treatment.

Most other classes of chemotherapeutic drug have been investigated in HCC (Table 21.1). Many drugs (including oral 5-FU, ifosfamide, paclitaxel and irinotecan) appear to be essentially inactive at least according to radiological response criteria. Other drugs have demonstrated some single-agent activity (cisplatin response rate 5–15%; etoposide 0–24%; intravenous 5-FU 0–28%; topotecan 14%) but few have been rigorously tested in randomized controlled trials [22, 23].

A randomized trial has compared the oral fluoropyrimidine, UFT, with supportive care. UFT comprises tegafur, an orally active 5-FU prodrug metabolized by the liver to 5-FU, and uracil, a biochemical modulator of 5-FU via inhibition of dihydropyrimidine dehydrogenase (DPD, the rate limiting enzyme of 5-FU metabolism). HCC is reported to have high levels of DPD, which may explain resistance to 5-FU and, therefore, DPD inhibition may enhance 5-FU activity. Although objective responses to UFT were uncommon, there was a significant prolongation of survival (median 51 vs. 27 weeks; $p < 0.01$). This was a small study with only 28 patients per arm and larger studies are required, but it does suggest that radiological response may not correlate with survival [24].

More recently, based on encouraging early phase data, two novel agents have been tested in larger phase III trials, both using doxorubicin as a comparator. T-138067 (Tularik Inc.) is a novel inhibitor of tubulin polymerization, which therefore inhibits cell division. Pre-clinical studies indicated activity against the hepatoblastoma cell line HepG2 and in a phase I dose-escalation study, one of the five HCC patients achieved a partial response [25]. In a 34 patient phase II study there were three partial responses and 13 patients with disease stability, prompting the randomized phase III trial. Disappointingly, this early promise failed to translate into a survival benefit, with median survival of 6 months in both arms [26].

Nolatrexed is a novel thymidylate synthase (TS) inhibitor rationally designed based on the three-dimensional structure of the target enzyme. Unlike other anti-folates, such as 5-FU, its lipophilic nature means that it does not require active uptake into cells and is orally available. Further, it does not require polygluta-mation for its activation. Both reduced cellular uptake and impaired glutamation can contribute to anti-folate resistance. Thus, nolatrexed has demonstrated in vitro activity even in HCC cell lines resistant to other anti-folates. In a phase II trial of 28 patients with HCC, there were two partial responses and a further 16 minor responses/disease stabilizations [27], prompting a 54 patient randomized phase II trial with doxorubicin as the comparator. Whilst there were no objective responses in either arm, there was a trend towards longer survival in those receiving nolatrexed (139 vs. 104 days) [28]. Being a small, randomized phase II trial, statistical com-parison of the two arms could not be made. Based on these data a phase III trial comparing nolatrexed with doxorubicin was conducted. Despite the encouraging evidence of activity in the earlier trials, in fact patients receiving nolatrexed survived significantly less long than those in the control arm (4.7 compared to 6.9 months, $p = 0.0068$) [29]. While the statistical assumptions used in the design of this trial were based on demonstrating superiority for nolatrexed, since there were no obvious nolatrexed-related early deaths, some have argued that this study provides evidence that doxorubicin may, in fact, positively influence survival in appropriately selected patients. Nevertheless, while conventional cytotoxic therapy has undoubted activity against HCC, whether or not this translates into a survival advantage has still not been rigorously demonstrated.

Combination Chemotherapy for Advanced Hepatocellular Carcinoma

On the basis of its modest activity as a single agent, doxorubicin has been investigated in combination with a variety of other drugs. A phase II study of a four-drug combination of cisplatin, interferon alpha-2b, doxorubicin and 5-fluorouracil (PIAF) was encouraging, and although the response rate was mod-est (26%), 9 of 13 partial responders had their disease rendered resectable and, in some of these cases, there was a complete pathological response, again demon-strating the limitations of radiological assessment of chemotherapy activity in HCC [30]. Despite this encouraging activity, a prospective randomized study comparing PIAF to doxorubicin failed to demonstrate any improvement in survival with the combination [31].

Non-doxorubicin-based chemotherapy combinations have not demonstrated any consistently improved activity over single agents, with a few notable exceptions. In a phase II study, the combination of etoposide plus epirubicin was well tolerated and a response rate of 39% was reported [32]. A phase II study of infusional 5-FU with cisplatin reported objective response rate of 47% [33].

An initial phase II study of gemcitabine reported an encouraging response rate (18%) [34] and its good safety profile lends it to combination with other agents, in particular there is evidence for synergy with platinum compounds. The combination of gemcitabine and oxaliplatin is active and tolerated well in a number of cancers. Further, the lack of renal and liver toxicity are attractive in the context of HCC and underlying cirrhosis. Phase II studies have reported encouraging efficacy (response rates 18–30%) with good tolerance, although it is important to be mindful of gemcitabine-induced thrombocytopenia in patients with cirrhosis and hypersplenism and of oxaliplatin-induced neurotoxicity in patients with alcoholic liver disease who may have pre-existing peripheral neuropathy [35].

These studies again suggest that HCC can be chemosensitive and that chemotherapy can be administered safely and with manageable toxicity in appropriately selected patients. However, randomized trials of combination chemotherapy have been conducted rarely and those that have been have mostly been statistically underpowered to detect significant improvements in survival and have not stratified according to known prognostic factors so that, in general, meaningful conclusions cannot be drawn.

Endocrine Therapy for Hepatocellular Carcinoma

Despite some encouraging data, there remains no convincing evidence of survival benefit for systemic chemotherapy for HCC and chemotherapy in this setting may be poorly tolerated due to co-existing chronic liver disease resulting in unpredictable drug metabolism. Thus, many non-cytotoxic systemic therapies have been investigated.

It is estimated that up to one-third of HCC express oestrogen receptors (ERs), and animal models of liver carcinogenesis, as well as epidemiological studies, suggest a role for sex steroids in its pathogenesis such that ER is a rational therapeutic target. Indeed, initial studies suggested promising activity for tamoxifen. For example, a small trial randomized 38 patients to tamoxifen or supportive care and reported 1-year survival rates of 22 and 5%, respectively [36]. A similar trial of 32 patients reported 1-year survival rates of 35 and 0%, favouring tamoxifen [37]. However, both trials were too small to detect any statistically significant difference in overall survival. Several larger studies have reported no benefit or, in the case of high-dose tamoxifen, a detrimental effect over placebo [38,39]. For example, the Italian CLIP study including almost 500 patients randomized to tamoxifen or placebo reported median survival of 15 and 16 months, respectively ($p = 0.54$) [40].

It is evident in the management of breast cancer that ER-negative tumours derive no benefit from endocrine therapy. However, these HCC studies did not select patients on the basis of ER status. Thus, it is possible that benefit for patients with ER-positive HCC may be diluted by a lack of effect against ER-negative tumours. A randomized trial of tamoxifen compared with placebo has attempted to address this question. Of 119 patients, the ER status was determined in 66 but there was no difference in survival between patients with ER-positive or ER-negative tumours [41].

A proposed explanation for the failure of tamoxifen even in ER-positive HCC is that the liver variant ER is resistant to tamoxifen due to an exon 5 deletion that alters the hormone binding domain whilst maintaining constitutive transcriptional activation. Megestrol is a progestin drug that acts at the post-transcriptional level and could, therefore, inhibit ER-dependent growth signalling independent of ER ligation. A randomized trial has examined megestrol vs. placebo in 45 patients with variant liver ER-positive HCC, with megestrol conferring a significant survival advantage in this selected group of patients (18 vs. 7 months; $p = 0.009$) [42]. Given the small size of this study, larger trials are required to corroborate these findings. Other studies have investigated luteinizing hormone-releasing hormone analogues and anti-androgens with no clear evidence of benefit [43, 44]. Similarly, endocrine therapy combined with other treatment modalities including systemic or hepatic arterial chemotherapy provides no clear additional benefit [45,46].

Somatostatin Analogues for Hepatocellular Carcinoma

Somatostatin analogues, such as octreotide, have revolutionized the management of symptomatic neuroendocrine tumours by suppressing the secretion of peptide hormones and ameliorating hormone-related symptoms. They may also exert a cytostatic effect by direct growth inhibition through somatostatin receptor (SSTR) ligation or by indirect effects through the suppression of trophic hormones such as insulin, insulin-like growth factor (IGF-1), cholecystokinin and gastrin [47]. Octreotide may also exert anti-angiogenic effects [48]. Overexpression of SSTR has been reported in up to 40% of HCC [49] and three clinical trials have addressed the role of octreotide in this setting. The first study investigated the expression of SSTR in hepatitic liver, cirrhotic liver and HCC in homogenates from needle biopsy specimens, demonstrating SSTR expression in all tumour samples to varying degrees. Fifty-eight HCC patients were then randomized to receive octreotide or no treatment, with median survival of 13 and 4 months, respectively ($p = 0.002$) [50]. A second study failed to corroborate these findings. In 70 patients receiving either a long-acting octreotide formulation (Lanreotide) or placebo, there was no difference in survival [51]. Median survival in both groups was very short (less than 2 months), suggesting this to be a population with a poor prognosis and, indeed, over a third of patients died before commencing therapy. Furthermore, the SSTR status of these patients was not known, such that octreotide therapy might be expected to be ineffective in many cases. More recently the HECTOR study prospectively randomized 120 patients with well-compensated liver disease between the long-acting Sandostatin LAR and placebo, but again there was no evidence of benefit [52].

Somatostatin acts through five receptors, SSTRs 1–5, and the anti-angiogenic effect is thought to be mediated primarily through SSTR3. Somatostatin analogues are available in short-acting and long-acting preparations and there are differences in their affinity for the different receptors. In particular, short-acting octreotide has a higher affinity for SSTR3. Since the first trial used short-acting octreotide, whereas the subsequent negative trials used long-acting preparations this might have contributed to the contrary results.

Adjuvant Therapy for Hepatocellular Carcinoma

Research studies for systemic therapy as an adjuvant to locoregional treatment have been restricted by a lack of clearly active agents in the advanced setting. At present, the only prospect of long-term survival for patients with HCC is through surgical resection, transplantation or local ablation. Where transplantation is available, its utility may be limited by a delay in donor organ availability during which time the tumour may progress. Pre-transplant neo-adjuvant therapy, most commonly using chemo-embolization, has been reported in several series but, to date, there have been no randomized controlled trials to support its routine use [53]. Similarly, there is no evidence for systemic therapy in this context. Successful transplant within current selection criteria is associated with a good prognosis, and tumour recurrence is seen in only a minority of patients. Thus, the impact of adjuvant systemic therapy would likely be modest and would require a clinical trial involving several thousand participants to demonstrate a significant improvement.

Following surgical resection and ablation, tumour recurrence and/or de novo tumour formation is common and adjuvant therapy has been investigated in the form of systemic therapy, hepatic arterial treatment, radiopharmaceuticals and immunotherapy. Trials of hepatic arterial chemotherapy (+/– embolization) in either the adjuvant or neo-adjuvant setting have not shown any survival benefit [54–57]. Studies using systemic chemotherapy (oral fluoropyrimidines or anthracyclines) have also failed to demonstrate a survival advantage in the adjuvant setting, although these studies have been small and not powered to detect modest differences [58–60].

The acyclic retinoid, polyprenoic acid, can induce differentiation and apoptosis of HCC cell lines in vitro and in vivo. A study randomized 89 patients to receive this agent for 12 months or to receive no additional therapy following resection. Recurrence in the treatment and control groups was 27 and 49%, respectively ($p = 0.04$). Based on an arbitrary definition of tumours appearing more than 6 months after surgery representing a new primary cancer rather than recurrence of the resected tumour, the majority of the benefit appeared to be in preventing de novo tumour recurrence, although this definition is not universally accepted and is probably too early a timepoint to differentiate from progression of existing micrometastases [61].

Another small study randomized 30 patients between adjuvant interferon alpha (IFN) or no further treatment after surgery. For IFN-treated patients 3-year disease-free survival was 67% compared with 20% in the control group ($p = 0.037$). It is not clear whether this apparent benefit was due to prevention of tumour recurrence or to prevention of new tumours in HCV-positive patients [62].

Degradation of heparan sulphate in the extracellular matrix by tumour heparanases contributes to invasion and metastasis, and possibly to angiogenesis. PI-88, a compound comprised of highly sulphated mannose oligosaccharides, inhibits heparanase activity and, thus, may attenuate these processes. A three-arm phase II study randomized 172 patients to receive one of two doses of PI-88 (160 mg or 250 mg per day) or no additional treatment following resection. Forty-eight weeks after randomization, patients receiving the lower dose of drug were more likely to be free from recurrence than those receiving no treatment (63% vs. 50%). However, there was no dose–response effect, the 48-week recurrence-free rate being 41% in patients receiving the higher dose. While there was a higher rate of treatment discontinuation due to toxicity in the higher dose group, this does not appear to fully account for their poorer outcome and a lack of stratification for risk factors for recurrence prior to randomization may have contributed to spurious differences between the treatment arms [63]. Nevertheless, on the basis of these data, a randomized phase III trial comparing PI-88 at a dose of 160 mg/day against no treatment was commenced but, unfortunately, was closed early for commercial reasons.

In summary, there is no convincing evidence to support the use of systemic or regional cytotoxic chemotherapy as an adjuvant to locoregional therapy for HCC. Novel approaches have shown promise in small trials, but larger trials with sufficient follow-up are required. Design of such studies raises interesting questions regarding the nature of HCC recurrence. On the one hand, like other cancers, recurrence may be mediated by micrometastatic spread occurring prior to the locoregional therapy and this typically becomes clinically apparent within the first 1–2 years of treatment. On the other, since patients still have underlying cirrhosis, so-called recurrence may reflect de novo tumour development and may occur later. Thus, the duration of adjuvant therapy may be difficult to determine and the ability to prevent progression of pre-malignant lesions to invasive carcinomas is unknown.

Novel Approaches to Cytotoxic Chemotherapy for Hepatocellular Carcinoma

Strategies to Overcome Drug Resistance

Conventional chemotherapy is often considered to be ineffective against HCC due to drug resistance. Chemoresistance can be intrinsic or acquired and is mediated through a variety of mechanisms. HCC cells are often intrinsically resistant to chemotherapy through the over-expression of drug transporter proteins including the multi-drug resistance gene, *MDR1*, encoding p-glycoprotein. In vitro studies have demonstrated that over-expression of *MDR1* leads to efflux of doxorubicin from the cell. A number of early phase clinical trials have investigated the role of p-glycoprotein inhibitors in combination with doxorubicin and other drugs without any clear signal to warrant their investigation in larger studies.

Cell replication pathways targeted by chemotherapy may be dysregulated in HCC. For example, topoisomerase 2a, an enzyme encoded by the *TOP2A* gene, is involved in DNA unwinding for replication and is the target for a number of chemotherapeutic agents. Mutations in the *TOP2A* gene are associated with doxorubicin resistance in HCC cell lines and its over-expression is reported to correlate with chemoresistance. In vitro studies have demonstrated that the topoisomerase 2 inhibitor, etoposide, can sensitize HCC cells to doxorubicin [64] and this may underpin the encouraging phase II data relating to etoposide in combination with the anthracycline epirubicin [32]. Nevertheless to confirm these data, phase III trials are required.

The proteosome is an intracellular enzyme complex responsible for degradation of ubiquitinated proteins and this process contributes to the regulation of transcription factors such as NFκB. NFκB coordinates many key cellular functions by regulating the expression of genes involved in cell survival and inflammation in response to a wide variety of stimuli and it has been implicated in acquired chemoresistance [65]. Bortezomib is a potent and selective proteosome inhibitor, which inhibits NFκB signalling. Anti-tumour activity of bortezomib as a single agent and in combination with chemotherapeutic agents has been demonstrated in pre-clinical models [65, 66] and a phase I/II trial demonstrated good tolerance in HCC patients, with 7 of 15 evaluable patients achieving disease stability [67]. Since proteosome inhibition attenuates pathways implicated in anthracycline and other cytotoxic drug resistance, combination studies are of interest. However, results from a phase II study of doxorubicin plus bortezomib were disappointing with a response rate of 2.3% and median survival of 5.7 months [68].

Pathways that are inhibited by novel targeted therapies (see Chapter 22), including MAP Kinase signalling (raf/mek/erk), may also contribute to drug resistance such that combination of these agents with chemotherapy may reverse this. Indeed, there is pre-clinical evidence of synergy between doxorubicin and raf inhibition. In a vascular endothelial model, resistance to doxorubicin is, at least in part, mediated via fibroblast growth factor (FGF)-mediated raf-dependent survival signals providing rationale for combining doxorubicin with the raf inhibitor, sorafenib, or inhibitors of FGF receptor tyrosine kinase such as brivanib [69]. A randomized phase II study has investigated the combination of sorafenib and doxorubicin compared to doxorubicin alone [70]. The overall survival in the combination arm was more than double the control arm (13.7 months compared to 6.5 months, HR 0.45). However, this being a randomized phase II study the aim was to determine whether or not the combination should be taken into a phase III setting rather than to allow statistically robust comparisons between treatment arms. To establish whether this benefit is attributable to synergy between the two agents or to sorafenib alone requires a further randomized trial of the combination using sorafenib as the control arm.

There is also clinical evidence of benefit from the combination of anti-angiogenic agents with conventional chemotherapy in other tumour types. For example, in patients with metastatic colorectal cancer the anti-VEGF monoclonal antibody, bevacizumab, significantly prolongs survival when added to chemotherapy [71]. Whilst the mechanism of action of bevacizumab is postulated to be anti-angiogenic, laboratory studies suggest that it may act through normalization of tortuous, highly permeable tumour neo-vasculature, reducing intra-tumoral interstitial pressure thereby increasing blood flow and improving chemotherapy delivery to the tumour [72]. A study has investigated the addition of bevacizumab to combination chemotherapy comprising gemcitabine and oxaliplatin, demonstrating some activity with a response rate of 20% and median survival of 9.5 months [73]. The significance of these results within the context of a single-arm phase II study is difficult to interpret but, whilst comparison across phase II studies is difficult due to potential imbalances in prognostic factors in the two groups of patients and different drug doses used, they do not appear to be significantly better than chemotherapy alone [35].

AFP as a Biomarker of Response to Chemotherapy

The development of effective chemotherapy for HCC has been hampered by traditional phase II trial design in which evidence for activity is based on small, single-arm studies usually with radiological response rate as the primary endpoint. This assumes that anti-cancer efficacy is reflected by changes in area assessed by cross-sectional imaging. However, there is evidence that this may not be the case in the context of HCC [30,74,75]. The utility of serum AFP as a marker of treatment response in HCC is uncertain. A study evaluated serial AFP measurements in patients participating in the phase III trial comparing PIAF with doxorubicin [76]. AFP response was defined as a greater than 20% fall following at least two cycles of chemotherapy. AFP response was associated with significantly improved survival (median 13.5 months in responders vs. 5.6 months in non-responders; $p < 0.0001$) and was commonly observed in patients with radiologically stable disease, again indicating that objective radiological response rate may tend to underestimate chemotherapy effect.

Hepatitis B Virus Reactivation and Chemotherapy

Hepatitis B virus (HBV) carriers are at risk of virus reactivation when receiving cytotoxic chemotherapy. A prospective study of 102 HBsAg-positive patients with HCC receiving doxorubicin-based chemotherapy showed that 32 patients developed hepatitis attributable to HBV reactivation of whom 30% died as a consequence [77]. Reactivation can be reduced by anti-viral therapy such as lamivudine [78]. A non-randomized comparison of HBV-positive patients receiving chemotherapy reported reactivation rates of 4% compared to 24% in patients receiving lamivudine or not, respectively. Since lamivudine prophylaxis was not routinely used prior to this, it is quite possible that HBV reactivation contributed to apparent toxicity in earlier chemotherapy studies, especially those conducted in HBV-endemic regions.

Discussion and Future Directions

Clinical trials of chemotherapeutic agents have mostly been conducted in patients with advanced disease, which may limit the scope for observing effective treatments. Furthermore, most patients with HCC have underlying cirrhosis and thus have two diseases with independent natural histories such that it may be difficult to determine whether failure to improve survival is related to failure to influence tumour progression or due to progressive liver disease. In general, patients with Child-Pugh class C cirrhosis should be excluded from clinical trials since their liver function will be the predominant factor influencing survival. Conversely, for patients with Childs A cirrhosis prognosis is more likely to be influenced by the cancer such that the effects of an active treatment on survival may be determined. Thus, recent large phase III trials have been restricted to patients with Child A cirrhosis.

The extent of underlying liver dysfunction is also important in influencing pharmacokinetics and drug toxicity. In phase I studies, impaired drug metabolism may affect the toxicity profile and dose intensity such that a sub-optimal dose may be selected for further study. Conversely, using patients with well-preserved liver function may select a dose which might be poorly tolerated by patients with less good function. Indeed, this raises issues about the application of trial data derived from fit and well patients to a more general population.

A key point in the development of anti-cancer drugs is the phase II trial. This is typically the point at which a decision must be taken to develop a compound further in large, time-consuming and costly phase III trials or to abandon. Historically, radiological response rate has been used as the primary endpoint. However, recent trials have suggested that changes in tumour size are not necessarily a good surrogate for clinical benefit. For example, in the PIAF study radiological partial responses, in some cases, correlated with complete pathological response in resection specimens [30] and the recent sorafenib trials, despite a radiological response rate of just 2%, did report significantly prolonged survival (see Chapter 22 and [74,75]). Since many phase II trials of chemotherapy relied on response rate as the primary measure of efficacy, it is quite possible that some active agents may have been inappropriately discarded.

Alternative phase II endpoints employ a time-dependent measure such as progression-free survival or time-to-progression. However, the natural history of HCC is difficult to predict as demonstrated by the two recent sorafenib trials. The median survival in the control group of the Asian study was 4 months compared to almost 8 months in the European group despite apparently similar eligibility criteria. Patient heterogeneity is clearly not captured by current disease staging systems such that single-arm phase II trials are particularly difficult to interpret in this disease setting and it is likely that agents tested in such trials may have been inappropriately discarded and, equally, this might explain the failure of apparently active agents to fulfil their early promise.

This problem may be solved by using a randomized phase II trial design with a contemporary comparator. However, although such studies may allow a more informed decision as to the activity of the agent, since they are not powered for formal statistical comparison, the decision to proceed to a phase III trial is still based on a subjective assessment.

For phase III trials, overall survival remains the most appropriate endpoint, but some measure of quality of life should also be included. Patients with HCC develop symptoms due to underlying liver disease and due to the cancer and these are highly interrelated and difficult for currently available quality of life tools to differentiate. Well-validated instruments for measuring quality of life have not been available until recently.

In conclusion, the assessment of cytotoxic chemotherapy in the setting of HCC has largely been limited by trials comprising of small, single-arm phase II studies with heterogeneous patient groups such that conclusions regarding efficacy have been difficult to determine. In particular, there are limitations to the application of radiological response rate as a surrogate for clinical benefit. In future, careful clinical trial design is required with particular reference to patient characteristics (notably performance status and liver function), the choice of endpoint and, in the phase II setting, randomization to an appropriate control arm.

The HCC clinical research agenda has recently moved on with advent of novel targeted therapies. However, conventional chemotherapy should not be disregarded and there is strong rationale for its combination with targeted agents.

References

1. Olweny CL, Toya T, Katongole-Mbidde E, Mugerwa J, Kyalwazi SK, Cohen H (1975) Treatment of hepatocellular carcinoma with adriamycin. Preliminary communication. Cancer 36:1250–1257
2. Vogel CL, Bayley AC, Brooker RJ, Anthony PP, Ziegler JL (1977) A phase II study of adriamycin (NSC 123127) in patients with hepatocellular carcinoma from Zambia and the United States. Cancer 39:1923–1929
3. Johnson PJ, Williams R, Thomas H, Sherlock S, Murray-Lyon IM (1978) Induction of remission in hepatocellular carcinoma with doxorubicin. Lancet 1:1006–1009
4. Falkson G, Moertel CG, Lavin P, Pretorius FJ, Carbone PP (1978) Chemotherapy studies in primary liver cancer: a prospective randomized clinical trial. Cancer 42:2149–2156
5. Olweny CL, Katongole-Mbidde E, Bahendeka S, Otim D, Mugerwa J, Kyalwazi SK (1980) Further experience in treating patients with hepatocellular carcinoma in Uganda. Cancer 46:2717–2722
6. Williams R, Melia WM (1980) Liver tumours and their management. Clin Radiol 31:1–11
7. Melia WM, Johnson PJ, Williams R (1983) Induction of remission in hepatocellular carcinoma. A comparison of VP 16 with adriamycin. Cancer 51:206–210
8. Chlebowski RT, Tong M, Weissman J, Block JB, Ramming KP, Weiner JM, Bateman JR, Chlebowski JS (1984) Hepatocellular carcinoma. Diagnostic and prognostic features in North American patients. Cancer 53:2701–2706

9. Choi TK, Lee NW, Wong J (1984) Chemotherapy for advanced hepatocellular carcinoma. Adriamycin versus quadruple chemotherapy. Cancer 53:401–405

10. Falkson G, MacIntyre JM, Schutt AJ, Coetzer B, Johnson LA, Simson IW, Douglass HO Jr (1984) Neocarzinostatin versus m-AMSA or doxorubicin in hepatocellular carcinoma. J Clin Oncol 2:581–584

11. Falkson G, MacIntyre JM, Moertel CG, Johnson LA, Scherman RC (1984) Primary liver cancer. An Eastern Cooperative Oncology Group Trial. Cancer 54:970–977

12. Colombo M, Tommasini MA, Del Ninno E, Rumi MG, De Fazio C, Dioguardi ML (1985) Hepatocellular carcinoma in Italy: report of a clinical trial with intravenous doxorubicin. Liver 5:336–341

13. Sciarrino E, Simonetti RG, Le Moli S, Pagliaro L (1985) Adriamycin treatment for hepatocellular carcinoma. Experience with 109 patients. Cancer 56:2751–2755

14. Melia WM, Johnson PJ, Williams R (1987) Controlled clinical trial of doxorubicin and tamoxifen versus doxorubicin alone in hepatocellular carcinoma. Cancer Treat Rep 71:5

15. Lai CL, Wu PC, Chan GC, Lok AS, Lin HJ (1988) Doxorubicin versus no antitumor therapy in inoperable hepatocellular carcinoma. A prospective randomized trial. Cancer 62:479–483

16. Johnson PJ, Dobbs N, Kalayci C, Aldous MC, Harper P, Metivier EM, Williams R (1992) Clinical efficacy and toxicity of standard dose adriamycin in hyperbilirubinaemic patients with hepatocellular carcinoma: relation to liver tests and pharmacokinetic parameters. Br J Cancer 65:751–755

17. Halm U, Etzrodt G, Schiefke I, Schmidt F, Witzigmann H, Mössner J, Berr F (2000) A phase II study of pegylated liposomal doxorubicin for treatment of advanced hepatocellular carcinoma. Ann Oncol 11:113–114

18. Hong RL, Tseng YL (2003) A phase II and pharmacokinetic study of pegylated liposomal doxorubicin in patients with advanced hepatocellular carcinoma. Cancer Chemother Pharmacol 51:433–438

19. Hochster HS, Green MD, Speyer J, Fazzini E, Blum R, Muggia FM (1985) 4'Epidoxorubicin (epirubicin): activity in hepatocellular carcinoma. J Clin Oncol 3:1535–1540

20. Pohl J, Zuna I, Stremmel W, Rudi J (2001) Systemic chemotherapy with epirubicin for treatment of advanced or multifocal hepatocellular carcinoma. Chemotherapy 47:359–365

21. Lai KH, Tsai YT, Lee SD, Ng WW, Teng HC, Tam TN, Lo GH, Lin HC, Lin HJ, Wu JC, et al (1989) Phase II study of mitoxantrone in unresectable primary hepatocellular carcinoma following hepatitis B infection. Cancer Chemother Pharmacol 23:54–56

22. Ravry MJ, Omura GA, Bartolucci AA, Einhorn L, Kramer B, Davila E (1986) Phase II evaluation of cisplatin in advanced hepatocellular carcinoma and cholangiocarcinoma: a Southeastern Cancer Study Group Trial. Cancer Treat Rep 70:311–312

23. Zaniboni A, Simoncini E, Marpicati P, Marini G (1988) Phase II study of 5-fluorouracil (5-FU) and high dose folinic acid (HDFA) in hepatocellular carcinoma. Br J Cancer 57:319

24. Ishikawa T, Ichida T, Sugitani S, Tsuboi Y, Genda T, Sugahara S, Uehara K, Inayoshi J, Yokoyama J, Ishimoto Y, Asakura H (2001) Improved survival with oral administration of enteric-coated tegafur/uracil for advanced stage IV-A hepatocellular carcinoma. J Gastroenterol Hepatol 16:452–459

25. Leung TW, Feun L, Posey J, Stagg RJ, Levy MD, Venook AP (2002) A phase II study of T138067-sodium in patients (pts) with unresectable hepatocellular carcinoma (HCC) [Abstract 572]. Proc Am Soc Clin Oncol 21

26. Posey J, Johnson P, Mok T, Hirmand M, Dahlberg S, Kwei L, Leung T (2005) Results of a phase 2/3 open-label, randomized trial of T138067 versus doxorubicin (DOX) in chemotherapy-naïve, unresectable hepatocellular carcinoma (HCC). J Clin Oncol, 2005 ASCO Annual Meeting Proceedings 23, No. 16S, Part I of II (June 1 Supplement): 4035

27. Stuart K, Tessitore J, Rudy J, Clendennin N, Johnston A (1999) A Phase II trial of nolatrexed dihydrochloride in patients with advanced hepatocellular carcinoma. Cancer 86:410–414

28. Mok TS, Leung TW, Lee SD, Chao Y, Chan AT, Huang A, Lui MC, Yeo W, Chak K, Johnston A, Johnson P (1999) A multi-centre randomized phase II study of nolatrexed versus

doxorubicin in treatment of Chinese patients with advanced hepatocellular carcinoma. Cancer Chemother Pharmacol 44:307–311

29. Gish RG, Porta C, Lazar L, Ruff P, Feld R, Croitoru A, Feun L, Jeziorski K, Leighton J, Gallo J, Kennealey GT (2007) Phase III randomized controlled trial comparing the survival of patients with unresectable hepatocellular carcinoma treated with nolatrexed or doxorubicin. J Clin Oncol 25:3069–3075

30. Leung TW, Patt YZ, Lau WY, Ho SK, Yu SC, Chan AT, Mok TS, Yeo W, Liew CT, Leung NW, Tang AM, Johnson PJ (1999) Complete pathological remission is possible with systemic combination chemotherapy for inoperable hepatocellular carcinoma. Clin Cancer Res 5: 1676–1681

31. Yeo W, Mok TS, Zee B, Leung TW, Lai PB, Lau WY, Koh J, Mo FK, Yu SC, Chan AT, Hui P, Ma B, Lam KC, Ho WM, Wong HT, Tang A, Johnson PJ (2005) A randomized phase III study of doxorubicin versus cisplatin/interferon alpha-2b/doxorubicin/fluorouracil (PIAF) combination chemotherapy for unresectable hepatocellular carcinoma. J Natl Cancer Inst 97:1532–1538

32. Bobbio-Pallavicini E, Porta C, Moroni M, Bertulezzi G, Civelli L, Pugliese P, Nastasi G (1997) Epirubicin and etoposide combination chemotherapy to treat hepatocellular carcinoma patients: a phase II study. Eur J Cancer 33:1784–1788

33. Tanioka H, Tsuji A, Morita S, Horimi T, Takamatsu M, Shirasaka T, Mizushima T, Ochi K, Kiura K, Tanimoto M (2003) Combination chemotherapy with continuous 5-fluorouracil and low-dose cisplatin infusion for advanced hepatocellular carcinoma. Anticancer Res 23: 1891–1897

34. Yang TS, Lin YC, Chen JS, Wang HM, Wang CH (2000) Phase II study of gemcitabine in patients with advanced hepatocellular carcinoma. Cancer 89:750–756

35. Louafi S, Boige V, Ducreux M, Bonyhay L, Mansourbakht T, de Baere T, Asnacios A, Hannoun L, Poynard T, Taïeb J (2007) Gemcitabine plus oxaliplatin (GEMOX) in patients with advanced hepatocellular carcinoma (HCC): results of a phase II study. Cancer 109: 1384–1390

36. Farinati F, Salvagnini M, de Maria N, Fornasiero A, Chiaramonte M, Rossaro L, Naccarato R (1990) Unresectable hepatocellular carcinoma: a prospective controlled trial with tamoxifen. J Hepatol 11:297–301

37. Farinati F, De Maria N, Fornasiero A, Salvagnini M, Fagiuoli S, Chiaramonte M, Naccarato R (1992) Prospective controlled trial with antiestrogen drug tamoxifen in patients with unresectable hepatocellular carcinoma. Dig Dis Sci 37:659–662

38. Castells A, Bruix J, Brú C, Ayuso C, Roca M, Boix L, Vilana R, Rodés J (1995) Treatment of hepatocellular carcinoma with tamoxifen: a double-blind placebo-controlled trial in 120 patients. Gastroenterology 109:917–922

39. Chow PK, Tai BC, Tan CK, Machin D, Win KM, Johnson PJ, Soo KC, Asian-Pacific Hepatocellular Carcinoma Trials Group (2002) High-dose tamoxifen in the treatment of inoperable hepatocellular carcinoma: a multicenter randomized controlled trial. Hepatology 36:1221–1226

40. CLIP Group (1998) Tamoxifen in treatment of hepatocellular carcinoma: a randomized controlled trial. CLIP Group (Cancer of the Liver Italian Programme). Lancet 352: 17–20

41. Liu CL, Fan ST, Ng IO, Lo CM, Poon RT, Wong J (2000) Treatment of advanced hepatocellular carcinoma with tamoxifen and the correlation with expression of hormone receptors: a prospective randomized study. Am J Gastroenterol 95:218–222

42. Villa E, Ferretti I, Grottola A, Buttafoco P, Buono MG, Giannini F, Manno M, Bertani H, Dugani A, Manenti F (2001) Hormonal therapy with megestrol in inoperable hepatocellular carcinoma characterized by variant oestrogen receptors. Br J Cancer 84:881–885

43. Manesis EK, Giannoulis G, Zoumboulis P, Vafiadou I, Hadziyannis SJ (1995) Treatment of hepatocellular carcinoma with combined suppression and inhibition of sex hormones: a randomized, controlled trial. Hepatology 21:1535–1542

44. Grimaldi C, Bleiberg H, Gay F, Messner M, Rougier P, Kok TC, Cirera L, Cervantes A, De Greve J, Paillot B, Buset M, Nitti D, Sahmoud T, Duez N, Wils J (1998) Evaluation of antiandrogen therapy in unresectable hepatocellular carcinoma: results of a European Organization for Research and Treatment of Cancer multicentric double-blind trial. J Clin Oncol 16:411–417

45. Melia WM, Johnson PJ, Williams R (1987) Controlled clinical trial of doxorubicin and tamoxifen versus doxorubicin alone in hepatocellular carcinoma. Cancer Treat Rep 71:1213–1216

46. Uchino J, Une Y, Sato Y, Gondo H, Nakajima Y, Sato N (1993) Chemohormonal therapy of unresectable hepatocellular carcinoma. Am J Clin Oncol 16:206–209

47. Rinke A, Müller HH, Schade-Brittinger C, Klose KJ, Barth P, Wied M, Mayer C, Aminossadati B, Pape UF, Bläker M, Harder J, Arnold C, Gress T, Arnold R (2009) PROMID Study Group. Placebo-controlled, double-blind, prospective, randomized study on the effect of octreotide LAR in the control of tumor growth in patients with metastatic neuroendocrine midgut tumors: a report from the PROMID Study Group. J Clin Oncol. 27(28):4656–4663.

48. Treiber G, Wex T, Röcken C, Fostitsch P, Malfertheiner P (2006) Impact of biomarkers on disease survival and progression in patients treated with octreotide for advanced hepatocellular carcinoma. J Cancer Res Clin Oncol 132:699–708

49. Reubi JC, Zimmermann A, Jonas S, Waser B, Neuhaus P, Läderach U, Wiedenmann B (1999) Regulatory peptide receptors in human hepatocellular carcinomas. Gut 45:766–774

50. Kouroumalis E, Skordilis P, Thermos K, Vasilaki A, Moschandrea J, Manousos ON (1998) Treatment of hepatocellular carcinoma with octreotide: a randomized controlled study. Gut 42:442–447

51. Yuen MF, Poon RT, Lai CL, Fan ST, Lo CM, Wong KW, Wong WM, Wong BC (2002) A randomized placebo-controlled study of long-acting octreotide for the treatment of advanced hepatocellular carcinoma. Hepatology 36:687–691

52. Becker G, Allgaier HP, Olschewski M, Zähringer A, Blum HE; HECTOR Study Group (2007) Long-acting octreotide versus placebo for treatment of advanced HCC: a randomized controlled double-blind study. Hepatology 45:9–15

53. Oldhafer KJ, Chavan A, Frühauf NR, Flemming P, Schlitt HJ, Kubicka S, Nashan B, Weimann A, Raab R, Manns MP, Galanski M (1998) Arterial chemoembolization before liver transplantation in patients with hepatocellular carcinoma: marked tumor necrosis, but no survival benefit? J Hepatol 29:953–959

54. Lai EC, Lo CM, Fan ST, Liu CL, Wong J (1998) Postoperative adjuvant chemotherapy after curative resection of hepatocellular carcinoma: a randomized controlled trial. Arch Surg 133:183–188

55. Wu CC, Ho YZ, Ho WL, Wu TC, Liu TJ, Peng FK (1995) Preoperative transcatheter arterial chemoembolization for resectable large hepatocellular carcinoma: a reappraisal. Br J Surg 82:122–126

56. Izumi R, Shimizu K, Iyobe T, Ii T, Yagi M, Matsui O, Nonomura A, Miyazaki I (1994) Postoperative adjuvant hepatic arterial infusion of Lipiodol containing anticancer drugs in patients with hepatocellular carcinoma. Hepatology 20:295–301

57. Yamasaki S, Hasegawa H, Kinoshita H, Furukawa M, Imaoka S, Takasaki K, Kakumoto Y, Saitsu H, Yamada R, Oosaki Y, Arii S, Okamoto E, Monden M, Ryu M, Kusano S, Kanematsu T, Ikeda K, Yamamoto M, Saoshiro T, Tsuzuki T. (1996) A prospective randomized trial of the preventive effect of pre-operative transcatheter arterial embolization against recurrence of hepatocellular carcinoma. Jpn J Cancer Res 87:206–211

58. Yamamoto M, Arii S, Sugahara K, Tobe T (1996) Adjuvant oral chemotherapy to prevent recurrence after curative resection for hepatocellular carcinoma. Br J Surg 83:336–340

59. Ono T, Nagasue N, Kohno H, Hayashi T, Uchida M, Yukaya H, Yamanoi A (1997) Adjuvant chemotherapy with epirubicin and carmofur after radical resection of hepatocellular carcinoma: a prospective randomized study. Semin Oncol 24(2 Suppl 6):S6–18–S6–25

60. Kohno H, Nagasue N, Hayashi T, Yamanoi A, Uchida M, Ono T, Yukaya H, Kimura N, Nakamura T (1996) Postoperative adjuvant chemotherapy after radical hepatic resection for hepatocellular carcinoma (HCC). Hepatogastroenterology 43:1405–1409
61. Muto Y, Moriwaki H, Ninomiya M, Adachi S, Saito A, Takasaki KT, Tanaka T, Tsurumi K, Okuno M, Tomita E, Nakamura T, Kojima T (1996) Prevention of second primary tumors by an acyclic retinoid, polyprenoic acid, in patients with hepatocellular carcinoma. Hepatoma Prevention Study Group. N Engl J Med 334:1561–1567
62. Kubo S, Nishiguchi S, Hirohashi K, Tanaka H, Shuto T, Yamazaki O, Shiomi S, Tamori A, Oka H, Igawa S, Kuroki T, Kinoshita H (2001) Effects of long-term postoperative interferon-alpha therapy on intrahepatic recurrence after resection of hepatitis C virus-related hepatocellular carcinoma. A randomized, controlled trial. Ann Intern Med 134: 963–967
63. Liu CJ, Lee PH, Lin DY, Wu CC, Jeng LB, Lin PW, Mok KT, Lee WC, Yeh HZ, Ho MC, Yang SS, Lee CC, Yu MC, Hu RH, Peng CY, Lai KL, Chang SS, Chen PJ (2009) Heparanase inhibitor PI-88 as adjuvant therapy for hepatocellular carcinoma after curative resection: a randomized phase II trial for safety and optimal dosage. J Hepatol 50:958–968
64. Wong N, Yeo W, Wong WL, Wong NL, Chan KY, Mo FK, Koh J, Chan SL, Chan AT, Lai PB, Ching AK, Tong JH, Ng HK, Johnson PJ, To KF (2009) TOP2A overexpression in hepatocellular carcinoma correlates with early age onset, shorter patient survival and chemoresistance. Int J Cancer 124:644–652
65. Hideshima T, Richardson P, Chauhan D, Palombella VJ, Elliott PJ, Adams J, Anderson KC (2001) The proteasome inhibitor PS-341 inhibits growth, induces apoptosis, and overcomes drug resistance in human multiple myeloma cells. Cancer Res 61:3071–3076
66. Cusack JC Jr, Liu R, Houston M, Abendroth K, Elliott PJ, Adams J, Baldwin AS Jr (2001) Enhanced chemosensitivity to CPT-11 with proteasome inhibitor PS-341: implications for systemic nuclear factor-kappaB inhibition. Cancer Res 61:3535–3540
67. Hegewisch-Becker S, Sterneck M, Schubert U, Rogiers X, Guerciolini R, Pierce JE, Hossfeld DK (2004) Phase I/II trial of bortezomib in patients with unresectable hepatocellular carcinoma (HCC). J Clin Oncol, 2004 ASCO Annual Meeting Proceedings (Post-Meeting Edition). 22(July 15 Suppl), 4089.
68. Berlin JD, Powell ME, Su Y, Horton L, Short S, Richmond A, Kauh JS, Staley CA, Mulcahy M, Benson AB (2008) Bortezomib (B) and doxorubicin (dox) in patients (pts) with hepatocellular cancer (HCC): a phase II trial of the Eastern Cooperative Oncology Group (ECOG 6202) with laboratory correlates [Abstract 4592]. Clin Oncol 26(May 20 Suppl)
69. Alavi A, Hood JD, Frausto R, Stupack DG, Cheresh DA (2003) Role of Raf in vascular protection from distinct apoptotic stimuli. Science 301:94–96
70. Abou-Alfa G, Johnson P, Knox J, et al (2007) Preliminary results from a Phase II, randomized, double-blind study of sorafenib plus doxorubicin versus placebo plus doxorubicin in patients with advanced hepatocellular carcinoma. Proceedings of the 2007 meeting of the European Cancer Organization. European Journal of Cancer Supplements [Abstract 3500]. 5:259
71. Hurwitz H, Fehrenbacher L, Novotny W, Cartwright T, Hainsworth J, Heim W, Berlin J, Baron A, Griffing S, Holmgren E, Ferrara N, Fyfe G, Rogers B, Ross R, Kabbinavar F (2004) Bevacizumab plus irinotecan, fluorouracil, and leucovorin for metastatic colorectal cancer. N Engl J Med 350:2335–2342
72. Jain RK (2005) Normalization of tumor vasculature: an emerging concept in antiangiogenic therapy. Science 307:58–62
73. Zhu AX, Blaszkowsky LS, Ryan DP, Clark JW, Muzikansky A, Horgan K, Sheehan S, Hale KE, Enzinger PC, Bhargava P, Stuart K (2006) Phase II study of gemcitabine and oxaliplatin in combination with bevacizumab in patients with advanced hepatocellular carcinoma. J Clin Oncol 24:1898–1903
74. Llovet JM, Ricci S, Mazzaferro V, Hilgard P, Gane E, Blanc JF, de Oliveira AC, Santoro A, Raoul JL, Forner A, Schwartz M, Porta C, Zeuzem S, Bolondi L, Greten TF, Galle PR, Seitz JF, Borbath I, Häussinger D, Giannaris T, Shan M, Moscovici M, Voliotis D, Bruix J; SHARP

Investigators Study Group (2008) Sorafenib in advanced hepatocellular carcinoma. N Engl J Med 359:378–390

75. Cheng AL, Kang YK, Chen Z, Tsao CJ, Qin S, Kim JS, Luo R, Feng J, Ye S, Yang TS, Xu J, Sun Y, Liang H, Liu J, Wang J, Tak WY, Pan H, Burock K, Zou J, Voliotis D, Guan Z (2009) Efficacy and safety of sorafenib in patients in the Asia-Pacific region with advanced hepatocellular carcinoma: a phase III randomized, double-blind, placebo-controlled trial. Lancet Oncol 10:25–34

76. Chan SL, Mo FK, Johnson PJ, Hui EP, Ma BB, Ho WM, Lam KC, Chan AT, Mok TS, Yeo W (2009) New utility of an old marker: serial alpha-fetoprotein measurement in predicting radiologic response and survival of patients with hepatocellular carcinoma undergoing systemic chemotherapy. J Clin Oncol 27:446–452

77. Yeo W, Lam KC, Zee B, Chan PS, Mo FK, Ho WM, Wong WL, Leung TW, Chan AT, Ma B, Mok TS, Johnson PJ (2004) Hepatitis B reactivation in patients with hepatocellular carcinoma undergoing systemic chemotherapy. Ann Oncol 15:1661–1666

78. Yeo W, Chan PK, Ho WM, Zee B, Lam KC, Lei KI, Chan AT, Mok TS, Lee JJ, Leung TW, Zhong S, Johnson PJ (2004) Lamivudine for the prevention of hepatitis B virus reactivation in hepatitis B s-antigen seropositive cancer patients undergoing cytotoxic chemotherapy. J Clin Oncol 22:927–934

Chapter 22
Targeted Therapies for Hepatocellular Carcinoma

Jonas W. Feilchenfeldt, Eileen M. O'Reilly, Costantine Albany, and Ghassan K. Abou-Alfa

Keywords HCC targeted therapies · Sorafenib · Bevacizumab · Sunitinib · Tyrosine kinase inhibitors (TKIs) · Erlotinib · HCC etiology

The liver's role in xenobiotic metabolism, i.e., the modification of drugs and toxic foreign compounds, has long served as a putative explanation for inherent drug resistance of hepatocellular carcinoma (HCC). Therefore, it does not come as a surprise that the initial discovery of the multiple-drug resistance gene (MDR) was in liver tissue [1], and hepatocyte cell lines are a natural reservoir for the study of drug resistance. Accordingly, liver cancer should be a disease where a therapeutic strategy based on an understanding of disease biology would prevail over a cytotoxic strategy where compounds are neutralized before reaching their target. Indeed while cytotoxic agents have failed to show a clinically meaningful impact [2] several clinical trials using targeted treatments such as tyrosine kinase inhibitors have demonstrated that in HCC overall survival may be favorably influenced [3]. In addition to the multikinase inhibitor, sorafenib, which has demonstrated an improvement in survival over placebo [4], over the past decade several different classes of targeted treatments have been clinically tested and can be sub-classified as tyrosine kinase inhibitors (e.g., sorafenib, sunitinib, erlotinib) or antibodies targeted to growth factors (e.g., bevacizumab) and their receptors (e.g., cetuximab) (Fig. 22.1).

As the historically evolved clinical expertise in the care for patients with liver disease traditionally has been in the domain of gastroenterologists, education regarding new therapies in HCC is critical to the wider range of medical disciplines currently involved in delivering care to these patients. The significance of this is illustrated by a thought-provoking study lead by Chen et al. from Taiwan, an area with high prevalence of HCC due to hepatitis B [5]. Comparing overall survival of 397 patients with HCC (all stages included) managed by high-volume physicians (70% patients

G.K. Abou-Alfa (✉)
Department of Gastrointestinal Oncology, Memorial Sloan-Kettering Cancer Center, New York, NY, USA

K.M. McMasters, J.-N. Vauthey (eds.), *Hepatocellular Carcinoma*,
DOI 10.1007/978-1-60327-522-4_22, © Springer Science+Business Media, LLC 2011

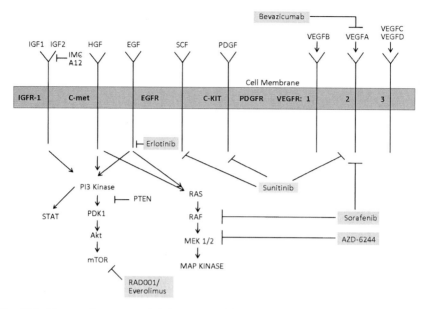

Fig. 22.1 Therapeutic targets and their corresponding pathways in HCC. Description of major signaling pathways in hepatocellular carcinoma and associated targets of drugs used in clinical practice respectively ongoing experimental studies. *Growth factors*: HGF, hepatocyte growth factor; EGF, epidermal growth factor; SCF, stem cell factor; PDGF, platelet-derived growth factor; VEGF, vascular endothelial growth factor; IGF-I, insulin-like growth factor-I. *Receptors*: IGF-I, insulin-like growth factor receptor 1 and 2; c-met, hepatocyte growth factor receptor. *Targets*: PI3 kinase, phosphatidylinositol 3-kinase; PDK1, 3-phosphoinositide-dependent protein kinase 1. *Experimental Compounds*: IMC-A12, insulin growth factor receptor inhibitor; AZD-6244, MEK1/2 inhibitor

with liver disease) versus low-volume physicians (less than 30%), a notable survival difference of 34 months versus 6 months was found (hazard ratio [HR] for survival, 1.94; 95% CI, 1.31–2.87; $p < 0.001$).

Despite proven clinical benefit of targeted treatment options, monitoring response to treatment and optimal patient selection based on prediction of treatment efficacy are unresolved questions and areas of ongoing research. This is in part a consequence of an incomplete understanding of the mechanism of action of the drugs, and also the difficulty in formally studying new imaging modalities, as well as validation of such modalities in a multicenter setting. Unexpectedly, the advances generated by targeted agents have created a renewed interest in standard chemotherapeutic agents which may ultimately reveal their potency in combination with biological agents [6]. The impact of liver function and the etiology of liver failure, whose etiologic spectrum comprises entities as diverse as viral, toxic, and metabolic origins, has been extensively studied as part of the development of sorafenib and related targeted agents. Given the multitude of clinically active compounds being assessed in phase II trials, further refinement of therapeutic monitoring, impacts on liver function, and etiology-driven clinical trials will be necessary to define the optimal clinical setting for such new agents.

Antiangiogenic Drugs

Sorafenib is a polyvalent molecule which has been shown in HCC cell lines to inhibit the serine–threonine kinase Raf-1 and several receptor tyrosine kinases such as vascular endothelial growth factor receptor (VEGFR2), platelet-derived growth factor receptor (PDGFR), FLT3, Ret, and c-Kit [7] (Fig. 22.1). Several of these pathways, e.g., ras-raf and VEGF, have been implicated in HCC carcinogenesis. Moreover, reduced angiogenesis along with increased apoptosis was observed in a human HCC xenograft tumor model when treated with sorafenib [8].

Following the initial observation of a partial response in a metastatic HCC patient in a phase I trial [9], a phase II study in HCC was undertaken to better assess efficacy, toxicity, and pharmacokinetics of sorafenib [10]. One hundred and thirty-seven patients were treated with sorafenib 400 mg twice daily. Seventy-two percent of patients had a Child-Pugh score of A and 28% a Child-Pugh score of B. The median time to progression was 4.2 months and the median overall survival was 9.2 months. The main drug-related grades 3 and 4 adverse effects were diarrhea (8%), hand-foot skin reaction (5.1%), and fatigue (9.5%). As clinical benefit does not routinely correlate with volume-based tumor response criteria such as WHO criteria in HCC, tumor necrosis was evaluated and quantified based on serial contrast-enhanced computed tomography (CT). In an exploratory analysis this mode of tumor assessment revealed that tumor necrosis may represent a marker of treatment efficacy despite a concomitant increase in tumor volume and potentially predict clinical benefit from treatment [10]. The current standard of care of sorafenib as systemic therapy for metastatic HCC is based on two phase III studies: the SHARP trial [4] and the Asia-Pacific trial [11]. The SHARP trial is an international, multicenter, phase III, double-blind trial randomly assigning 602 patients to either sorafenib 400 mg twice daily or placebo, with a primary endpoint of overall survival. Patients were recruited from the Western hemisphere, with main etiologies for HCC being hepatitis C (26%), hepatitis B (19%), and alcohol (26%). Median overall survival was 10.7 months in the sorafenib group and 7.9 months in the placebo group (hazard ratio in the sorafenib group, 0.69; 95% CI, 0.55–0.87; $p < 0.001$). The median time to radiologic progression was 5.5 months in the sorafenib group and 2.8 months in the placebo group ($p < 0.001$). Seven patients in the sorafenib group (2%) and two patients in the placebo group (1%) had a partial response and with no complete response in either study arm. Grades 3 and 4 side effects included diarrhea (8%) and hand-foot syndrome (8%). Bleeding was a rare event.

The Asia-Pacific trial is a multicenter phase III, double-blind trial randomly assigning 226 patients in a 2:1 ratio to either sorafenib 400 mg twice daily ($n = 150$) versus placebo ($n = 76$) [11]. As the name implies, patients were recruited mainly in Asia, where the highest prevalent etiology is hepatitis B for HCC. Median overall survival was 6.5 months (95% CI, 5.56–7.56) in patients treated with sorafenib compared with 4.2 months (3.75–5.46) in those who received placebo (hazard ratio [HR] 0.68; 95% CI, 0.50–0.93; $p = 0.014$). Median time to progression was 2.8 months (2.63–3.58) in the sorafenib group compared with 1.4 months (1.35–1.55) in the placebo group (HR 0.57 [0.42–0.79]; $p = 0.0005$). The commonest grades 3 and 4 side effects were hand-foot syndrome, diarrhea, and fatigue. Despite the similar hazard ratios of survival improvement, the disproportionate magnitude of survival improvement between the SHARP and the Asia-Pacific studies is noteworthy and will be discussed later in view of the implication for sorafenib and other agents regarding the underlying cause of the HCC.

The improvement in overall survival, the manageable toxicity, and the targeted action of sorafenib motivated further studies to improve its clinical efficacy. A recently completed randomized phase II trial assessing sorafenib in combination with doxorubicin in HCC demonstrated significant improvement in time to progression, progression-free survival, and overall survival in favor of the combination therapy [6]. This study is discussed in detail in the combination therapy chapter.

Vascular endothelial growth factor (VEGF) plays a prognostic [12, 13] and possibly a pathogenetic role in HCC. As a single agent, bevacizumab, an anti-VEGF A antibody (Fig. 22.1), has previously demonstrated significant clinical activity in metastatic renal cancer [14]. Based on the aforementioned biological rationale, 30 patients with advanced HCC were treated with bevacizumab initially at a dosage of 5 mg/kg. As 12 patients progressed with 16 weeks of treatment, the dose was subsequently increased to 10 mg/kg. Main reported adverse events were bleeding from varices, transient ischemic attack, hemorrhagic ascites, and proteinuria. Among the 24 patients evaluable for efficacy, 3 patients had a partial response and 13 had stable disease [15]. In a similar study, 46 patients with unresectable HCC were treated with bevacizumab at a dosage of 5–10 mg/kg once every 2 weeks [16]. One complete response and five partial responses were observed; the median overall survival was 12.4 months. Grades 3 and 4 adverse events included hypertension (15%), thrombosis (6%), and hemorrhage (11%). The improved overall survival compares favorably with a standard of care, sorafenib. Given EGFR-dependent regulation of VEGF and conversely the existence of VEGF-mediated resistance to EGFR-inhibition [17], the anti-VEGFR, bevacizumab, has been explored in combination with the tyrosine kinase inhibitor, erlotinib, in HCC [18] and this study will be reviewed in the next chapter.

Sunitinib is a multikinase inhibitor targeting VEGF and PDGF receptor pathways [19] both of which play a role in HCC (Fig. 22.1). A phase II study recruited 37 patients with unresectable HCC from Europe and Asia. Sunitinib was dosed at 50 mg daily for 4 weeks followed by a 2 weeks break cycle [20]. Median overall survival was 9.9 months (95% CI, 7.5–11.7). Thrombocytopenia (43%), neutropenia (24%), CNS symptoms (24%), asthenia (22%), and hemorrhage (14%) were the most common grades 3 and 4 adverse events. Four patients died due to "ascites, edema, bleeding, drowsiness, and hepatic encephalopathy." The detailed causes of deaths are as yet not fully reported. Treatment efficacy analysis showed one confirmed partial response and stability of disease in 39% of the patients. A median treatment time of approximately 12 weeks likely reflects a too toxic regimen at the chosen drug level.

In another phase II study 34 patients with unresectable HCC received sunitinib at lower dose of 37.5 mg daily for 4 weeks followed by 2 weeks off [21]. Median overall survival was 9.9 months (95% CI, 7.5–11.7). Grades 3 and 4 adverse events included elevated SGOT (18%); lymphopenia (15%); neutropenia, thrombocytopenia, and fatigue (12%); elevated SGPT (9%); and hand-foot syndrome, rash, hyperbilirubinemia, and hypertension (6%). Nonetheless, the overall survival data of those two studies do not suggest superiority compared to sorafenib.

Brivanib is a selective inhibitor of vascular endothelial growth factor receptor (VEGFR) and fibroblast growth factor receptor (FGFR) and has been shown to decrease HCC xenograft tumor models in mice [22]. This dual inhibition is particularly attractive as fibroblast growth factor has been postulated to confer resistance to VEGF inhibition [17]. In a study evaluating brivanib as first- and second-line therapy in 96 patients with advanced HCC, there were limited responses. Median survival was 10 months in the treatment naïve cohort and was not reached in the second-line cohort [23]. Progression-free survival was 2.7 months in the treatment naïve group versus 2 months in the second-line group. The drug was well tolerated in the second-line setting [24].

ABT-869, a VEGF and PDGF inhibitor. ABT-869 was evaluated in a phase II study of 44 patients with HCC. Of the 44 patients, 38 were Child-Pugh A and 6 were Child-Pugh B. The Child-Pugh A patients median overall survival was 9.7 months and time-to-progression was 5.4 months.

Tyrosine Kinase Inhibitors (TKIs)

Epidermal growth factor receptor (EGF) signaling is active in precursor lesions of HCC such as fibrosis and cirrhosis. Varied EGFR ligands such as EGF, hepatocyte growth factor (HGF), transforming growth factor beta, and insulin growth factor (IGF) are involved in hepatocarcinogenesis making this pathway an attractive target for the treatment of HCC (Fig. 22.1). Several trials have explored the role of TKIs in HCC.

Gefitinib is an oral EGFR tyrosine kinase inhibitor that blocks EGF-receptor 1, while lapatinib inhibits both EGFR-1 and EGFR-2 receptor. Both compounds have been studied in phase II trial, but given their limited efficacy further development as monotherapy is unlikely [25, 26]. Cetuximab, a monoclonal antibody targeted against the EGFR-1 receptor, has been studied in two phase II studies. While one study has reported an encouraging overall survival of 9.6 months [27], the earlier trial reported an unimpressive median TTP of 8 weeks [28].

Erlotinib is a selective inhibitor of the EGFR/HER-1-related tyrosine kinase enzyme. In an initial study, 38 patients with unresectable HCC were treated with erlotinib 150 mg daily on a continuous basis [29]. Median overall survival was 13 months. Grades 3 and 4 skin toxicity and diarrhea were the most notable adverse events. A second independent phase II study treated 40 patients with erlotinib 150 mg with a median overall survival of 10.7 months [30]. Most notable side effects were diarrhea, fatigue, and AST elevation. As mentioned above, erlotinib has been explored in combination with bevacizumab in HCC [18] and this study will be reviewed in the next chapter.

Management Issues

Etiology

In the Asia-Pacific study comparing sorafenib versus placebo described above [11], the statistically significant improvement ($p = 0.014$) did not reach the same magnitude of benefit as in the SHARP trial [4], despite the similarity in the hazard ratios of overall survival, progression-free survival, and time to progression. A possible explanation for these observed differences may be related to more advanced disease stage and lower performance status in patients from the Asia-Pacific study as compared to the SHARP trial [31]. Another explanation for the difference in outcome revolves around the etiology of HCC in those two studies. The majority of patients (73%) accrued on the Asia-Pacific study had hepatitis B as an underlying risk factor versus 18% of patients on the SHARP trial. In a retrospective evaluation of the large phase II trial evaluating sorafenib in patients with advanced HCC [9], $N = 137$, it was noted that hepatitis C positive patients had a longer time to progression of 6.5 months compared to 4 months ($p = 0.05$) for the patients with hepatitis B etiology [32]. Again there was a trend toward a survival advantage ($p = 0.29$) for the hepatitis C (12.4 months) versus hepatitis B patients (7.3 months). Similarly, a sub-group analysis from the SHARP has shown that patients with hepatitis C-based HCC treated with sorafenib ($n = 93$) had a median survival advantage of 14 months compared to the whole sorafenib treated group of 10.7 months, while the overall survival of the hepatitis C placebo arm compared to the placebo arm of the whole studied population was similar (7.9 months) [33]. These collective observations and in vitro data linking HCV infection to increased raf activity [34, 35] may explain a possible added advantage for patients with hepatitis C treated with sorafenib by addressing the root cause of the underlying liver dysfunction and predisposition to HCC. The outcome of the 18% of patients with hepatitis B-related HCC in the SHARP trial remains to be reported [36]. Overall for now, sorafenib has become a standard of care for patients with advanced HCC regardless of the etiology of their cancer; however, recognition exists for subsets potentially deriving greater or lesser benefit.

Impact of Liver Function

The results of the SHARP trial apply to patients with good to excellent performance status and Child-Pugh A score [4]; however, the safety and efficacy of sorafenib in patients with Child-Pugh B or C cirrhosis have yet to be defined. In a phase II study evaluating sorafenib in HCC [9], 28% of patients had Child-Pugh B cirrhosis. Pharmacokinetics for sorafenib were evaluated in 28 patients on the study and the AUC (0–8) (mg h/L) was comparable between the Child-Pugh A (25.4) and Child-Pugh B (30.3) patients. Cmax (mg/L) were 4.9 and 6 Child-Pugh A and B patients, respectively, with similar drug-related toxicity profiles. However, it was observed that the Child-Pugh B patients had worsening of their liver function more frequently [37]. An increase in bilirubin was reported in 40% of Child-Pugh B patients compared to 18% of Child-Pugh A. Eighteen percent of Child-Pugh B patients developed or had worsening ascites compared to 11% of Child-Pugh A. Emerging or worsening encephalopathy was reported in 11% of Child-Pugh B patients compared to 2% of Child-Pugh A. As sorafenib acts as a substrate for the UDP-glucuronosyltransferase UGT1A1, it remains unclear if the total bilirubin elevation observed is due to worsening liver function caused by a direct toxic effect of sorafenib, by a benign inhibitory effect of UGT1A1, or simply due to disease progression, or combination of these potential explanations. Direct bilirubin levels were not obtained in the original phase II study. Despite a shorter course of therapy for Child-Pugh B patients (12.9 weeks) compared to Child-Pugh A (24.9 weeks), sorafenib was discontinued or dose reduced at the same rates. Median time to progression for Child-Pugh A was 21 weeks (95% CI: 16–25 weeks) and Child-Pugh B 13 weeks (95% CI: 9–18 weeks). Overall survival for Child-Pugh A was 41 weeks (95% CI: 37–64 weeks) and 14 weeks for Child-Pugh B (95% CI: 12–26 weeks). Thus, Child-Pugh B patients fared worse than Child-Pugh A patients and had more frequent worsening of their cirrhosis. More data are needed to appropriately define the safety and efficacy of sorafenib in patients with HCC and Child-Pugh B liver function.

In a phase I study evaluating two different doses of sorafenib in Japanese patients with advanced HCC [38], there were no substantial differences in the incidence of adverse events between Child-Pugh A and B groups. However, geometric means of AUC_{0-12} and Cmax at steady state were slightly lower in patients with Child-Pugh B cirrhosis compared with Child-Pugh A.

In 51 patients with solid and hematologic tumors and compromised liver or renal function, a phase I study of sorafenib did not report any apparent correlation with age or body weight [39]. More importantly deteriorating functional status of liver and renal parameters did not herald decreased clearance underscoring today's empiric standard of practice as regards dosing of sorafenib. Suggested recommendations regarding dosing of sorafenib from this study are 400 mg twice per day for bilirubin up to 1.5 × upper limit of normal (ULN); 200 mg twice per day for bilirubin 1.5–3 × ULN; while no safe dose of sorafenib was established for bilirubin levels above 3 × ULN.

In a recent manuscript detailing the FDA process of approval of sorafenib in HCC, Kane et al. referred to "the paucity of treatment options and variability in Child-Pugh scoring" as a reason for the broad approval for therapy by the FDA [40]; however, there has been a clear trend toward a restricted use of sorafenib for patient with Child-Pugh A and low B only [41–43] also highlighted by the recent more restricted approval of sorafenib solely for HCC patients with Child-Pugh A by the Canadian authorities [44].

Tumor Assessment

The importance of complete and partial tumor response is based on the assumption that volume reduction is a surrogate for treatment efficacy, i.e., prolongation of overall survival. RECIST and WHO classification are two commonly employed systems designed to quantitate tumor volume [45]. With the clinical success of targeted therapy achieving meaningful clinical benefit even in absence of tumor volume alterations, classic evaluation parameters may seem inadequate to assess treatment efficacy. True objective responses in HCC patients treated with sorafenib are rare [4, 9, 11]. In the phase II trial with sorafenib [9], 33.6% of patients had stable disease (SD) for ≥ 16 weeks, and central "tumor necrosis" in response to sorafenib was frequently noted (Fig. 22.2). In a subset of 12 patients, tumor necrosis was evaluated based on analysis of computed tomography (CT) scans and correlated to treatment response [10]. The ratio of tumor necrosis and volume (TV/TN) was significantly associated with response, with responders (including stable disease) having greater increases in the ratio between necrosis and tumor volume relative to baseline, as compared to non-responders ($p = 0.02$), N/T was not significantly associated with overall survival. N/T as part of evaluating response needs to be prospectively evaluated and validated as part of a large clinical study.

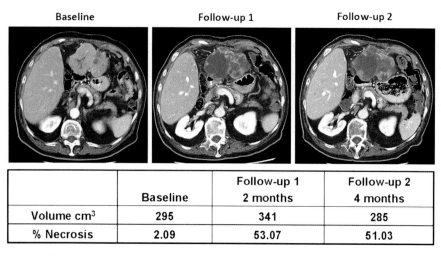

	Baseline	Follow-up 1 2 months	Follow-up 2 4 months
Volume cm^3	295	341	285
% Necrosis	2.09	53.07	51.03

Fig. 22.2 Tumor necrosis (TN) was quantified with a semiautomated computerized technique on intravenous contrast-enhanced scans in 11 of 16 patients with HCC treated with sorafenib. Among the parameters studies, i.e., tumor volume (TV), necrosis (TN), and the TV/TN ratio solely TV/TN was correlated significantly to treatment response but not survival. Modified after Abou-Alfa GK et al. [7]

This concept was further explored in a phase II study with the sunitinib [20]. Thirty-seven patients with unresectable HCC underwent assessment of antitumor activity using experimental parameters such as tumor density, volumetric measurement of percent tumor necrosis (VMTN), and intratumoral blood perfusion on monthly CT scan as compared to RECIST criteria. Decreased tumor density was observed in 68% of patients and activity assessed by VMTN showed minor (<50%) and major (= 50%) post-treatment tumor necrosis in 25 and 46% of patients, respectively. The authors concluded that tumor necrosis equal to 50% observed in 46% of patients receiving sunitinib suggested significant antitumor activity. These findings highlight the potential value of using tumor necrosis as a therapeutic monitoring tool which is feasibly translated to routine clinical practice.

Contrast-enhanced imaging techniques such as dynamic contrast enhanced (DCE)-MRI may provide additional information to better characterize and differentiate responders from non-responders. In the previously discussed phase II trial of sunitinib in HCC [21], DCE-MRI analyses were performed serially to measure modifications in vascular permeability (K^{trans}). There were reported decreases in this surrogate marker of angiogenic activity; however, correlation to response and outcome is awaited. Similarly, as part of the phase II trial studying the anti-VEGFR agent, bevacizumab in HCC patients, DCE-MRI was performed before and after 8 weeks of treatment in eight patients and a significant decrease in enhancement was noted in seven out of eight patients [16]. The fact that a significant correlation was reported with reduction in tumor diameter speaks, however, against a representative effect in a disease where tumor reduction is a very rare event. Larger studies are required to evaluate the significance of the observed findings.

Ultrasound, a non-invasive imaging modality which allows dynamic assessment of blood flow in a quantitative manner and in combination with contrast agents such as micro-bubbles, has further refined quantification of blood flow [46]. Exploiting this technology, 48 patients with HCC treated with bevacizumab every 2 weeks were followed by dynamic contrast enhanced (DCE)-US. DCE-US was performed pre-treatment and at days 3, 7, 15, and 2 months after SonoVue R (Bracco) bolus injection. Predefined flow parameters were measured [47]. Patients were categorized into good and poor responders according to the clinical benefit after 4 months based on RECIST criteria (good responders = partial response plus stable disease). Quantitative functional evaluation by DCE-US performed at day 3 and day 8 reportedly predicted the response to treatment at 4 months. Although preliminary these results, if validated in a multicenter setting, might constitute an attractive tool to tailor treatment to responders and shield patients from unwanted and sometimes significant side effects right at the start of therapy.

Computed tomographic (CT) perfusion is a similar technology that allows quantitative assessment of tumor blood flow (BF), blood volume (BV), mean transit time (MTT), and permeability surface area product (PS) [48]. In a feasibility study, 30 patients with unresectable or metastatic HCC underwent two CT perfusion imaging examinations within 30 h. The observed difference in perfusion between tumor tissue and normal liver was significantly different and there was a good correlation between repeated exams ($r = 0.9$, $p < 0.01$), underscoring the reproducibility of this new technology. Perfusion CT was further explored in a phase II trial of HCC patients with bevacizumab in combination with oxaliplatin and gemcitabine [49]. CT scans were performed at baseline and 10–12 days thereafter. Among the parameters studied, mean transit time (MTT) allowed prediction of clinical outcome. Responders were separated from non-responders on the basis of stable disease or response versus disease progression. When comparing baseline perfusion parameters to outcome, MTT was decreased in the group with worse clinical outcome. Studies exploring this technology further in HCC patients undergoing treatment are eagerly awaited to better evaluate the clinical use of this technology.

New Drug Development

As we continue to learn more about the molecular pathogenesis of HCC, new drugs for new targets continue to be developed.

Up-regulation of IGF-II, which occurs in 40% of HCC, has stimulated interest in its role as a potential target in HCC. IGF-II may target to the tyrosine kinase IGF-I receptor or the insulin receptor isoform A [50]. An IGF-1R antagonist is currently being studied in a phase II clinical trials in HCC.

Angiopoietin-2 (Ang-2) has been reported to be overexpressed in HCC [51]. This and other recent observations suggest the study of angiopoietin-2 inhibiting strategies in HCC. A phase II study evaluating AMG-386, an antiangiogenic therapy that provides potent and selective inhibition of angiopoietins [52], in HCC is planned.

The reported role of hepatocyte growth factor in HCC and its interaction with other relevant pathways in hepatocellular carcinogenesis such as EGF or IGF pathway have stimulated interest in this growth factor. In an exploratory study, RNA expression of HGF and its receptor c-met were measured in resected HCC tumor tissue and corresponding normal tissue. Despite a preferential overexpression of c-met in this early-stage resected disease setting, there was no correlation with overall survival [53]. Given persuasive animal data using NK4, a hepatocyte growth factor antagonist which showed antitumoral activity in an HCC xenograft model [54], clinical trials with c-met inhibitors in humans are ongoing to define its role in HCC.

Hedgehog (Hh) responsive tumors have been shown to spontaneously arise under circumstances where chronic liver injury and cirrhosis occur [55]. Exploratory studies of this pathway and its inhibitors, e.g., GDC0446 [56] are underway.

This is to name a few. On the other hand, several large randomized clinical trial efforts are underway evaluating new targeted therapies' single agents against the standard of care sorafenib. These include the evaluation of brivanib versus sorafenib, ABT-869 versus sorafenib, and sunitinib versus sorafenib. The latter phase III trial comparing sunitinib to sorafenib was closed prematurely, because of higher incidence of adverse events in the sunitinib arm. The study also did not meet criteria to demonstrate survival superiority or non-inferiority to sorafenib [57].

Summary

Single-agent therapies for advanced HCC have been studied extensively. Thus far, sorafenib has been approved as a standard of care. Several studies evaluating other antiangiogenic agents, tyrosine kinase inhibitors, and multi other targets are at varied phases in their development. Other than defining the clinical activity of these agents, several studies are also contributing to a better understanding of HCC in regard to etiology, extent of liver failure, and radiologic tumor assessment.

References

1. Thorgeirsson SS, Huber BE, Sorrell S, Fojo A, Pastan I, Gottesman MM (1987) Expression of the multidrug-resistant gene in hepatocarcinogenesis and regenerating rat liver. Science 236:1120–1122
2. Lopez PM, Villanueva A, Llovet JM (2006) Systematic review: evidence-based management of hepatocellular carcinoma—an updated analysis of randomized controlled trials. Aliment Pharmacol Ther 23:1535–1547
3. Llovet JM, Bruix J (2009) Testing molecular therapies in hepatocellular carcinoma: the need for randomized Phase II trials. J Clin Oncol 27:833–835
4. Llovet JM, Ricci S, Mazzaferro V, Hilgard P, Gane E, Blanc JF, de Oliveira AC et al (2008) Sorafenib in advanced hepatocellular carcinoma. N Engl J Med 359:378–390
5. Chen TM, Chang TM, Huang PT, Tsai MH, Lin LF, Liu CC, Ho KS et al (2008) Management and patient survival in hepatocellular carcinoma: does the physician's level of experience matter? J Gastroenterol Hepatol 23(7 Pt 2):e179–188
6. Abou-Alfa GK, Johnson P, Knox J, Davidenko I, Lacava J, Leung T et al (2008) Final results from a phase II (PhII), randomized, double-blind study of sorafenib plus doxorubicin (S+D) versus placebo plus doxorubicin (P+D) in patients (pts) with advanced hepatocellular carcinoma (AHCC). Gastrointestinal Cancer Symposium, Orlando, FL [Abstract 128] http://www.asco.org/ASCOv2/Meetings/Abstracts?&vmview=abst_detail_view&confID=53&abstractID=10215
7. Abou-Alfa GK, Zhao B, Capanu M, Guo P, Liu F, Jacobs G et al (2008) Tumor necrosis as a correlate for response in subgroup of patients with advanced hepatocellular carcinoma (HCC) treated with sorafenib. Ann Oncol 19(Suppl 8):viii178 [Abstract]
8. Liu L, Cao Y, Chen C, Zhang X, McNabola A, Wilkie D et al (2006) Sorafenib blocks the RAF/MEK/ERK pathway, inhibits tumor angiogenesis, and induces tumor cell apoptosis in hepatocellular carcinoma model PLC/PRF/5. Cancer Res 66:11851–11858
9. Strumberg D, Richly H, Hilger RA, Schleucher N, Korfee S, Tewes M et al (2005) Phase I clinical and pharmacokinetic study of the Novel Raf kinase and vascular endothelial growth factor receptor inhibitor BAY 43-9006 in patients with advanced refractory solid tumors. J Clin Oncol 23:965–972
10. Abou-Alfa GK, Schwartz L, Ricci S, Amadori D, Santoro A, Figer A et al (2006) Phase II study of sorafenib in patients with advanced hepatocellular carcinoma. J Clin Oncol 24:4293–4300
11. Cheng AL, Kang YK, Chen Z, Tsao CJ, Qin S, Kim JS et al (2009) Efficacy and safety of sorafenib in patients in the Asia-Pacific region with advanced hepatocellular carcinoma: a phase III randomised, double-blind, placebo-controlled trial. Lancet Oncol 10:25–34
12. Poon RT, Ng IO, Lau C, Zhu LX, Yu WC, Lo CM et al (2001) Serum vascular endothelial growth factor predicts venous invasion in hepatocellular carcinoma: a prospective study. Ann Surg 233:227–235

13. Lee TK, Poon RT, Yuen AP, Man K, Yang ZF, Guan XY et al (2006) Rac activation is associated with hepatocellular carcinoma metastasis by up-regulation of vascular endothelial growth factor expression. Clin Cancer Res 12:5082–5089

14. Yang JC, Haworth L, Sherry RM, Hwu P, Schwartzentruber DJ, Topalian SL et al (2003). A randomized trial of bevacizumab, an anti-vascular endothelial growth factor antibody for metastatic renal cancer. N Engl J Med 349:427–434

15. Malka D, Dromain C, Farace F, Horn S, Pignon J, Ducreux M et al (2007) Bevacizumab in patients (pts) with advanced hepatocellular carcinoma (HCC): Preliminary results of a phase II study with circulating endothelial cell (CEC) monitoring. J Clin Oncol 25(Suppl 18S): 4570

16. Siegel AB, Cohen EI, Ocean A, Lehrer D, Goldenberg A, Knox JJ et al (2008) Phase II trial evaluating the clinical and biologic effects of bevacizumab in unresectable hepatocellular carcinoma. J Clin Oncol 262:992–998

17. Tabernero J (2007) The role of VEGF and EGFR inhibition: implications for combining anti-VEGF and anti-EGFR agents. Mol Cancer Res 5:203–220

18. Thomas MB, Morris JS, Chadha R, Iwasaki M, Kaur H, Lin E et al (2009) Phase II trial of the combination of bevacizumab and erlotinib in patients who have advanced hepatocellular carcinoma. J Clin Oncol 27:833–835

19. Mendel DB, Laird AD, Xin X, Louie SG, Christensen JG, Li G, Schreck RE, Abrams TJ, Ngai TJ, Lee LB, Murray LJ, Carver J, Chan E et al (2003) In vivo antitumor activity of SU11248, a novel tyrosine kinase inhibitor targeting vascular endothelial growth factor and platelet-derived growth factor receptors: determination of a pharmacokinetic/pharmacodynamic relationship. Clin Cancer Res 9:327–337

20. Faivre SJ, Raymond E, Douillard J, Boucher E, Lim HY, Kim JS et al (2007) Assessment of safety and drug-induced tumor necrosis with sunitinib in patients (pts) with unresectable hepatocellular carcinoma (HCC). J Clin Oncol 25(Suppl 18S):3546

21. Zhu AX, Sahani DV, di Tomaso E, Duda DG, Catalano OA, Ancukiewicz M et al (2008) Sunitinib monotherapy in patients with advanced hepatocellular carcinoma (HCC): insights from a multidisciplinary phase II study. J Clin Oncol 26 (Suppl 15S):4521 [Abstract]

22. Huynh H, Ngo VC, Fargnoli J, Ayers M, Soo KC, Koong HN et al (2008) Brivanib alaninate, a dual inhibitor of vascular endothelial growth factor receptor and fibroblast growth factor receptor tyrosine kinases, induces growth inhibition in mouse models of human hepatocellular carcinoma. Clin Cancer Res 14:6146–6153

23. Raoul JL, Finn RS, Kang YK, Park JW, Harris R, Coric V, et al. (2009) An open-label phase II study of first- and second-line treatment with brivanib in patients with hepatocellular carcinoma (HCC). J Clin Oncol 27:15s [suppl; abstr 4577]

24. Finn RS, Kang Y, Park J, Harris R, Donica M, Walters I (2009) Phase II, open label study of brivanib alaninate in patients (pts) with hepatocellular carcinoma (HCC) who failed prior antiangiogenic therapy. Gastrointestinal Cancer Symposium, San Francisco, CA [Abstract No 200]

25. O'Dwyer PJ, Giantonio BJ, Levy DE, Kauh JS, Fitzgerald DB, Benson AB (2006) Gefitinib in advanced unresectable hepatocellular carcinoma: results from the Eastern Cooperative Oncology Group's Study E1203. J Clin Oncol 24(Suppl, 18S):4143

26. Ramanathan RK, Belani CP, Singh DA, Tanaka M, Lenz HJ, Yen Y, et al. (2009) A phase II study of lapatinib in patients with advanced biliary tree and hepatocellular cancer. Cancer Chemother Pharmacol 64(4):777–783

27. Zhu AX, Stuart K, Blaszkowsky LS, Muzikansky A, Reitberg DP, Clark JW et al (2007) Phase 2 study of cetuximab in patients with advanced hepatocellular carcinoma. Cancer 110: 581–589

28. Gruenwald V, Wilkens L, Gebel M, Greten TF, Kubicka S, Ganser A,Manns MP, Malek NP (2007) A phase II open-label study of cetuximab in unresectable hepatocellular carcinoma: final results. J Clin Oncol 25(Suppl 18S):4598

29. Philip PA, Mahoney MR, Allmer C, Thomas J, Pitot HC, Kim G et al (2005) Phase II study of Erlotinib (OSI-774) in patients with advanced hepatocellular cancer. J Clin Oncol 23: 6657–6663

30. Thomas MB, Chadha R, Glover K, Wang X, Morris J, Brown T et al (2007) Phase 2 study of erlotinib in patients with unresectable hepatocellular carcinoma. Cancer 110:1059–1067

31. Llovet J, ASCO 2008, Chicago, IL [Commentary]

32. Huitzil FD, Saltz LS, Song J, Capanu M, Jacobs G, Moscovici M et al (2007) Retrospective analysis of outcome in hepatocellular carcinoma (HCC) patients (pts) with Hepatitis C (C+) versus B (B+) treated with Sorafenib (S). ASCO GI Oncology Symposium, Orlando, FL [Abstract 173]

33. Bolondi L, Caspary W, Bennouna J, Thomson B, Van Steenbergen WF et al (2008) Clinical benefit of sorafenib in hepatitis C patient with hepatocellular carcinoma (HCC): subgroup analysis of the SHARP trial. ASCO Gastrointestinal Cancer Symposium, Orlando, FL [Abstract 129]

34. Bürckstümmer T, Kriegs M, Lupberger J, Pauli EK, Schmittel S, Hildt E (2006) Raf-1 kinase associates with Hepatitis C virus NS5A and regulates viral replication. FEBS Lett 580: 575–580

35. Giambartolomei S, Covone F, Levrero M, Balsano C (2001) Sustained activation of the Raf/MEK/Erk pathway in response to EGF in stable cell lines expressing the Hepatitis C Virus (HCV) core protein. Oncogene 20:2606–2610

36. Kelley RK, Venook AP (2008) Sorafenib in hepatocellular carcinoma: separating the hype from the hope. J Clin Oncol 26:5845–5848

37. Abou-Alfa GK, Amadori D, Santoro A, Figer A, De Greve J, Lathia C et al (2008) Is sorafenib (S) safe and effective in patients (pts) with hepatocellular carcinoma (HCC) and Child-Pugh B (CPB) cirrhosis? J Clin Oncol 26(Suppl):4518 [Abstract]

38. Furuse J, Ishii H, Nakachi K, Suzuki E, Shimizu S, Nakajima K (2008) Phase I study of sorafenib in Japanese patients with hepatocellular carcinoma. Cancer Sci 99:159–165

39. Miller AA, Murry DJ, Owzar K, Hollis DR, Kennedy EB, Abou-Alfa G et al (2009) Phase I and pharmacokinetic study of sorafenib in patients with hepatic or renal dysfunction: CALGB 60301. J Clin Oncol 27:1800–1805

40. Kane RC, Farrell AT, Madabushi R, Booth B, Chattopadhyay S, Sridhara R et al (2009) Sorafenib for the treatment of unresectable hepatocellular carcinoma. Oncologist 14:95–100

41. Abou-Alfa GK (2009) Commentary: sorafenib – the end of a long journey in search of systemic therapy for hepatocellular carcinoma, or the beginning? Oncologist 14:92–94

42. Pinter M, Sieghart W, Graziadei I, Vogel W, Maieron A, Königsberg R et al (2009) Sorafenib in unresectable hepatocellular carcinoma from mild to advanced stage liver cirrhosis. Oncologist 14:70–76

43. Zhu AX, Clark JW (2009) Commentary: sorafenib use in patients with advanced hepatocellular carcinoma and underlying Child-Pugh B cirrhosis: evidence and controversy. Oncologist 14:67–69

44. Cancer Care Ontario, Ontario, Canada, http://www.cancercare.on.ca/pdfdrugs/Sorafenib.pdf. Accessed May 2009

45. Eisenhauer EA, Therasse P, Bogaerts J, Schwartz LH, Sargent D, Ford R, Dancey J et al (2009) New response evaluation criteria in solid tumours: revised RECIST guideline (version 1.1). Eur J Cancer 45:228–247

46. Lamuraglia M, Escudier B, Chami L, Schwartz B, Leclère J, Roche A, Lassau N (2006) To predict progression-free survival and overall survival in metastatic renal cancer treated with sorafenib: pilot study using dynamic contrast-enhanced Doppler ultrasound. Eur J Cancer 42:2472–2479

47. Benatsou B, Lassau N, Chami L, Koscielny S, Roche A, Ducreux M et al (2008) Dynamic contrast-enhanced ultrasonography (DCE-US) with quantification for the early evaluation of hepato cellular carcinoma treated by bevacizumab in phase II. J Clin Oncol 26(Suppl):4588 [Abstract]

48. Sahani DV, Holalkere NS, Mueller PR, Zhu AX (2007) Advanced hepatocellular carcinoma: CT perfusion of liver and tumor tissue–initial experience. Radiology 243:736–743

49. Zhu AX, Holalkere NS, Muzikansky A, Horgan K, Sahani DV (2008) Early antiangiogenic activity of bevacizumab evaluated by computed tomography perfusion scan in patients with advanced hepatocellular carcinoma. Oncologist 13:120–125

50. Nussbaum T, Samarin J, Ehemann V, Bissinger M, Ryschich E, Khamidjanov A et al (2008) Autocrine insulin-like growth factor-II stimulation of tumor cell migration is a progression step in human hepatocarcinogenesis. Hepatology 48:146–156

51. Tanaka S, Mori M, Sakamoto Y, Makuuchi M, Sugimachi K, Wands JR (1999) Biologic significance of angiopoietin-2 expression in human hepatocellular carcinoma. J Clin Invest 103:341–345

52. Hong D, Gordon M, Appleman L, Kurzrock R, Sun Y., Rasmussen E et al (2008) Interim results from a phase 1b study of safety, pharmacokinetics (PK) and tumor response of the angiopoietin1/2-neutralizing peptibody AMG 386 in combination with AMG 706, bevacizumab (b) or sorafenib (s) in advanced solid tumors. Ann Oncol 19(Suppl 8), viii154 [Abstract]

53. Huitzil FD, Sun MY, Capanu M, Blumgart LH, Jarnagin WR, Fong Y et al (2008) Expression of the c-met and HGF in resected hepatocellular carcinoma (rHCC): Correlation with clinicopathological features (CP) and overall survival (OS). J Clin Oncol 26(Suppl 15S):4599 [Abstract]

54. Heideman DA, Overmeer RM, van Beusechem VW, Lamers WH, Hakvoort TB, Snijders PJ et al (2005) Inhibition of angiogenesis and HGF-cMET-elicited malignant processes in human hepatocellular carcinoma cells using adenoviral vector-mediated NK4 gene therapy. Cancer Gene Ther 12:954–962

55. Sicklick JK, Li YX, Jayaraman A, Kannangai R, Qi Y, Vivekanandan P et al (2006) Regulation of the Hedgehog pathway in human hepatocarcinogenesis. Carcinogenesis 27:748–757

56. LoRusso PM, Rudin CM, Borad MJ, Vernillet L, Darbonne WC, Mackey H et al. (2008) First-in-human, first-in-class, phase (ph) I study of systemic Hedgehog (Hh) pathway antagonist, GDC-0449, in patients (pts) with advanced solid tumors. J Clin Oncol 26(Suppl 15S):3516 [Abstract]

57. http://media.pfizer.com/files/news/press_releases/2010/sun_1170_042210.pdf

Chapter 23
The Future: Combination Systemic Therapy for Hepatocellular Carcinoma

Ahmed O. Kaseb and Melanie B. Thomas

Keywords HCC systemic therapy · Carcinogenic pathways in HCC · Growth factors · Combination systemic therapy · SHARP trial · EGFR and VEGF pathways · Sorafenib

Introduction

Hepatocellular carcinoma (HCC) is a potentially curable tumor by surgical resection, local ablation, or liver transplantation. However, the majority of patients with HCC present with advanced stage disease, which is most commonly, accompanied by severe background liver disease. Hence, curative treatments are feasible for only a small fraction of patients with localized disease. The emergence of chemotherapy in the 1950s has led to the availability of systemic therapies for patients with hematologic malignancies and advanced solid tumors. However, systemic cytotoxic therapies have demonstrated a very limited impact on the natural history of advanced HCC. In addition, molecular characterization of hepatocarcinogenesis has led to the recognition of defined aberrant signaling pathways which helped in subsequent development of targeted agents as potential choices for the treatment of HCC, when used alone or in combination.

The approval of the oral anti-cancer agent sorafenib (Nexavar®) for the treatment of patients with HCC in 2007 in both the United States and the European Union [1] represented a significant step forward in providing effective therapeutic options for the many individuals with advanced HCC. Prior to this exciting paradigm shift, HCC was regarded as a chemo-refractory, resistant tumor, and a sense of skepticism of ever developing effective systemic therapy for HCC, pervaded the field. Over the course of the previous decades, numerous clinical trials

A.O. Kaseb (✉)
Department of Gastrointestinal Medical Oncology, The University of Texas MD Anderson Cancer Center, Houston, TX, USA

of a wide variety of chemotherapeutic and hormonal agents had shown little or no activity in this complex malignancy [2]. Despite the fact that sorafenib does not yield radiographic tumor shrinkage, the traditional measure of anti-tumor activity, it clearly does impact carcinogenic activity in HCC, based on prolongation of both time to tumor progression and overall survival [3]. The demonstration of improved patient outcome of a targeted chemotherapeutic agent in this very challenging malignancy has also generated renewed enthusiasm in the field and an explosion of clinical research efforts in HCC worldwide.

Sorafenib also provides a platform on which to build future comparative, adjuvant, and combination clinical trials to further improve patient outcome. The challenge going forward is to identify those agents that in combination with sorafenib have the greatest potential for improved efficacy while ensuring patient safety.

Combination Systemic Therapy for Hepatocellular Carcinoma

In recent years, several molecular "targets" including oncogenes, oncoproteins, and cellular receptors have been identified in a variety of cancers as being key elements in carcinogenic pathways. Hepatocarcinogenesis is a complex multistep process, which results in a large number of heterogeneous molecular abnormalities [4–8], and thus offers numerous potential targets for existing therapeutic agents. Consequently several agents that target a variety of pathways are rational choices for combination therapy in HCC. Clearly sorafenib is now established as an effective targeted agent in HCC. The future of successful systemic therapy in HCC is to improve upon the survival benefit of sorafenib by developing rational, effective combination regimens. Possible regimens include combining traditional cytotoxic agents, biologic agents that target other carcinogenic pathways, or both, with sorafenib. Ideally, preclinical data exist or will be developed, that confirms additive anti-cancer activity, to provide rationale for designing clinical trials of combinations. Further, development of strategies to "validate" the role of a particular molecular target in HCC, and surrogate markers of whether binding that target results in clinical efficacy, are desirable. Unfortunately, such data are elusive in even much more well-characterized tumors. Notably, angiogenesis is an essential step in the growth and spread of HCC. Inhibiting angiogenesis would therefore seem to be a reasonable approach to prevent or treat HCC. However, tumor neovessels differ from normal vasculature in that they are tortuous, irregular, and hyperpermeable. These abnormalities result in irregular blood flow and increased interstitial pressure inside the tumor, which can impair the delivery of oxygen (a known radiation sensitizer) and drugs to cancer cells. Emerging evidence suggests that antiangiogenic therapy can normalize the structure and function of the tumor neovasculature, thereby improving drug delivery. This normalization effect may underlie the therapeutic benefit of combined antiangiogenic and cytotoxic therapies as evident in colorectal cancer studies [9].

In some malignancies, the molecular target–targeted agent relationship is well understood, for example, the monoclonal antibody trastuzumab (Herceptin®) is only effective in tumors in which the her-2/neu oncoprotein is amplified. Conversely, there are several agents that target the transmembrane epidermal growth factor receptor (EGFR) and have demonstrated survival benefit in a broad range of tumor types, yet little is understood regarding the relationship between "target" expression and agent efficacy or lack thereof. Further, bevacizumab is a recombinant humanized monoclonal antibody that binds VEGF-A and targets tumor-associated angiogenesis by preventing receptor binding and has shown improved patient survival in multiple tumor types, yet a confirmed measurable relationship between target expression, binding, and activity remains to be described. Table 23.1 summarizes evidence that describes the status of target "validation" in a variety of malignancies.

Key Carcinogenic Pathways in HCC

The PI3K/Akt/mTOR pathway (phosphoinositide-3 kinase/protein kinase B/mammalian target of rapamycin) is responsible for cellular proliferation and apoptosis and is closely linked to cell cycle. PI3K is associated with cell surface growth factor receptors and upon ligand binding can trigger formation of PIP3, which in turn activates Akt and leads to a number of downstream events (mTOR being one of the targets) [10, 11]. This pathway is upregulated in a subset of HCC patients. Molecular targeted therapy such as rapamycin, a naturally occurring mTOR inhibitor, showed promising results in HCC cell lines [12, 13–15]. However, published results from clinical trials of agents that target MTOR in HCC patients are available in abstract form only [16–19].

The Ras–raf kinase pathway is also dysregulated in HCC and Ras-pathway activation is nearly ubiquitous in human HCC. This is an important regulatory pathway for cell growth, survival, and migration and is highly regulated by activators and inhibitors. The related Jak/Stat pathway is also activated by growth factors and cytokines involved in cell differentiation, proliferation, apoptosis. Both pathways are activated in majority of HCC tissue compared to non-cancerous liver, possibly by loss of inhibition. The protein RKIP (Raf kinase inhibitory protein) is downregulated in human HCC.

Growth Factors as Therapeutic Targets in HCC

There is extensive evidence for growth factor dysregulation in HCC (Table 23.2). The epidermal growth factor receptor (EGFR) is frequently expressed in human HCC cell cultures and EGF may be one of the mitogens that are needed for cellular proliferation. Several agents that inhibit EGF signaling are clinically available, including gefitinib, cetuximab, erlotinib and panitumumab. Erlotinib is an orally

Table 23.1 Select targeted anti-cancer agents

Agent	Target	Tumor type	Effect	Target Validated?
Trastuzumab Lapatinib	HER2 receptor HER1-2 heterodimers	HER2-overexpressing breast cancer	Improves survival Decreases recurrence as adjuvant therapy	Yes
Bevacizumab	mAB binds serum VEGF-A ligand	Metastatic colorectal, lung, breast cancers	Improves survival, TTP in metastatic colon, lung, breast cancers	No
Cetuximab (EGFR mAb)	Extra-cellular domain EGFR	Irinotecan-refractory colorectal cancer	Improves survival, TTP in metastatic colon	Yes: Kras mutants do not benefit from EGFR mAb
Gefitinib Erlotinib (EGFR TKI)	Intracellular phosphorylation site	NSCLC pancreatic	Improves survival NSCLC, 2nd line Improves PFS in pancreatic ca by <2 wks	EGFR mutations in minority of NSCLC patients predict benefit
Sorafenib	Raf–ras pathway, VEGF	RCC, HCC	Improves survival, TTP	No
Sunitinib	Raf–ras pathway, VEGF	GIST RCC	Improves survival and TTP	No
Bortezomib	mTOR	Myeloma	Improves survival Decreases transfusions	No
Imatinib	C-kit, PDGF	GIST CML	Improves RR, survival Decreases recurrence	Yes

HER, human epidermal growth factor receptor; mAB, monoclonal antibody; VEGF, vascular endothelial growth factor receptor; TTP, time to progression; EGFR, epithelial growth factor receptor; NSCLC, non-small cell lung cancer; RCC, renal cell carcinoma; HCC, hepatocellular carcinoma; mTOR, mammalian target of rapamycin; RR, response rate; PDGF, platelet-derived growth factor; GIST, gastrointestinal stromal tumor; CML, chronic myelocytic leukemia

active and selective inhibitor of the EGFR/HER1-related tyrosine kinase enzyme. EGFR/HER1 expression was detected in 88% of the patients in a Phase II study of erlotinib [20]. In two Phase II studies of this agent, the response rates were less than 10% but the disease control rate was more than 50%, and median survival times were 10.7 and 13 months, respectively [20, 21].

Table 23.2 Potential therapeutic targets in HCC

Factor	Mechanism	Expression in HCC
VEGF (angiogenesis)	• HCC highly vascular tumors • Early vascular invasion; negative prognostic factor • VEGF – known mitogen for hepatocytes • Frequency of vascular invasion is higher in HCC patient with high serum VEGF levels than low VEGF levels	• Highly prevalent in HCC • Increases with cell differentiation • VEGF gene is transcribed by HCC cells • VEGF protein produced by HCC cells • Neovascularization begins with precursor dysplastic nodules, progresses through HCC
IGF family	Common in fetal liver; declines after birth	Highly prevalent in HCC
Platelet-derived growth factor (PDGF)	Cell membrane receptor involved in proliferation, migration, blood vessel formation	• Highly expressed in liver • Induces fibrosis, steatosis, HCC • Links TGFβ to β-catenin accumulation
Fibroblast growth factor (FGF)	Involved in tumor neoangiogenesis	Over expression common in fibrosis, cirrhosis, HCC
HGF (hepatocyte growth factor)	Known pro-angiogenic growth factor, acts via c-met	• Common in hepatocyte regeneration • Expressed by hepatic stellate cells and myofibroblasts
EGF (epidermal growth factor receptor)	• Known mitogen in multiple tumor types Increases HCC cell line proliferation	• Common in chronic hepatitis, cirrhosis and HCC (40–80%) • erbB2 expression variable (11–80%)
TGFα (transforming growth factor) TGFβ/EGFR	Upregulates DNA synthesis Mitogenic for hepatocytes Interacts with EGFR Up regulated in 40%	• Frequent in hepatitis, cirrhosis, HCC; not in normal liver. • Expression in 80% of all HCCs • Potent stimulator of hepatocellular DNA synthesis, mitogenic

HCCs are generally hypervascular, and vascular endothelial growth factor (VEGF) promotes HCC development and metastasis. Various agents targeting the VEGF circulating ligand or transmembrane receptor, including bevacizumab (Avastin®), sorafenib (Nexavar®), and TSU-68, have been studied in patients with HCC. Bevacizumab, a monoclonal antibody inhibitor of VEGF ligand, has been investigated in Phase II studies alone or in combination with other agents.

These studies showed a high disease control rate of over 80% and a median PFS of more than 6 months [22, 23]. Sorafenib, an oral multikinase inhibitor, blocks tumor cell proliferation mainly by targeting Raf/MEK/ERK signaling at the level of Raf kinase and exerts an antiangiogenic effect by targeting VEGFR-2/-3. TSU-68 is an oral antiangiogenesis compound that blocks VEGFR-2 (vascular endothelial growth factor receptor), PDGFR (platelet-derived growth factor receptor), and FGFR (fibroblast growth factor receptor); a Phase I/II study has been conducted in Japan.

Existing Evidence for Benefit from Combination Systemic Therapy in HCC

There is much to be learned from the recent history of the development of combination targeted therapy in other solid tumors. For example, early Phase II clinical trials of the combination of bevacizumab and erlotinib in advanced renal cell carcinoma (RCC) showed improved survival; however, in a larger randomized trial the difference in outcome from the combination therapy did not provide additional clinical benefit compared with bevacizumab alone [24–29]. Among the most efficacious combination therapies in solid tumors are those that have been developed in metastatic colorectal cancer. The addition of cetuximab (Erbitux®) to irinotecan-based chemotherapy and bevacizumab to 5-fluorouracil-based chemotherapy substantially prolonged patient survival in multiple studies [30–35]. Following the success of combination cytotoxic and biologic therapies in colorectal cancer, several trials were designed to assess the benefits of combining both biologics, erbitux and bevacizumab, with cytotoxic chemotherapy. Unfortunately, it was found that the combination resulted in excess toxicity and the trial was stopped early [36]. Similarly a Phase I clinical trial of the combination of sorafenib and bevacizumab in patients with solid tumor showed promising clinical activity, even in patients with refractory tumors, but significant toxicity requiring dose reductions in a significant majority of patients [37]. While the side effect profile of targeted agents in general is more favorable than traditional cytotoxic therapy, these agents are not benign and combinations must be studied in a step-wise fashion to maintain safety.

Notably, interaction between the EGFR and the VEGF pathways is well known. EGFR and VEGF share common downstream signaling pathways, and several preclinical studies have provided evidence for either direct or indirect angiogenic effects of EGFR signaling. In addition, direct EGFR angiogenic effects have been demonstrated by Hirata et al. [38]. Furthermore, in preclinical models, upregulation of VEGF has been implicated in resistance to EGFR inhibition [39]. Therefore, several clinical trials in different types of cancers combined anti-VEGF plus anti-EGFR [40]. Our trial was the first to report the clinical activity and confirm the tolerability

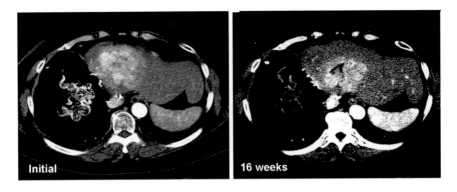

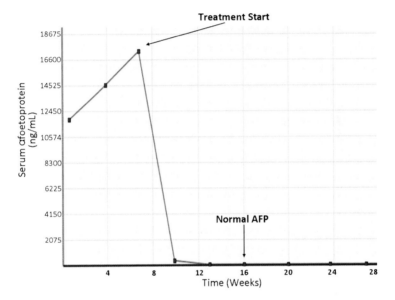

Fig. 23.1 Computed tomography images of the abdomen using four-phase imaging technique. Patient is a 59-year-old woman with right lobar moderately differentiated HCC, treated with right hepatectomy, and found to have a recurrence per her liver remnant a year later with serum AFP above 16,000 ng/mL. *Top figure* shows baseline CT with a restaging image after 16 weeks of treatment with bevacizumab and erlotinib; it shows decreased tumor size, increased central necrosis indicating anti-tumor effect. *Bottom figure* shows serum AFP level sharply declining to normal level after 16 weeks of treatment

of this combination in patients with HCC. Ten patients achieved a partial response for a confirmed overall response rate (intent-to-treat) of 25% (sorafenib = 2.7%). The median progression-free survival (PFS) was 39 weeks (95% CI, 26–45 weeks; 9.0 months) (sorafenib 5.5 months), and the median overall survival was 68 weeks (95% CI, 48–78 weeks; 15.6 months) (sorafenib 10.7 months) (Fig. 23.1).

Table 23.3 Selected clinical trials of systemic therapy combinations in patients with advanced HCC

Study	Regimen	Phase	Sample size	Response rate%	Median survival (mos)
Pastorelli et al. [41]	Pegylated adriamycin + gemcitabine	II	35	23	8.8 mos
Thomas et al. [42]	Bevacizumab + erlotinib	II	40	20.6	15.6 (PFS 9 mos)
Sun et al. [43]	Capecitabine + oxaliplatin + bevacizumab	II	30	11	PFS 5.4 mos
Zhu et al. [44]	GEMOX + bevacizumab	II	33	20	9.6 mos
Louafi et al. [45]	GEMOX + cetuximab	2	43	23	9.2
O'Neil et al. [46]	Capecitabine + oxaliplatin + cetuximab	2	25	11	TTP 4.3
Abou-Alfa et al. [47]	Doxorubicin + sorafenib vs doxorubicin	2	47/49	4 vs 2	13.8 vs 6.5
Hsu et al. [48]	Capecitabine + bevacizumab	2	34 (CLIP≤3)	9	8.2
Shen et al. [49]	Sorafenib + UFT (Tegafur/Uracil)	2	24	12	PFS 3.7

Several targeted agents have been recently tested in patients with advanced HCC in combination with other systemic therapies (see Table 23.3) [41–49].

Current Challenges to Combination Systemic Therapy in HCC Management

Perhaps the most significant recent advance in oncology therapeutics has been the approval of various "molecularly targeted" anti-cancer drugs, including antiangiogenic agents, either alone or in combination. However, clinical development of such drugs suffers from several handicaps, including a lack of effective ways to choose patients who are likely to respond, and monitoring the biologic activity as measured by tumor response.

Traditional systemic chemotherapies target mitotic events in proliferating cells. By exploiting the growth fraction differential between tumor cells and those of normal cells, tumor reduction might be eventually achieved. Furthermore, resistance to systemic chemotherapies may emerge as a result of tumor cellular changes, such as gene mutations, increased gene expression regulating drug efflux pumps, or downregulation of mutations in drug targets [50]. Notably, resistance mechanisms are often specific to the drug or drug class. Therefore, when using a multiagent regimen, the emergence of resistance to one agent might not apply to others. One of the major challenges in this clinical setting is to develop a mechanism to discern sensitivity to the individual components of a treatment regimen once progression occurs, which may aid in reserving drugs for which there remains sensitivity for further use. Unlike the mutational mechanisms that underlie resistance with systemic chemotherapies, resistance to targeted agents probably emerges via the activation of alternate pathways involved with hepatocarcinogenesis. Several mechanisms of resistance to antiangiogenesis therapy in HCC have been proposed, including signaling via alternative pathways, an increase in pericytes of the tumor neovessels that could reduce VEGF dependency, and activation and recruitment of bone-marrow-derived proangiogenic cells [51]. Thus, resistance to targeted agents may be related to activation of existing processes, rather than genetic mutations.

Another area of challenge is assessing response to targeted therapy combinations. For many years, the standard way to assess a patient's response to treatment has been to measure tumor size on longitudinal computed tomography (CT) or magnetic resonance imaging (MRI) scans, using bidimensional (World Health Organization [WHO]) or unidimensional (response evaluation criteria for solid tumor [RECIST]) criteria. However, because targeted agents inhibit molecular components of cellular proliferation and angiogenesis and thus abrogate tumor growth, they are more likely to delay disease progression and stabilize tumor size. This might explain the observed survival benefit despite the low incidence of objective responses as defined by RECIST criteria. Indeed, there is a potential for a transient increase in tumor volume or bidimensional area, the traditional endpoint for the determination of efficacy in clinical trials and in clinical practice. In clinical trials, even transient progression in tumor size is an indication to remove a patient from a study and consider the investigational agent of no benefit. Thus, the long-term effects may never be seen. Therefore, development of surrogate endpoints, either circulating or image-based, to evaluate any possible efficacy became a major challenge for clinical investigators developing targeted agents and for clinicians treating patients under treatment with targeted agents either alone or in combination with other systemic therapies. Changes in tumor microvasculature, as measured by changes in blood flow and volume and transit time, have been recommended as standards for describing the kinetics of a given dynamic or functional imaging modality in antiangiogenic studies. However, these observations will need to be validated prospectively.

Clinical Trial Design for Combination Systemic Therapy in HCC

As noted previously, the availability in the clinic of several novel biologic agents and the urgent need for effective therapies for advanced hepatocellular carcinoma has led to the evaluation of many of these agents in HCC, principally in Phase II trials. The SHARP trial is the first to demonstrate a statistically significant survival benefit for any chemotherapy agent in patients with HCC. This trial was, however, conducted in patients with excellent performance status and well-preserved (Childs A) liver function. The efficacy and safety of sorafenib in patients with poorer performance status and more advanced hepatic dysfunction is yet to be established. Assessment of patient safety and tolerance is essential to combination therapy trials in HCC given the prevalence of hepatic dysfunction in this population. This can be accomplished by conducting separate Phase I (dose-escalation) trials or combination Phase I–II trials. A key objective going forward is to continue assessing new biologic agents in combination with sorafenib, across the broad spectrum of HCC patients seen in the community. The traditional approach in oncology research has been to evaluate new agents in single-arm Phase II studies using classic radiological response criteria such as WHO or RECIST [52–55] as a measure of anti-tumor activity. A "favorable" rate of radiographic response would be considered a biologic signal that supports transitioning promising agents forward into randomized, controlled Phase III clinical trials. This approach, however, is being questioned since traditional radiographic tumor shrinkage is uncommon with biologic agents, although they clearly lead to meaningful patient benefit in a wide variety of malignancies [56]. This is clearly the case in HCC where radiological assessment is notoriously difficult due to poor delineation of tumors in the liver and tumor necrosis may occur without any change in overall tumor dimensions [57]. These observations have led some investigators to develop Phase II studies with a major focus on correlative studies that may help delineate a mechanism of action for a particular drug (e.g., a kinase inhibitor along one of the different cell cycle pathways) such as downregulation of a downstream kinase which may predict response or by using novel radiological techniques that use changes in blood flow as criteria by which to assess biologic activity of antiangiogenic therapies [58–61]. Another option is to use the randomized Phase II trial design that by providing a contemporary control group may permit a more confident assessment of the likelihood that a particular agent is worthy to progress to Phase III [62–64]. Clinical trials are costly, time consuming, and use precious patient resources, and there is inevitable tension between designing trials based on empirically combining agents based on "rational" targets vs the longer process of first developing preclinical data that support combinations, which may or may not be confirmed in human trials.

Key considerations in the planning and design of clinical trials of combination agents in HCC include as follows:

- There is no lack of new agents to study in HCC.
- Nearly all major carcinogenic mechanisms are "candidates" for targeted therapy in HCC.
- It is critical to avoid "shotgun" approach of doing Phase II studies of every new available agent, in the absence of preclinical supporting evidence.
- Conduct rational, evidenced-based drug selection. and preclinical "target validation" if possible.
- Combination regimens must be both efficacious and safe in HCC patients, especially in those with hepatic dysfunction.

- Patient selection in Phase II clinical trials can be challenging due to lack of consistent definition of what constitutes "advanced disease."
- Assessing clinically meaningful anti-cancer activity. Currently the RECIST criteria used to evaluate changes in unidimensional tumor size are inadequate to capture changes in tumor vascularity commonly seen with biologic agents in HCC. Future clinical trials should include validated functional imaging techniques to truly capture the anti-tumor activity targeted agents.

Conclusions

Conducting controlled clinical trials of systemic chemotherapy regimens in HCC patients is challenging. Obstacles include the multiple comorbidities of patients with cirrhosis, the intrinsic chemo-resistance of HCC, the advanced nature of HCC at presentation in a majority of patients, patients selection, lack of biomarkers, both circulating and image-based, to response or resistance to therapy, pharmacotherapeutic challenges of treating a cancer that arises in an already-damaged liver, and the distribution of the majority of patients primarily in developing nations where multi-disciplinary treatment of HCC may not be available. Hepatocellular cancer is a heterogeneous disease in terms of its etiology, underlying associations, and biologic and clinical behavior, which further complicates clinical trial design. The recent approval of sorafenib for advanced HCC is encouraging progress and is expected to pave the way for additional trials in the adjuvant setting. The need for effective systemic therapies for HCC patients remains evident, and making continued progress in this disease requires the talent and expertise of all the medical disciplines involved in the care of HCC patients.

References

1. Lang L (2008) FDA approves sorafenib for patients with inoperable liver cancer. Gastroenterology 134:379
2. Simonetti RG, Liberati A, Angiolini C et al (1997) Treatment of hepatocellular carcinoma: a systematic review of randomized controlled trials. Ann Oncol 8:117–136
3. Llovet JM, Ricci S, Mazzaferro V et al (2008) Sorafenib in advanced hepatocellular carcinoma. N Engl J Med 359:378–390
4. Yao DF, Dong ZZ, Yao M (2007) Specific molecular markers in hepatocellular carcinoma. Hepatobiliary Pancreat Dis Int 6:241–247
5. Marongiu F, Doratiotto S, Montisci S et al (2008) Liver repopulation and carcinogenesis: two sides of the same coin? Am J Pathol 172:857–864
6. Varnholt H (2008) The role of microRNAs in primary liver cancer. Ann Hepatol 7:104–113
7. McGivern DR, Lemon SM (2009) Tumor suppressors, chromosomal instability, and hepatitis C virus-associated liver cancer. Annu Rev Pathol 4:399–415
8. Pang RW, Poon RT (2007) From molecular biology to targeted therapies for hepatocellular carcinoma: the future is now. Oncology 72(Suppl 1):30–44
9. Jain RK (2005) Antiangiogenic therapy for cancer: current and emerging concepts. Oncology (Williston Park) 19:7–16

10. Tovar V, Villanueva A, Llovet JM (2007) [Cell biology and genetics in liver cancer]. Gastroenterol Hepatol 30:360–369
11. Calvisi DF, Pinna F, Ladu S et al (2008) Aberrant iNOS signaling is under genetic control in rodent liver cancer and potentially prognostic for the human disease. Carcinogenesis 29:1639–1647
12. Tam KH, Yang ZF, Lau CK et al (2009) Inhibition of mTOR enhances chemosensitivity in hepatocellular carcinoma. Cancer Lett 273:201–209
13. Ladu S, Calvisi DF, Conner EA et al (2008) E2F1 inhibits c-Myc-driven apoptosis via PIK3CA/Akt/mTOR and COX-2 in a mouse model of human liver cancer. Gastroenterology 135:1322–1332
14. Lang SA, Moser C, Fichnter-Feigl S et al (2009) Targeting heat-shock protein 90 improves efficacy of rapamycin in a model of hepatocellular carcinoma in mice. Hepatology 49:523–532
15. Huynh H, Ngo VC, Koong HN et al (2009) Sorafenib and rapamycin induce growth suppression in mouse models of hepatocellular carcinoma. J Cell Mol Med
16. Treiber G (2009) mTOR inhibitors for hepatocellular cancer: a forward-moving target. Expert Rev Anticancer Ther 9: 247–261
17. Tanaka S, Arii S (2009) Molecularly targeted therapy for hepatocellular carcinoma. Cancer Sci 100:1–8
18. Rizell M, Andersson M, Cahlin C et al (2008) Effects of the mTOR inhibitor sirolimus in patients with hepatocellular and cholangiocellular cancer. Int J Clin Oncol 13:66–70
19. Monaco AP (2009) The role of mTOR inhibitors in the management of posttransplant malignancy. Transplantation 87:157–163
20. Thomas MB, Chadha R, Glover K et al (2007) Phase 2 study of erlotinib in patients with unresectable hepatocellular carcinoma. Cancer 110:1059–1067
21. Philip PA, Mahoney MR, Allmer C et al (2005) Phase II study of Erlotinib (OSI-774) in patients with advanced hepatocellular cancer. J Clin Oncol 23:6657–6663
22. Finn RS, Zhu AX (2009) Targeting angiogenesis in hepatocellular carcinoma: focus on VEGF and bevacizumab. Expert Rev Anticancer Ther 9: 503–509
23. Siegel AB, Cohen EI, Ocean A et al (2008) Phase II trial evaluating the clinical and biologic effects of bevacizumab in unresectable hepatocellular carcinoma. J Clin Oncol 26:2992–2998
24. Bukowski RM (2008) What role do combinations of interferon and targeted agents play in the first-line therapy of metastatic renal cell carcinoma? Clin Genitourin Cancer 6:S14–S21
25. Chowdhury S, Larkin JM, Gore ME (2008) Recent advances in the treatment of renal cell carcinoma and the role of targeted therapies. Eur J Cancer 44:2152–2161
26. Kruck S, Kuczyk MA, Gakis G et al (2008) Novel therapeutic options in metastatic renal cancer – review and post ASCO 2007 update. Rev Recent Clin Trials 3:212–216
27. Papaetis GS, Karapanagiotou LM, Pandha H et al (2008) Targeted therapy for advanced renal cell cancer: cytokines and beyond. Curr Pharm Des 14:2229–2251
28. Rini BI, Flaherty K (2008) Clinical effect and future considerations for molecularly-targeted therapy in renal cell carcinoma. Urol Oncol 26:543–549
29. Wysocki PJ, Zolnierek J, Szczylik C et al (2008) Targeted therapy of renal cell cancer. Curr Opin Investig Drugs 9:570–575
30. Wong SF (2005) Cetuximab: an epidermal growth factor receptor monoclonal antibody for the treatment of colorectal cancer. Clin Ther 27:684–694
31. Folprecht G, Lutz MP, Schoffski P et al (2006) Cetuximab and irinotecan/5-fluorouracil/folinic acid is a safe combination for the first-line treatment of patients with epidermal growth factor receptor expressing metastatic colorectal carcinoma. Ann Oncol 17:450–456
32. Rougier P, Lepere C (2005) Second-line treatment of patients with metastatic colorectal cancer. Semin Oncol 32:S48–S54
33. Hurwitz H, Fehrenbacher L, Novotny W et al (2004) Bevacizumab plus irinotecan, fluorouracil, and leucovorin for metastatic colorectal cancer. N Engl J Med 350:2335–2342

34. Fernando NH, Hurwitz HI (2004) Targeted therapy of colorectal cancer: clinical experience with bevacizumab. Oncologist 9(Suppl 1):11–18

35. Hurwitz HI, Fehrenbacher L, Hainsworth JD et al (2005) Bevacizumab in combination with fluorouracil and leucovorin: an active regimen for first-line metastatic colorectal cancer. J Clin Oncol 23:3502–3508

36. Simkens L, Tol J, Koopman M et al (2008) Current questions in the treatment of advanced colorectal cancer: the CAIRO studies of the Dutch Colorectal Cancer Group. Clin Colorectal Cancer 7:105–109

37. Azad NS, Posadas EM, Kwitkowski VE et al (2008) Combination targeted therapy with sorafenib and bevacizumab results in enhanced toxicity and antitumor activity. J Clin Oncol 26:3709–3714

38. Hirata A, Ogawa S, Kometani T et al (2002) ZD1839 (Iressa) induces antiangiogenic effects through inhibition of epidermal growth factor receptor tyrosine kinase. Cancer Res 62: 2554–2560

39. Viloria-Petit A, Crombet T, Jothy S et al (2001) Acquired resistance to the antitumor effect of epidermal growth factor receptor-blocking antibodies in vivo: a role for altered tumor angiogenesis. Cancer Res 61:5090–5101

40. Ciardiello F, Troiani T, Bianco R et al (2006) Interaction between the epidermal growth factor receptor (EGFR) and the vascular endothelial growth factor (VEGF) pathways: a rational approach for multi-target anticancer therapy. Ann Oncol 17(Suppl 7):vii109–vii114

41. Pastorelli D, Cartei G, Zustovich F et al (2006) Gemcitabine and liposomal doxorubicin in biliary and hepatic carcinoma (HCC) chemotherapy: preliminary results and review of the literature. Ann Oncol 17(Suppl 5): v153–v157

42. Thomas MB, Morris JS, Chadha R et al (2009) Phase II trial of the combination of beva-cizumab and erlotinib in patients who have advanced hepatocellular carcinoma. J Clin Oncol 27:843–850

43. Sun W, Haller DG, Mykulowycz K et al (2007) Combination of capecitabine, oxaliplatin with bevacizumab in treatment of advanced hepatocellular carcinoma (HCC): a phase II study. J Clin Oncol, 2007 ASCO Annual Meeting Proceedings Part I, vol 25, No. 18S (June 20 Supplement), Abstract No. 4574

44. Zhu AX, Blaszkowsky LS, Ryan DP et al (2006) Phase II study of gemcitabine and oxaliplatin in combination with bevacizumab in patients with advanced hepatocellular carcinoma. J Clin Oncol 24:1898–1903

45. Louafi S, Boige V, Ducreux M et al (2007) Gemcitabine plus oxaliplatin (GEMOX) in patients with advanced hepatocellular carcinoma (HCC): results of a phase II study. Cancer 109: 1384–1390

46. O'Neil BH, Bernard SA, Goldberg RM et al (2008) Phase II study of oxaliplatin, capecitabine, and cetuximab in advanced hepatocellular carcinoma. J Clin Oncol, 2008 Gastrointestinal Cancers Symposium, Abstract No. 228

47. Abou-Alfa GK, Johnson P, Knox J et al (2008) Final results from a phase II (PhII), random-ized, double-blind study of sorafenib plus doxorubicin (S+D) versus placebo plus doxorubicin (P+D) in patients (pts) with advanced hepatocellular carcinoma (AHCC). J Clin Oncol, 2008 ASCO Annual Meeting, vol 26:(May 20 Suppl), Abstract No. 4603

48. Hsu C, Yang T, Hsu C et al (2008) Phase II study of bevacizumab (A) plus capecitabine (X) in patients (pts) with advanced/metastatic hepatocellular carcinoma (HCC): final report. J Clin Oncol, 2008 Gastrointestinal Cancers Symposium, Abstract No. 128

49. Mellor HR, Callaghan R (2008) Resistance to chemotherapy in cancer: a complex and integrated cellular response. Pharmacology 81:275–300

50. Bergers G, Hanahan D (2008) Modes of resistance to anti-angiogenic therapy. Nat Rev Cancer 8:592–603

51. Suzuki C, Jacobsson H, Hatschek T et al (2008) Radiologic measurements of tumor response to treatment: practical approaches and limitations. Radiographics 28:329–344

52. Kharuzhyk S, Fabel M, von Tengg-Kobligk H et al (2008) Image-based evaluation of tumor response to treatment: where is radiology today? Exp Oncol 30:181–189
53. Therasse P, Eisenhauer EA, Verweij J (2006) RECIST revisited: a review of validation studies on tumour assessment. Eur J Cancer 42:1031–1039
54. Therasse P, Arbuck SG, Eisenhauer EA et al (2000) New guidelines to evaluate the response to treatment in solid tumors. European Organization for Research and Treatment of Cancer, National Cancer Institute of the United States, National Cancer Institute of Canada.[see comment]. J Natl Cancer Inst 92:205–216
55. Barros Costa RL (2009) Targeted therapy: comprehensive review. Am J Hosp Palliat Care 26:137–146
56. Gervais DA, Kalva S, Thabet A (2009) Percutaneous image-guided therapy of intra-abdominal malignancy: imaging evaluation of treatment response. Abdom Imaging 34:593–609
57. Chen K, Li ZB, Wang H et al (2008) Dual-modality optical and positron emission tomography imaging of vascular endothelial growth factor receptor on tumor vasculature using quantum dots. Eur J Nucl Med Mol Imaging 35:2235–2244
58. Jiang HJ, Zhang ZR, Shen BZ et al (2008) Functional CT for assessment of early vascular physiology in liver tumors. Hepatobiliary Pancreat Dis Int 7:497–502
59. Juanyin J, Tracy K, Zhang L et al (2009) Noninvasive imaging of the functional effects of anti-VEGF therapy on tumor cell extravasation and regional blood volume in an experimental brain metastasis model. Clin Exp Metastasis, 2009
60. Frangioni JV (2008) New technologies for human cancer imaging. J Clin Oncol 26:4012–4021
61. Stadler WM (2007) The randomized discontinuation trial: a phase II design to assess growth-inhibitory agents. Mol Cancer Ther 6:1180–1185
62. Karrison TG, Maitland ML, Stadler WM et al (2007) Design of phase II cancer trials using a continuous endpoint of change in tumor size: application to a study of sorafenib and erlotinib in non small-cell lung cancer. J Natl Cancer Inst 99:1455–1461
63. Rubinstein L, Crowley J, Ivy P et al (2009) Randomized phase II designs. Clin Cancer Res 15:1883–1890
64. Shen Y, Hsu C, Hsu C et al (2008) Phase II study of sorafenib plus tegafur/uracil (UFT) in patients with advanced hepatocellular carcinoma (HCC). J Clin Oncol, 2008 ASCO Annual Meeting, vol 26:(May 20 Suppl), Abstract No. 15664

Chapter 24
Follow-Up and Salvage Therapy for Recurrent Hepatocellular Carcinoma

Kelly M. McMasters and Jean-Nicolas Vauthey

Keywords HCC · Hepatic resection · Salvage therapy HCC · HCC Recurrence · Molecular markers

Introduction

Although liver transplantation has become a viable option for treatment of many patients with hepatocellular carcinoma (HCC), the limited availability of donor organs and the strict criteria for organ transplantation limit the use of transplantation for this disease. Hepatic resection remains the gold standard nontransplant treatment modality and is still the first-line treatment in many centers. For patients with unresectable disease, radiofrequency ablation and other ablative techniques are often now used with curative intent for patients with limited hepatic disease amenable to such strategies. Although advances in surgical technique and perioperative care have reduced operative mortality for patients with HCC dramatically, and several series have reported a 40–50% 5-year survival rate after resection for HCC, recurrence is the rule rather than the exception, and many patients succumb to this disease even after surviving 5 years. Recurrence after liver resection has been reported in the range of 75–100% in several series. Indeed, the first site of recurrence is most commonly the liver in 78–96% of cases, either as a result of intrahepatic metastasis or as a multicentric disease arising in the liver remnant [1]. Recurrence after ablation also remains exceedingly high.

Poon et al. [2] performed a systematic review of the English literature from 1980 until 1999 to evaluate risk factors associated with recurrence after resection for HCC. The authors found that pathologic factors that were significant in predicting tumor recurrence included vascular invasion, presence of satellite nodules, large tumor size (especially >5 cm), and advanced TNM stage; active hepatitis also was a

K.M. McMasters (✉)
Department of Surgery, University of Louisville, Louisville, KY, USA

K.M. McMasters, J.-N. Vauthey (eds.), *Hepatocellular Carcinoma*,
DOI 10.1007/978-1-60327-522-4_24, © Springer Science+Business Media, LLC 2011

significant factor predisposing patients to recurrence. Other pathologic factors such as tumor encapsulation, histologic differentiation, and DNA ploidy have not been shown to predict recurrence consistently. Molecular markers such as proliferating cell nuclear antigen (PCNA), telomerase activity, and various angiogenesis markers may also predict recurrence. Whether cirrhosis is a predictor of recurrence is also controversial. In terms of surgical factors affecting recurrence of HCC, certainly resection margins, intraoperative blood loss, and perioperative transfusion have been associated with a higher risk of postoperative recurrence. The number of tumors is also a predictor of recurrence-free survival. Unfortunately, to date, there are no proven effective adjuvant therapies to reduce the risk of recurrence after resection or ablation. Given the high-risk of recurrence after resection or ablation for HCC and the potential for salvage therapy, careful postoperative surveillance is warranted.

Follow-Up After Resection or Ablation for HCC

Although many centers use slightly different surveillance strategies after resection or ablation for HCC, all utilize a combination of tumor markers and imaging studies. The liver is the most common site of metastatic or recurrent disease; common sites of extrahepatic disease, in order of prevalence, include lung, abdominal lymph nodes, bone, and adrenal gland. The United States National Comprehensive Cancer Network (NCCN) recommends high-quality cross-sectional imaging every 3–6 months for 2 years, then annually [3]. This can include multi-slice triple phase CT scanning or magnetic resonance imaging (MRI). In many centers around the world, however, ultrasound is used as the principal imaging modality for follow-up, although its sensitivity is somewhat less for detection of recurrence. Alpha-fetoprotein (AFP) levels, if initially elevated, should be checked every 3 months for 2 years, then every 6 months thereafter. The role of other tumor markers, such as des-gamma carboxyprothrombin (DCP), AFP-L3, glypican-3, IGF-1, and HGF, remains unclear in this setting. Because pulmonary metastasis is the most common site of extrahepatic metastatic disease for HCC, chest x-ray or CT scan of the chest should also be evaluated at regular intervals. A bone scan for patients with symptoms of bone metastases is also warranted, but is not generally ordered routinely for surveillance.

Salvage Therapy for Patients with Hepatic Recurrence of HCC

Treatment modalities for patients with hepatic recurrence of HCC include liver transplantation, repeat resection, ablation, intra-arterial therapy, and systemic therapy. Transarterial chemoembolization (TACE) and intra-arterial drug-eluting bead therapy are discussed in Chapters 19 and 20, respectively; little is known about the use of these modalities for patients with recurrent HCC in the liver. Similarly, the use of radiofrequency (Chapter 17) or microwave (Chapter 18) ablation for recurrent HCC has not been well studied. Therefore, we will focus on transplantation, repeat resection, and TACE as salvage therapy for liver recurrence.

Poon et al. [1] evaluated their experience with 105 patients who developed intrahepatic recurrence. These patients were treated with repeat resection ($n = 11$), TACE ($n = 71$), percutaneous ethanol injection ($n = 6$), systemic chemotherapy ($n = 8$), or palliative treatment ($n = 9$). The overall 1-, 3-, and 5-year survival rates from the time of recurrence were 65, 35, and 20%, respectively. The 1-, 3-, and 5-year survival rates for the 11 patients who underwent repeat resection after recurrence were 81, 69, and 69%, respectively. Five of these patients were alive and disease free for a range of 9–56 months after repeat resection, three were alive with recurrence, and four had died of recurrent disease. Of the 71 patients who underwent TACE for treatment for liver recurrence, the 1-, 3-, and 5-year survival rates were 72, 38, and 21%, respectively. The survival of these patients was significantly worse than those who underwent repeat resection. The 1-, 3-, and 5-year survival rates for the six patients who underwent percutaneous ethanol ablation were 67, 22, and 0%, respectively. Eight patients underwent systemic chemotherapy with a 1-year survival rate of 38%, but no patient survived 3 years. The nine patients who underwent palliative care only had a median survival rate of 2.7 months and there were no 1-year survivors. On multivariate analysis, Child's Classification at the time of recurrence, serum albumin level at the time of recurrence, interval between initial hepatectomy and recurrence, the number of recurrent tumors, the presence of extrahepatic recurrence, and type of treatment for recurrence were all statistically significant factors predicting survival. The authors concluded that aggressive multimodality treatment can result in prolonged survival for patients with intraheptic recurrence after curative resection for HCC. However, the optimal guidelines for patient management in this situation remain to be clarified.

Shah et al. [4] reviewed their experience with 193 consecutive patients who underwent hepatic resection with curative intent for HCC. A total of 98 patients (51%) experienced recurrent cancer; initial tumor recurrence was confined to the liver in 86 patients (88%). Of the 98 patients who experienced tumor recurrence, 53 patients (54%) underwent additional therapy, including ablation ($n = 31$), repeat resection ($n = 11$), TACE ($n = 8$), and liver transplantation ($n = 3$). The patients who did not undergo any therapy either had a large tumor burden of recurrent multifocal disease, extrahepatic disease, or refused further therapy. The overall survival rate for patients who underwent additional therapy was 45 months vs. 9 months for those that did not undergo further therapy. On multivariate analysis, vascular invasion, time to recurrence less than 12 months, and lack of additional therapy were all independent prognostic factors predictive of poor survival after hepatic recurrence of HCC. The authors proposed the algorithm for treatment of recurrence after hepatic resection for HCC, as seen in Fig. 24.1.

Poon et al. [2] reviewed the world literature regarding management of recurrent hepatocellular carcinoma after resection. Multiple series have documented 5-year survival rates between 37 and 87% for repeat resection after hepatic recurrence of HCC. In multiple studies, repeat resection was shown to result in improved survival

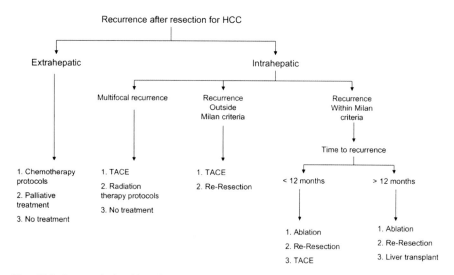

Fig. 24.1 Proposed algorithm for treatment of recurrence after resection for HCC. TACE, transarterial chemoembolization. Reproduced from Surgery 2007 with permission from Elsevier/Mosby/Saunders [4]

compared to nonsurgical therapy (Table 24.1) [1, 5–17]. In some studies, it has been shown that the overall survival rates of patients with recurrence managed by repeat resection, calculated from the time of first hepatic resection, were similar to those without recurrence. This certainly suggests that repeat resection is a valuable treatment modality for patients with hepatic recurrence. There are no prospective randomized trials to compare treatment modalities for patients with hepatic recurrence; however, the data strongly suggest that repeat hepatic resection is an effective treatment for such patients.

Poon et al. [2] also reviewed the results of TACE for recurrent hepatocellular carcinoma after resection. Several series have reported 3-year survival rates of between 24 and 48% and 5-year survival rates between 0 and 27% for patients treated with TACE after recurrence. However, there is no level I evidence to suggest that TACE is superior to other therapies for patients with recurrent HCC in the liver (Table 24.2) [1, 11, 18–24]. Another study of the use of bland particle embolization after intrahepatic recurrence of HCC demonstrated a median survival after embolization of 46 months, with actuarial survival rates at 1 year, 2 years, and 5 years after recurrence of 86, 74, and 47%, respectively [25].

Belghiti et al. [26] initially evaluated the feasibility and postoperative course of liver resection prior to liver transplantation for HCC in 18 patients, showing equivalent disease-free and overall survival for primary and secondary liver transplantation. They also reported similar overall incidence of complications in both groups. Vennarecci et al. [27] reviewed their experience with salvage liver transplantation in nine patients who experienced recurrent HCC in the liver after resection.

Table 24.1 Repeat hepatic resection for recurrent hepatocellular carcinoma [4–17]

Author (year [ref])	No. of patients	Re-resection rate[a] (%)	Surgical death rate[b] (%)	Survival after recurrence			Re-resection compared with nonsurgical treatments[c]
				1 year (%)	3 years (%)	5 years (%)	
Nakajima (1993 [5])	14	25	0	100	87	87	Better survival
Matsuda (1993 [6])	16	44	0	93	21	–	Better survival
Zhou (1993 [7])	65	35	0	87	54	42	Better survival
Kakazu (1993 [8])	24	17	0	–	82	82	–
Suenaga (1994 [9])	18	24	0	88	37	37	Better survival
Shimada (1994 [10])	21	–	0	90	78	58	–
Lee (1995 [11])	25	31	0	72	45	–	Better survival
Nagasue (1996 [12])	50	30	8	–	–	50	Better survival
Hu (1996 [13])	59	48	0	69	44	–	Better survival
Shuto (1996 [14])	31	19	0	96	71	52	Better survival
Shimada (1998 [15])	41	–	0	100	68	45	–
Arii (1998 [16])	22	–	0	95	50	–	–
Farges (1998 [17])	15	17	0	86	75	60	Better survival
Poon (1999 [1])	11	10	0	81	69	69	Better survival

[a]Percentage of patient with intrahepatic recurrence undergoing re-resection
[b]30-day death rate
[c]Nonsurgical treatments included transarterial chemoembolization, percutaneous ethanol injection, systemic or oral chemotherapy, and symptomatic treatment
With permission from [2]

Table 24.2 Transarterial chemoembolization for recurrent hepatocellular carcinoma

Author (year [ref])	No. of patients	TACE rate[a] (%)	Survival after recurrence		
			1 year (%)	3 years (%)	5 years (%)
Sasaki (1987 [18])	30	70	84	25	–
Nagao (1990 [19])	17	41	88	35	–
Nakao (1991 [20])	66	81	88	42	27
Takayasu (1992 [21])	50	42	64	24	5
Ouchi (1993 [22])	12	63	75	75	27
Park (1993 [23])	87	–	75	–	–
Okazaki (1993 [24])	68	–	87	34	0
Lee (1995 [11])	12	–	75	48	–
Poon (1999 [1])	71	68	72	38	21

TACE, transarterial chemoembolization
[a]Percentage of patients with intrahepatic recurrence treated with TACE
With permission from [2]

They found that the post transplant 1-, 3-, and 5-year survival rates for salvage liver transplantation were 89, 89, and 89%, respectively, similar to those who underwent primary liver transplantation (78, 63, and 63%, respectively). The 1-, 3-, 5-year disease-free survival rates for salvage liver transplantation were 100, 100 and 100%, respectively vs. 89, 74, and 74% for those that underwent primary liver transplantation for HCC. They also found that the operative mortality rates, perioperative bleeding complications, operative times, intensive care unit stays, hospital stay, and overall incidence of postoperative complications were similar among patients who underwent salvage liver transplantation after prior resection vs. those who underwent primary liver transplantation for HCC. Facciuto et al. [28] also reported on a small series of five patients who underwent salvage liver transplantation for recurrence after resection. At a median of 18 months after salvage transplant, all five patients were alive, four were free of disease, and one had developed recurrent HCC. Although there are limited data on the use of transplantation as salvage therapy after resection for HCC, the available evidence suggests that this is a potentially curative strategy with results that may be comparable to primary liver transplantation for selected patients. Del Gaudio et al. [29] compared the results of 10 patients who underwent salvage liver transplantation after prior resection for HCC to 80 patients who underwent primary liver transplantation. Only 26% of resected patients were candidates for transplantation. The 5-year overall rates were 62% vs. 73% and disease-free survival rates were 48% vs. 71% comparing patients who underwent salvage transplantation vs. primary liver transplantation, respectively. While these results were not statistically different, the small number of patients in the salvage transplantation group may indicate the possibility of a type II statistical error. Whether resection followed by salvage transplantation is truly comparable to primary liver transplantation remains an open question. However, the shortage of available donor organs and the strict selection criteria for transplantation candidates limit this approach for most patients with recurrent HCC. Furthermore, the majority of patients who recur after liver resection were not transplantation candidates at the time of their initial therapy.

A few studies have evaluated the role of resection for extrahepatic recurrence of HCC. Lo et al. [30] reviewed their experience with surgical resection of solitary lesions in the lung or abdomen in 12 patients, with a mean survival of 20 months; six patients survived disease free for more than 1 year. Another study from the same group [31] reported long-term survival ranging from 33 to 168 months after resection of solitary lung metastases from HCC in six patients. Other studies have documented prolonged survival after surgical resection of isolated recurrences in the adrenal gland, peritoneal cavity, or other extrahepatic sites [32, 33].

Conclusions

There are no prospective randomized trials to compare the results of various therapies for patients with intrahepatic recurrence after potentially curative resection or ablation for HCC. However, the available evidence suggests that liver transplantation should be considered in those patients who are eligible. Retrospective data support the use of repeat resection in patients with intrahepatic recurrence. For patients who are not candidates for transplantation or repeat resection because of the size and distribution of recurrent tumors, the presence of concomitant extrahepatic disease, age, overall medical condition, or poor liver function, ablative therapy should be considered when feasible. Radiofrequency, microwave, or percutaneous ethanol ablation can be considered in patients with relatively small tumors amenable to such therapy. TACE and drug-eluting bead chemoembolization, intraarterial radiotherapy, and systemic therapy should be considered as salvage therapy for those that cannot undergo resection or ablation; however, the data in support of such treatments are somewhat limited. Selected patients with resectable extrahepatic metastases from HCC may benefit from surgical extirpation. Further studies are necessary to define the role of salvage therapy in the treatment of recurrent HCC.

References

1. Poon RT, Fan ST, Lo CM, Liu CL, Wong J (1999) Intrahepatic recurrence after curative resection of hepatocellular carcinoma: long-term results of treatment and prognostic factors. Ann Surg 229:216–222
2. Poon RT, Fan S-T, and Wong J (2000) Risk factors, prevention, and management of postoperative recurrence after resection of hepatocellular carcinoma. Ann Surg 232:10–24
3. NCCN (2009) Clinical Practice Guidelines in Oncology™. Hepatobiliary Cancers 2. www.NCCN.org. Accessed June 2, 2010
4. Shah SA, Cleary SP, Wei AC et al (2007) Recurrence after liver resection for hepatocellular carcinoma: risk factors, treatment, and outcomes. Surgery 141:330–339
5. Nakajima Y, Ohmura T, Kimura J et al (1993) Role of surgical treatment for recurrent hepatocellular carcinoma after hepatic resection. World J Surg 17:792–795

6. Matsuda Y, Ito T, Oguchi Y et al (1993) Rationale of surgical management for recurrent hepatocellular carcinoma. Ann Surg 217:28–34
7. Zhou XD, Yu YQ, Tang ZY et al (1993) Surgical treatment of recurrent hepatocellular carcinoma. Hepatogastroenterology 40:333–336
8. Kakazu T, Makuuchi M, Kawasaki S et al (1993) Repeat hepatic resection for recurrent hepatocellular carcinoma. Hepatogastroenterology 40:337–341
9. Suenaga M, Sugiura H, Kokuba Y et al (1994) Repeated hepatic resection for recurrent hepatocellular carcinoma in eighteen cases. Surgery 115:452–457
10. Shimada M, Matsumata T, Taketomi A et al (1994) Repeat hepatectomy for recurrent hepatocellular carcinoma. Surgery 115:703–706
11. Lee PH, Lin WJ, Tsang YM et al (1995) Clinical management of recurrent hepatocellular carcinoma. Ann Surg 222:670–676
12. Nagasue N, Kohno T, Hayashi M et al (1996) Repeat hepatectomy for recurrent hepatocellular carcinoma. Br J Surg 83:127–131
13. Hu RH, Lee PH, Yu SC et al (1996) Surgical resection for recurrent hepatocellular carcinoma: prognosis and analysis of risk factors. Surgery 120:23–29
14. Shuto T, Kinoshita H, Hirohashi K et al (1996) Indication for, and effectiveness of, a second hepatic resection for recurrent hepatocellular carcinoma. Hepatogastroenterology 43:932–937
15. Shimada M, Takenaka K, Taguchi K et al (1998) Prognostic factors after repeat hepatectomy for recurrent hepatocellular carcinoma. Ann Surg 227:80–85
16. Arii S, Monden K, Niwano M et al (1998) Results of surgical treatment for recurrent hepatocellular carcinoma: comparison of outcome among patients with multicentric carcinogenesis, intrahepatic metastasis and extraheptic recurrence. J Hepatobiliary Pancreat Surg 5:86–92
17. Farges O, Regimbeau JM, Belghiti J (1998) Aggressive management of recurrence following surgical resection of hepatocellular carcinoma. Hepatogastroenterology 45:1275–1280
18. Sasaki Y, Imaoka S, Fujita M et al (1987) Regional therapy in the management of intraheptic recurrence after surgery for hepatoma. Ann Surg 206:40–47
19. Nagao T, Inoue S, Yoshimi F et al (1990) Postoperative recurrence of hepatocellular carcinoma. Ann Surg 211:28–33
20. Nakao N, Kamino K, Miura K et al (1991) Recurrent hepatocellular carcinoma after partial hepatectomy: value of treatment with transcatheter arterial chemoembolization. AJR Am J Roentgenol 156:1177–1179
21. Takayasu K, Wakao F, Moriyama N et al (1992) Postresection recurrence of hepatocellular carcinoma treated by arterial embolization: analysis of prognostic factors. Hepatology 16:906–911
22. Ouchi K, Matsubara S, Fukuhara K et al (1993) Recurrence of hepatocellular carcinoma in the liver remnant after hepatic resection. Am J Surg 166:270–273
23. Park JH, Han JK, Chung JW et al (1993) Postoperative recurrence of hepatocellular carcinoma: results of transcatheter arterial chemoembolization. Cardiovasc Intervent Radiol 16:21–24
24. Okazaki M, Yamasaki S, Ono H et al (1993) Chemoembolotherapy for recurrent hepatocellular carcinoma in the residual liver after hepatectomy. Hepatogastroenterology 40:320–323
25. Covey AM, Maluccio MA, Schubert J et al (2006) Particle embolization of recurrent hepatocellular carcinoma after hepatectomy. Cancer 106:2181–2189
26. Belghiti J, Cortes A, Abdalla EK, et al (2005) Resection prior to liver transplantation for hepatocellular carcinoma. Ann Surg 241:671–672
27. Vennarecci G, Ettorre GM, Antonini M et al (2007) First-line liver resection and salvage liver transplantation are increasing therapeutic strategies for patients with hepatocellular carcinoma and child a cirrhosis. Transplant Proc 39:1857–1860
28. Facciuto ME, Koneru B, Rocca JP et al. (2008) Surgical treatment of hepatocellular carcinoma beyond Milan criteria. Results of liver resection, salvage transplantation, and primary liver transplantation. Ann Surg Oncol 15:1383–1391

29. Del Gaudio M, Ercolani G, Ravaioli M et al (2008) Liver transplantation for recurrent hepatocellular carcinoma on cirrhosis after liver resection: University of Bologna experience. Am J Transplant 8:1177–1185
30. Lo CM, Lai EC, Fan ST, Choi TK, Wong J (1994) Resection for extrahepatic recurrence of hepatocellular carcinoma. Br J Surg 81:1019–1021
31. Lam CM, Lo CM, Yuen WK, Liu CL, Fan ST (1998) Prolonged survival in selected patients following surgical resection for pulmonary metastasis from hepatocellular carcinoma. Br J Surg 85:1198–1200
32. Park JS, Yoon DS, Kim KS et al (2007) What is the best treatment modality for adrenal metastasis from hepatocellular carcinoma? J Surg Oncol 96:32–36
33. Uka K, Aikata H, Takaki S et al (2007) Clinical features and prognosis of patients with extrahepatic metastases from hepatocellular carcinoma. World J Gastroenterol 13:414–420

Index

Note: The letters 'f' and 't' following locators refer to figures and tables respectively.

K.M. McMasters, J.-N. Vauthey (eds.), *Hepatocellular Carcinoma*,
DOI 10.1007/978-1-60327-522-4, © Springer Science+Business Media, LLC 2011